PRAISE FOR *THE TRUTH PILL*

Truth, they say, is often a bitter pill. This book, not an easy read, lives up to the saying. It is also a deeply disturbing book for a country which is supposed to be the pharmacy of the world and where the pharmaceutical sector is growing at a fast clip.

—*National Herald*

In *The Truth Pill: The Myth of Drug Regulation in India*, Dinesh S. Thakur and Prashant Reddy T. not only expose episodes of immorality among drug regulatory bodies in India (manufacturing and trade), but lay bare flaws in the judicial structure and a complicit establishment that plays along.

—*Hindustan Times*

Thakur and Reddy have painstakingly drawn rich elements from a mix of judicial, executive, legislative, and media documents to weave artfully the first of its kind cogent big-picture public policy history of drug regulation which is extremely valuable, and a must read for anyone remotely interested in the pharma sector...

—*The Financial Express*

More of us should read [this] book...

—Bibek Debroy,
The New Indian Express

The Truth Pill is an excellent and thoroughly researched book that is a valuable addition to the shelves of even those who track and write on the problems of the Indian pharma sector and its regulation regularly.

—*Business Standard*

The book points to the constantly evolving and innovating pharmaceutical industry and the need for a regularly upgraded regulatory system, armed with qualified personnel...

—*The Hindu BusinessLine*

A fascinating and authoritative book on the opaque structure of India's drug regulations.

—*Frontline Magazine*

...this is a well-structured, well researched book that highlights issues that are not common knowledge...Thakur and Reddy have used their research to give us a must-read account of how long a road we still have to travel.

—*India Today*

...it is a timely book and a wake-up call for all those interested in the well-being of Indian citizens and anyone in the world using these drugs.

—*The Tribune*

Drawing on in-depth legal and regulatory analyses, numerous case studies and responses to hundreds of Freedom of Information requests, they exhaustively document glaring gaps in India's legal framework and severe shortcomings in regulatory oversight and enforcement.

—*BMJ Global Health Blog*

The book examines how pharmaceutical brands have escaped scrutiny despite serious lapses resulting in fatal outcomes.

—*Scroll.in*

THE TRUTH PILL

The Myth of Drug Regulation in India

DINESH S. THAKUR

PRASHANT REDDY T.

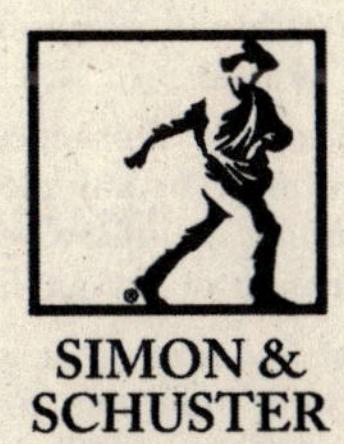

SIMON & SCHUSTER

London · New York · Sydney · Toronto · New Delhi

First published in India by Simon & Schuster India, 2022
This edition published by Simon & Schuster India, 2025

1 3 5 7 9 10 8 6 4 2

Simon & Schuster India
818, Indraprakash Building,
21, Barakhamba Road,
New Delhi 110001.

www.simonandschuster.co.in

Paperback ISBN: 978-81-979492-6-5
eBook ISBN: 978-93-92099-22-9

Typeset in India by SÜRYA, New Delhi
Printed and bound in India by Replika Press Pvt. Ltd.

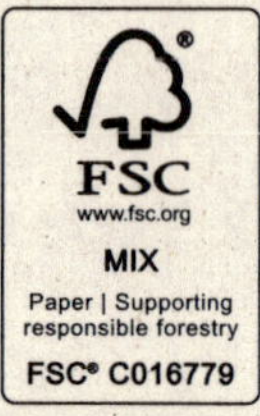

To Dr Raj Kumar,
who is a mentor and a role model to me

—Dinesh S. Thakur

~

For my friend and mentor,
the Late Dr Shamnad Basheer

—Prashant Reddy T.

CONTENTS

Prologue

An Epidemic of DEG Poisoning and Regulatory Failure

As the year 2019 drew to a close, doctors at two North Indian hospitals were grappling with a mysterious condition that had affected approximately 21 children, several of whom were infants. The weather had started to turn as winter began to set in and all of these children had been suffering from a cough or a cold which were typical for this time of the year; but they then progressed to vomiting and ultimately suffering from kidney failure. Most of these children came from Ramnagar in Jammu.[1]

It is a remarkable medical event for a cluster of otherwise healthy children from the same neighbourhood to suddenly suffer from acute kidney failure. The first response of the government in such circumstances is to put together a team of doctors, microbiologists and epidemiologists from various institutions to conduct an epidemiological investigation.[2] The Government of India rushed a group of experts to trace the source of the mystery affliction before it affected even more children in the area. At the time, the media reported that the children had died of a "mystery disease" and the government was looking at the usual suspects such as contaminated water to establish the cause of death.[3]

At the highly regarded Post-Graduate Institute of Medical Education & Research (PGIMER), Chandigarh, where many of the sick children had been admitted for treatment, doctors ran a battery of tests on their young patients to diagnose their ailments. The medication consumed by the children prior to their admission to the hospital was also sent for testing. One of these medications was a cough syrup called COLDBEST, which is a fixed dose combination of Paracetamol, Phenylephrine Hydrochloride and Chlorpheniramine Maleate manufactured by Digital Vision, a pharmaceutical company with its manufacturing base in Himachal Pradesh, which is the national hub for most pharmaceutical companies due to a generous tax exemption policy introduced by the Government of India to bolster industrial development in the hilly region. The parents of the children in Jammu had bought this cough syrup from a local pharmacy after their children had exhibited signs of a fever along with either a cough or a cold.

The Regional Drug Testing Laboratory, Chandigarh, which tested three different samples of the same batch of COLDBEST alleged that the samples of the cough syrup tested positive for 34.24%, 34.97% and 35.87% of Diethylene Glycol (DEG) which is a powerful industrial solvent that is used in the manufacture of anti-freeze, brake fluid, etc.[4] It is never used in the manufacture of medicine and can be fatal to humans who consume it.[5] It causes the kidneys to fail and that can eventually lead to death. In cases of DEG poisoning due to manufacturing errors, children tend to suffer the most because their smaller body size causes them to be more vulnerable to the toxic effects of DEG when compared to adults. As one academic paper put it "...children often seem to be the sentinels in this cruel and unintended form of toxic surveillance".[6] Finally, the doctors at PGIMER had a probable answer to explain the renal failure leading to death of the children from Ramnagar.

By the time the mystery was solved by the doctors at PGIMER, approximately 11 children from Ramnagar between the ages of two months and six years died due to renal failure. The youngest was not yet named. The names of the remaining were Annirudh, Akshu Kumar, Ashish, Pranav, Amit Kumar, Surabhi Sharma, Kanishk Dogra, Varuni, Jannu Kumar and Shriyansh. They were born to parents who were daily wage labourers, a truck driver, a school teacher and a soldier in the Indian Army. One of the parents was so distraught upon hearing the news of the death of his child he reportedly demolished his own house.[7]

Though these children were all equal citizens of a democratic India, the news of their deaths struggled to get the attention of the Delhi-centric English-language media that often sets the national agenda. It is virtually guaranteed that these deaths would have received far more media attention and perhaps even some public outrage if they were from the middle class and residing in New Delhi. Ultimately, just two English-language Indian newspapers, *The Tribune* and *The Indian Express* gave the story the required attention.[8]

The larger tragedy was the fact that the deaths of these children from Jammu were entirely preventable. After all, DEG poisoning is a well-known and well-documented problem within the pharmaceutical industry since 1937, when the first mass DEG poisoning event took place in the United States. At the time, a company called S.E. Massengill of Bristol, Tennessee, was just getting into the business of selling a new wonder drug called Sulfanilamide, which was one of the first antibiotics that could treat a broad spectrum of bacterial infections. Massengill wanted to sell Sulfanilamide in liquid form, as a sweetened syrup because it anticipated that such a formulation would lead to higher sales in the pediatric market. The chief chemist at the company experimented with various solvents that could dissolve Sulfanilamide into a syrup and ultimately ended up using DEG as a solvent without being aware that DEG was toxic for humans. The formulation had not been tested for toxicity because it was not mandatory to do so under the law at the time.[9]

The first batch of "Elixir Sulfanilamide" entered the American market in October 1937, and in a matter of a few days, doctors reported the death of six patients who consumed Massengill's drug. Despite a frantic recall effort, a total of 105 patients, including 34 children, were killed in the United States after consuming Massengill's cough syrup. An additional "victim", was the Chief Chemist at Massengill who killed himself while awaiting a trial before a court of law for his role in the incident.[10] The deaths of those patients provoked an overhaul of the Federal Food, Drug and Cosmetics Act in 1938 with an increased focus on safety.[11] The United States has never experienced another mass DEG poisoning event after 1937.

The rest of the world, especially countries in the developing world, have however experienced several DEG poisoning events: seven children died in South Africa in 1969,[12] 47 children died in Nigeria in 1990[13] and another 84 children died in 2008,[14] 236 children died in Bangladesh between 1990–92,[15] 29 people died in Argentina in 1992, 88 children died in Haiti in 1996[16] and 365 people died in Panama in 2007.[17]

India has the uniquely depressing record of having had at least five major DEG poisoning events. The first took place in Madras in 1972, killing 15 children after they consumed a cough syrup called Pipmol C that had been adulterated with DEG.[18] The second event took place in Mumbai in 1986 at the famous J.J. Hospital killing 14 patients after they consumed glycerin that had been adulterated with DEG.[19] The third mass DEG poisoning event took place in Bihar in 1988 killing 11 patients.[20] The fourth event took place in Gurgaon, a district neighbouring Delhi in 1998 when 33 children between the ages of two months and six years died after consuming a cough syrup adulterated with DEG.[21] The event in Jammu in December 2019 was therefore the fifth such mass-poisoning event in India.

In each of the above cases, the actual death toll is most certainly higher than what has been publicly reported since DEG poisoning is difficult to diagnose. For example, the doctors probing the 33 deaths of children in Gurgaon, remarked in their study that, "At the beginning of the investigation we never imagined that contaminated medicine was causing acute renal failure in children."[22] Only when deaths take place in a cluster are doctors more likely to study common medications taken by all of the deceased and have them tested.

So, why does DEG adulteration recur with such frequency in India?

The simple answer is that Indian pharmaceutical companies quite often fail to test either the raw materials or the final formulation before shipping it to the market. This is despite Good Manufacturing Practices (GMP) as prescribed in Indian law requiring mandatory testing of both the raw material before it is used in production and the final formulation before it is shipped to the market. Such testing is required to ensure that the company has in fact received the correct solvent from the supplier and that it is of the correct purity. In many of these disasters, traders responsible for supplying chemicals such as propylene glycol have either mislabeled DEG as Propylene Glycol by mistake or have adulterated Propylene Glycol with DEG, either on purpose to reduce costs or by mistake due to poor quality control measures.

In the case of the mass poisoning event in Jammu, the Himachal Pradesh Drug Control Administration (HPDCA) that has jurisdiction over the manufacturer of the alleged adulterated cough syrup—Digital Vision—alleged before the Himachal Pradesh High Court that Digital Vision lacked an appropriate facility to test the finished formulation for DEG contamination and that the analysis report from Digital Vision's quality control department indicating the absence of DEG in dangerous quantities was "misleading". Digital Vision itself has completely refuted all these allegations and has claimed that an independent laboratory, as well as government laboratories concluded that its samples were of standard quality and not adulterated.[23]

If these allegations about the lack of an adequate testing facility are established to be true, it is necessary to question the HPDCA on its failure to notice such deep-rooted egregious violations during its previous inspections of Digital Vision's manufacturing facility. How could it have missed the lack of testing equipment in past inspections? Going by Digital Vision's past record, it is obvious that the HPDCA had multiple opportunities to inspect the firm's manufacturing facilities.

According to a government-maintained database called XLN, Digital Vision had been cited at least 13 times for violation of quality standards by just three state drug controllers in Maharashtra, Gujarat and Kerala between 2012 and 2019 prior to the tragedy in Jammu, due to its drugs failing quality testing standards during random sampling and testing conducted by drug inspectors from those states.[24] The national drug regulator, CDSCO's drug alerts, which report testing by central government laboratories mention another five instances of Digital Vision's drugs failing quality testing in the years prior to the tragedy in Jammu.[25] An investigation by a journalist alleged that, as per available data, the company's drugs failed quality testing on 19 occasions in total![26]

Thus, by a conservative estimate, the HPDCA must have received at least 19 notices across a decade from other state drug controllers or its own drug inspectors informing it that Digital Vision's drugs had failed quality testing. This also meant that the HPDCA had 19 different opportunities to conduct inspections of Digital Vision's manufacturing facilities. In addition, the HPDCA would have also had to conduct yearly inspections of Digital Vision's facility as required under the law. Since the HPDCA, is not required to proactively publish reports of its inspections on its website, we simply do not know whether HPDCA ever inspected Digital Vision's facility on those 19 occasions. In an ideal scenario, the lack of quality control equipment to test for DEG poisoning at Digital Vision's facility, as alleged before the High Court, should have been spotted during these inspections, leading to an immediate cancellation of the company's manufacturing licence for failing to comply with GMP standards prescribed in the law. Why did that not happen? Did the drug inspectors look the other way due to political pressure? Or did the HPDCA not take any serious action because of good old-fashioned corruption? While there is no specific evidence of corruption in this case, the Indian press regularly reports about rampant corruption amongst drug inspectors.[27]

Separate and apart from the question of why exactly the drug regulatory system missed the warning signs at Digital Vision, is the response of the Indian state to the death of the 11 young children from Ramnagar. Historically, the Indian state responds to such incidents in one of two ways. The first is the criminal prosecution of the persons responsible for manufacturing and selling the adulterated drugs in question. This is a question of delivering justice to the deceased and their families. It took three years for the local police to file a chargesheet against Digital Vision in the December of 2022. [28] Whether this prosecution results in convictions remains to be seen.

The second response by the State should ideally involve a broader investigation into the failure of the regulator and the shortcomings in the law, so that policy can be reformed in order to prevent a similar tragedy in the future. Unfortunately, neither the state government nor the central government thought it necessary to commission a deeper investigation into the regulatory failure that led to the fifth mass death event due to DEG poisoning in the history of independent India. It is not like there was no such demand for an investigation. In August 2020, one of us petitioned the Minister of Health, requesting the Ministry to conduct a transparent investigation into the entire incident.[29]

The Minister did not even bother acknowledging the petition, let alone act on it.

We then followed up with a request for information under the RTI Act, asking the Ministry of Health whether it had conducted any investigation into the regulatory failures that led to the deaths of those 11 children.[30] The Ministry did not bother answering the question. It preferred to simply transfer the request for information to the Central Drug Standards Control Organisation (CDSCO) which is India's national drug regulator. The CDSCO in turn transferred the blame for the entire issue to the state drug controller on the grounds that it was the latter's responsibility to regulate Digital Vision.[31] Technically speaking, it was not an incorrect response but it is also a fact that only the Ministry of Health can initiate any amendment to the Drugs & Cosmetics Act, 1940, and the rules therein. State governments cannot affect policy changes at the national level. Under India's convoluted drug regulatory law, the Government of India is responsible for imports and approving new drugs based on safety and efficacy data but the licensing of manufacturing units and prosecutions of pharmaceutical companies is primarily the responsibility of the state governments. Thus, for a policy reform exercise to be undertaken, the Ministry of Health needed to understand what exactly went wrong in this case from a regulatory perspective. The Ministry however was not interested in getting to the bottom of the issue. There can be no cure without a diagnosis.

Governance in India has not always been this incompetent. Back in 1986, after the deaths of 14 patients at the J.J. Hospital in Mumbai due to DEG poisoning, the Chief Minister of Maharashtra appointed Justice Lentin, a sitting judge of the Bombay High Court, to head a Commission of Inquiry into the events leading to the deaths of the 14 patients. The resulting report of this Commission of Inquiry is the stuff of legend.

To begin with, Justice Lentin held rigorous, marathon hearings in an open courtroom, something that is seldom seen today. Justifying the need for holding a public inquiry, Justice Lentin wrote:

> Secrecy breeds suspicion, and suspicion breeds contempt. A public inquiry would therefore ensure public confidence in the work of the commission to arrive at the truth without fear or favour, regardless of power, position, influence and importance of witnesses.[32]

In less than a year, Justice Lentin produced a report that ran into 300 pages, holding a powerful Joint Commissioner of the Maharashtra Food & Drug Administration (FDA) and even the Health Minister of the State of Maharashtra accountable for a dysfunctional regulatory system that created the environment for the tragedy at J.J. Hospital. The foreword to his scathing report was as follows[33]:

> These pages describe and illustrate the ugly facets of the human mind and human nature, projecting

> errors of judgment, misuse of ministerial power and authority, apathy towards human life, corruption, nexus and quid pro quo between unscrupulous license holders, analytical laboratories, elements in the Industries department controlling the awarding of rate contracts, manufacturers, traders, merchants, suppliers, the FDA and persons holding ministerial rank. None of this will be palatable in the affected quarters. But that cannot be helped.

In the pages that followed, Justice Lentin laid out reams of evidence painting a picture of an utterly broken system of drug regulation within the State of Maharashtra. Since Justice Lentin had held public hearings, the proceedings and the final report received widespread media coverage, thereby focusing public attention on the issue.

Documenting what it described as "amazing facts" dug out by Justice Lentin, the *India Today* news magazine described the manner in which the Maharashtra FDA failed to take action against the 582 formulations that were found to be substandard in the year 1986, the fact that 250 drug manufacturing units in Maharashtra were operating without any analytical laboratories, the manner in which Health Ministers regularly intervened to prevent honest bureaucrats at the State FDA from prosecuting erring pharmaceutical companies; evidence of doctors at J.J. Hospital and Ministers receiving money from pharmaceutical companies and finally, concrete evidence on how family members of Dolas—the powerful Joint Commissioner of the Maharashtra FDA responsible for much of drug regulation in Maharashtra—acquired a stake in pharmaceutical companies in Maharashtra.[34]

Summarizing the commission's report, *India Today* concluded:

> The commission's investigations have uncovered the horrifying spectacle of a watchdog health agency totally surrendering to the manipulations of people like Dolas. ... And the FDA has continued its lawless reign even after agencies from other states like Gujarat and Tamil Nadu complained about the quality of drugs emanating from the FDA's fiefdom.

Daily newspapers like *The Indian Express*, *The Times of India* and the *Sunday Observer* were the ones that maintained constant pressure on the government to act on the findings of the report. These newspapers published reports under the following headlines: "FDA still shielding guilty", "Name of game is favouritism", "Of ministerial incompetence, graft and neglect", "Labs hand-in-glove with FDA", "Sinister gangs of merchants of death", "Proxy payment behind glycerol contract", "Never before such lies", "Criminal silence".[35]

The media pressure worked and Bhai Sawant, the Health Minister of the State of Maharashtra resigned from the state cabinet on 10 March 1988. The State Government suspended senior doctors of J.J. Hospital and three officials from the state FDA, including the powerful Joint Commissioner S.M. Dolas who was severely indicted by Justice Lentin. The State

Government also endorsed most of the points made in the Commission's report.[36]

Recognizing the monumental work done by Justice Lentin, one doctor called upon the medical profession to "build upon Justice Lentin's labours" and "convince politicians and bureaucrats that the recommendations made by the learned judge can be neglected only at our peril".[37] Unfortunately, those lessons from 1988 were never learnt by the Indian drug regulatory framework at the national level.

More shockingly, it came to light in 2022, that the prosecution against 24 people was still pending, 36 years after the deaths caused by the adulterated medicine at J.J. Hospital in 1986. In fact, the reporter discovered that charges were never framed by the court, as a result of which the trial never began![38]

While corruption likely had a role to play in the tragedy at J.J. Hospital, it is also important to understand that the problem with India's drug regulatory framework is not limited to corruption, as was the focus of the Lentin Commission in 1988. There is also the question of poor regulatory design. These range from the lack of regulatory transparency to the absurdly complex distribution of regulatory powers in India across 38 authorities spread across each state and union territory plus the CDSCO which works under the Union Government. For example, inspection reports of pharmaceutical facilities are not made publicly available without which there is no way to assess whether drug inspectors are actually doing their job as required. On the jurisdictional issue, since each state and union territory has its own drug regulator who issues licences to manufacturing facilities, there is often little information sharing and coordination amongst them. Further, inter-state investigations are extremely difficult because a drug inspector working for the Maharashtra FDA lacks jurisdiction to enter and inspect Digital Vision's facility in Himachal Pradesh unless accompanied by a drug inspector from the HPDCA. The HPDCA however has its own reasons to not permit such inspections, the most important of which is the fact that the state government wants to continue pitching the state as a hub for pharmaceutical manufacturing. Together these various flaws cause catastrophes like the deaths of these 11 young children.

For a country like India, which has earned itself the moniker of being "the developing world's pharmacy," the failure of its national regulator to function efficiently impacts not just Indian citizens but also the citizens of all its trading partners who are purchasing Indian drugs. This became evident in October 2022, when cough syrups exported from India and allegedly contaminated with DEG were blamed for the deaths of approximately 70 children in The Gambia located in West Africa. This time around, since the World Health Organization (WHO) was involved in issuing global alerts, the issue got attention in the global media. Maiden Pharmaceuticals, the company blamed for the tragedy in The Gambia had a spotty track record with different state drug regulators and state procurement agencies in India accusing it of manufacturing substandard drugs. Despite the company's poor track record, the Government of India came to the defence of the company with no less an authority than the Drug Controller General of India (DCGI) that heads the CDSCO, publicly accusing the WHO of drawing a "premature" link between the cough syrups exported from India and the deaths of the children.[39] This despite overwhelming evidence that the cough syrups were the cause of the deaths.

Two months later, in December 2022, cough syrup manufactured by a different pharmaceutical company allegedly caused the deaths of 20 children in Uzbekistan, once again due to DEG contamination. This time, the manufacturer was arrested but the Ministry of Health was yet to announce any steps to tackle the larger problem, which was the continued operation of pharmaceutical companies that were not complying with GMPs.

In June 2023, the Ministry of Commerce, worried about the reputational crisis facing the Indian pharmaceutical industry, introduced a new rule under a trade law, mandating that all exports of cough syrups from India would have to clear quality testing in government laboratories. This despite the fact that the Ministry of Commerce had no mandate to regulate the pharmaceutical industry.

By the end of the year 2023, sources within the CDSCO leaked to the press that cough syrups of 54 pharmaceutical companies failed quality testing. Around the same time, Cameroon blamed the deaths of 12 children in the country on contaminated cough syrups exported from India. By July 2024, the media reported that cough syrups manufactured by 100 pharmaceutical companies failed testing, many of them contaminated with DEG. Although the exports of the contaminated batches were presumably blocked, the government never published the names of the pharmaceutical companies whose cough syrups failed testing. The government also did not reveal whether these same companies were selling their product within India and the actions taken to restrain them from continuing to sell them in India.

We began this book with the DEG poisoning cases in order to highlight the worst possible consequences of the lackadaisical, if not negligent approach of the Ministry of Health, the CDSCO and the state drug regulators, all of whom were more interested in protecting themselves and the pharmaceutical industry instead of the citizens of this country. However, what worries us more than the cough syrups are the consequences of regulatory lethargy on the more mundane aspects of drug regulation; where although regulatory failures may not cause deaths, but could still lead to a significant adverse impact on public health in a manner where it is difficult to draw direct connection between poor regulation and its consequences. Take for example, the approval of dubious new drugs with little to no evidence to justify the therapeutic claims made by the manufacturer or when the drug lacks sufficient active ingredient or fails to properly dissolve in the bloodstream of a patient. These are issues that do not necessarily lead to deaths but contribute in the long term to poor outcomes for individual patients and ultimately for public health.

The primary challenge in discussing many of these regulatory issues is that drug regulation as a policy issue lies at the intersection of regulatory science and public law, two areas that are not exactly popular amongst the common citizenry or politicians.

The secondary challenge is the difficulty in measuring and explaining the harm caused to patients due to poor regulatory policies and ineffective practices. The consequences of an inadequate scheme of drug regulation are much like climate change—not everybody can see the linkages in real time; its consequences cannot be easily measured but it is most definitely causing harm to public health.

In this book, we take a stab at explaining some of these crucial regulatory issues in a prose that is hopefully palatable to the ordinary consumer of "Made in India" medicine.

Notes

1. Deepanker Gupta, "6 infants die due to unknown illness" *The Tribune* (Ramnagar/Udhampur, 16 January 2020) <https://www.tribuneindia.com/news/j-k/6-infants-die-due-to-unknown-illness-27436> accessed 28 May 2021; Prabha Raghavan and Arun Sharma, "Behind killer cough syrup Coldbest: Glaring gaps in regulation and its manufacture" *The Indian Express* (Jammu, 12 March 2020) <https://indianexpress.com/article/india/behind-killer-cough-syrup-

glaring-gaps-in-regulation-and-its-manufacture-6310065/> accessed 28 May 2021.

2. "Central team to probe kids' death" *The Tribune* (Jammu, 18 January 2020) <https://www.tribuneindia.com/news/j-k/central-team-to-probe-kids%E2%80%99-death-28309> accessed 28 May 2021.
3. Press Trust of India, "10 Children Die Of 'Mysterious Disease' In J&K's Udhampur, Say Officials" *NDTV* (Jammu, 18 January 2020) <https://www.ndtv.com/india-news/10-children-die-of-mysterious-disease-in-jammu-and-kashmirs-udhampur-say-officials-2166041> accessed 28 May 2021.
4. CDSCO Drug Alerts for March 2020 <https://cdsco.gov.in/opencms/opencms/en/Notifications/Alerts/>
5. HT Correspondents, "HP pharma unit booked for infants' death due to contaminated syrup" *Hindustan Times* (Shimla/Jammu, 3 March 2020) <https://www.hindustantimes.com/cities/hp-pharma-unit-booked-for-infants-death-due-to-contaminated-syrup/story-K02StB2Byi2OupRrT2CVTI.html> accessed on 28 May 2021.
6. Alan D. Woolf, "The Haitian Diethylene Glycol Poisoning Tragedy: A Dark Wood Revisited" (1998) 279 *JAMA* 1215.
7. Arun Sharma, "Killer chemical' in cough syrup: Udhampur parents got medicine from local chemist", *The Indian Express* (Ramnagar, 26 February 2020) <https://indianexpress.com/article/india/jammu-cough-syrup-children-death-digital-vision-local-chemist-6286929/> accessed 28 May 2021. Replies from PGIMER to RTI Application No. APC/2021/550 dated 23.06.2021.
8. ibid.
9. William Rosen, *Miracle Cure: The Creation of Antibiotics and the Birth of Modern* (Penguin 2017) 76.
10. ibid 75.
11. Peter Barton Hutt, "Drug Regulation in The United States" (1986) 2 *Intl J of Technology Assessment in Health Care* 619, 621.
12. Paul M. Wax, "It's Happening Again- Another Diethylene Glycol Mass Poisoning" (1996) 34 *Clinical Toxicology* 517.

13. HO Okuonghae and others, “Diethylene Glycol Poisoning in Nigerian Children” (1992) 12 *Annals of Tropical Pediatrics* 235.
14. Lydia Polgreen, “84 Children Are Killed by Medicine in Nigeria” *The New York Times* (Dakar, 6 February 2009) <https://www.nytimes.com/2009/02/07/world/africa/07nigeria.html> accessed 28 May 2021.
15. Mohammed Hanif and others, “Fatal renal failure caused by diethylene glycol in paracetamol elixir: the Bangladesh epidemic” (1995) 311 BMJ 88.
16. Woolf (n 6).
17. Walt Bogdanich and Jake Hooker, “From China to Panama, a Trail of Poisoned Medicine” *The New York Times* (6 May 2007) <https://www.nytimes.com/2007/05/06/world/americas/06poison.html> accessed 28 May 2021.
18. V.R. Ravi Kumar, “When a Drug Turned Killer” *The Hindu* (9 February 2020) <https://www.thehindu.com/opinion/open-page/when-a-drug-turned-killer/article30770710.ece> accessed 28 May 2021.
19. M. Rahman, “Investigation exposes corruption in drug control in Bombay” *India Today* (31 August 1987) <https://www.indiatoday.in/magazine/living/story/19870831-investigation-exposes-corruption-in-drug-control-in-bombay-799245-1987-08-31> accessed 28 May 2021.
20. Salil Tripathi, “Justice Lentin Commission report indicts Maharashtra public health administration” *India Today* (30 April 1988) <https://www.indiatoday.in/magazine/indiascope/story/19880430-justice-lentin-commission-report-indicts-maharashtra-public-health-administration-797183-1988-04-30> accessed 28 May 2021.
21. Jagvir Singh and others, “Diethylene glycol poisoning in Gurgaon, India, 1998” (2001) 79 *Bull World Health Organ* 88.
22. ibid 92.
23. *M/S Digital Vision vs State of Himachal Pradesh And Others* CWP No.2572 of 2020 (14 August 2020) [para

4(ii)(b)] <https://indiankanoon.org/doc/115798745/> accessed 30 May 2021.

24. "XLN-Xtended Licensing, Laboratory & Legal Node" <https://xlnindia.gov.in/> accessed 30 May 2021.
25. CDSCO Drug Alerts for June, 2014; January, 2017; September, 2018; March, 2019; December, 2019; March, 2020.
26. Priyanka Pulla, "How weak drug laws are costing lives", *Mint* (27 September 2021) < https://www.livemint.com/politics/policy/how-weak-drug-laws-are-costing-lives-11632761831130.html> accessed 29 September 2021.
27. Divya Rajagopal, "CBI Arrests Deputy Drug Controller over Graft Charges" *The Economic Times* (18 August 2019) <https://economictimes.indiatimes.com/news/politics-and-nation/cbi-arrests-deputy-drug-controller-over-graft-charges/articleshow/70728107.cms> accessed 30 May 2021.
28. Aditi Tandon, "Owners of Himachal's Digital Vision among give chargesheeted", *The Tribune* (22 December, 2022) <https://www.tribuneindia.com/news/himachal/owners-of-himachals-digital-vision-among-five-chargesheeted-463274/>
29. Petition requesting transparency in the investigation and recall of DEG contaminated cough syrup that has killed 12 children from Dinesh Thakur to Union Minister of Health, Government of India, 29 August 2020 <https://casemindia.org/wp-content/uploads/2020/08/Recall-Petition-For-Coldbest-Final.pdf> accessed on 23 September 2021.
30. Reply dated 1 June 2021 by the Ministry of Health to Application no. MOHFW/R/T/21/02075 filed under the Right to Information Act 2005 on 1 June 2021.
31. Reply dated 6 July 2021 by CDSCO to Application no. CDSCO/R/T/21/00410 filed under the Right to Information Act on 1 June 2021.
32. Justice B. Lentin, *Report of the Commission of Inquiry (Re. Deaths of Patients in J. J. Hospital at Bombay in January-February 1986 due to alleged reaction of drugs)* (1988) v.

33. ibid iii.
34. Rahman (n 19).
35. Sunil K. Pandya, "Letter from Bombay: An Unmitigated Tragedy" (1988) 297 *BMJ* 117.
36. ibid.
37. Sunil K. Pandya, "Medicine and Society: A Review of the Lentin Commission Report on the Glycerol Tragedy at the J.J. Hospital, Bombay" (1988) 1 *The National Medical Journal of India* 144.
38. Tabassum Barnagarwala, "Mumbai's JJ Hospital to The Gambia: 36 years apart but a familiar story of deadly toxic drugs", *Scroll* (11 November 2022) <https://scroll.in/article/1036860/mumbais-jj-hospital-to-the-gambia-36-years-apart-but-a-familiar-story-of-deadly-toxic-drugs> accessed 1 October 2024.
39. "WHO drew premature link between children deaths in Gambia, India-made cough syrups: DCGI", *Times of India* (15 December 2022) <https://timesofindia.indiatimes.com/india/who-drew-premature-link-between-children-deaths-in-gambia-india-made-cough-syrups-dcgi/articleshow/96259541.cms> accessed 1 October 2024.

CHAPTER ONE

The Birth of Modern Medicine and Drug Regulation

Until the 19th century, the theory and practice of medicine, whether in the East or the West, was based on theories propounded more than 2,000 years ago. Western medicine was based mostly on the humoral theory. This theory, attributed to Hippocrates (approx. 4th BCE to 3rd BCE) and widely popularized by Galen (129–210 AD)[1] theorized that all illness in humans was caused due to an imbalance of the four main humours in the human body—black bile, yellow bile, phlegm, and blood, each of which were individually associated with four elements—earth, fire, water, and air.[2] For example, local inflammations in any part of the body were presumed to be caused by excess blood and hence the remedy of "blood-letting", where the presumed "excess" blood was drained from the body through "medical intervention" in an effort to restore the humoural balance.[3]

At the time, there was a limited understanding of human anatomy because of cultural and legal restrictions against the dissection of human bodies.[4] Later, French doctors like Giovanni Battusta Morgagni and Xavier Bichat began conducting autopsies identifying specific organs and tissues affected by disease. This vastly improved the depth of knowledge about the functioning of the human body. However, despite these advances, there was little scientific consensus in the West on the cause and nature of diseases.[5]

Even in the early 19th century, when Europe was facing outbreaks of cholera, the prevailing theory about the cause of the disease was the primitive Miasma theory. It attributed the spread of diseases like cholera to the inhalation of noxious forms of "bad air", especially the air polluted by decomposing matter.[6] This conclusion was possibly influenced by the observation that epidemics and the plague tended to occur during hot summer months in European cities which had rotting garbage and waste. Maintaining cleanliness and avoiding "bad air" was seen as key to avoiding illnesses.[7]

In the East, where Ayurveda was one of the prevalent medicinal systems in the Indian sub-continent over several centuries, the main underlying theory was that of tri-doshas. The three doshas—vata, pita, and kapha—are presumed to be the energy centers of the human body. One interpretation presumes each dosha to draw its energy from a combination of the elements that constitute the pancha bhoota—space, air, water, fire, and earth.[8] Another interpretation presumes vata to be wind, pitta to be bile, and kapha to be phlegm.[9]

These three doshas were presumed to be influenced by environmental factors, age, and food.[10] As with the humoural theory, an imbalance of doshas was presumed in Ayurveda, to be the cause of most illnesses. In fact, there are Ayurvedic practitioners who insist that Greek theory of humoural medicine was in fact inspired by Ayurveda. Some therapeutic strategies underlying Ayurveda are similar to ancient Greek medicine and include enemas, blood-letting, emesis, purgation, and nasal purging as means to restore the balance.[11]

Needless to say, ancient medicine, whether in the East or the West, was not particularly effective in curing humans of painful diseases.

The birth of the cell theory and germ theory

The theory of medicine was finally transformed only in the late 19th century, less than 200 years ago, when pioneering research by European scientists laid the foundations of the "Cell Theory" and the "Germ Theory of Disease."

While the discovery and naming of "cells" per se is attributed to English scientist Robert Hooke who described "cells" in 1665 in his book *Micrographia,*[12] the "Cell Theory" by itself owes its existence to German scientists Mathias Schleiden and Theodor Schwann, who in the 1830s proposed that cells were the basic constituent building blocks for all plants and animals. The theory contributed to the understanding that all diseases were caused by an alteration of cells in organisms.[13]

The ultimate breakthrough that revolutionized medical science was the conception of the "Germ Theory." This theory postulated that diseases were caused by bacteria, many of them present in the air as proved by Louis Pasteur through his experiments. After being called upon to investigate an outbreak of an infectious disease in the silk industry, he was able to identify two microorganisms that were causing the disease. This led him to believe that microorganisms could cause disease and for that era, this was a revolutionary theory.[14]

Soon thereafter, the German scientist, Robert Koch, was able to prove in a scientifically rigorous manner the infectious nature of disease-causing bacteria in living organisms. He first infected lab mice with fluids extracted from the spleen of cows and sheep that had died of anthrax poisoning. When the mice contracted the disease, he had proof that something in the blood of the dead animals was carrying the disease. He then managed to isolate and purify the element from the blood, by culturing it and injecting it into healthy animals leading them to contract the disease thereby proving the link between a specific pathogen and a particular disease.[15] This experimental research by Koch firmly established the "Germ Theory" and led to him laying down what are known as "Koch's postulates" to establish whether a disease was in fact caused by microorganisms. In the years that followed, Koch identified the specific bacteria responsible for causing tuberculosis (tubercle bacillus) in 1882 and cholera in 1884, thereby transforming scientific understanding of these diseases which had claimed a large number of lives in Europe and the rest of the world.[16] These breakthroughs would change the way mankind searched for possible cures.

The birth of modern medicine

Historically, various civilizations across the earth have been known to experiment with plants and herbs to find cures for diseases and other medical conditions. Many of these civilizations documented in various herbal pharmacopeia, the herbs and plants that had the potential to cure various diseases. In ancient Greece, Dioscorides wrote a treatise called *De material medica*, in which he compiled a list of plants with medical properties that were discovered in the past and through his own research. Ancient Rome had a similar text called *Natural History*, written by Pliny, which compiled an extensive list of herbal and other natural remedies. The Chinese too had several herbal pharmacopeias. The earliest of which, called *Shen-Nung Pen T'sao Ching,* published during the time of the Han dynasty in the 2nd century CE, listed over 365 herbal medicines.[17] Similarly, India has ancient Ayurvedic texts which list the potential medicinal properties of certain herbs and plants.[18]

Humanity's eternal search for medical cures changed in the 19th century after the "Germ Theory" led to breakthroughs in the understanding of disease-causing bacteria, as well as advances in understanding the functioning of the human immune system. These theoretical breakthroughs combined with other scientific breakthroughs by German chemists opened a new door beyond just plants and herbs in the search for new cures. This new world of medical research evolved into two different branches of science—biologicals and chemicals.

In the 19th century, biologicals consisted of only vaccines, which could prevent infections and anti-sera which could for the first-time cure otherwise life-threatening diseases. Until the discovery of the "Germ Theory", the only vaccine that existed was Edward Jenner's smallpox vaccine which he had developed in 1796 by inoculating a child with material taken from a cowpox sore on the hand of a milkmaid. Prior to Jenner's vaccine, there existed a practice called variolation which was used widely across the world, which involved infecting people with small quantities of the smallpox virus, a process which worked to confer immunity on the recipient but was dangerous, often leading to deaths.[19] These were medical innovations that resulted from the powers of observation and correlation without a deep understanding of the science of causation. However, a better understanding of infections and human immunology helped scientists like Pasteur to lead the way in creating a new line of vaccines.

The first of these vaccines were developed in 1880 after Pasteur discovered that the virulence of a pathogen could decrease on its exposure to air or other elements and that injecting such weaker pathogens into healthy humans would stimulate a long-lasting immune response from the human body. Pasteur's theory was proved through his much-publicized experiment in which he administered on some animals a new anthrax vaccine that he had developed. Animals that he had inoculated with his vaccine survived anthrax infections while those in the control group that did not receive the vaccine were infected and perished. Soon Pasteur used the same theory to make the first rabies vaccine, which if administered soon after a dog bite could significantly reduce the chance of infection.[20]

Apart from the development of vaccines, there was also the development of the first antiserum that could cure diphtheria by Emil Behring and Kitasato Shibasaburo, both scientists at Koch's institute. They were able to demonstrate that animals infected with weakened diphtheria toxins were able to produce antibodies which when injected in an infected animal could neutralize the diphtheria toxins in the latter. The first antiserum for diphtheria, cultured in horses and then administered on humans, was an exceptional medical success story. A clinical trial in 1894 with this antiserum on 220 children suffering from diphtheria demonstrated a 77% cure rate. These were extraordinary test results for a disease which at the time was called the "strangling angel" in Europe because of the high toll it took on children and infants.[21] In 1901, Behring was awarded the first ever Nobel Prize in Physiology for his work on the diphtheria and tetanus antiserum.

A second new source of medicines that was tapped into by the Germans were chemicals and dyes. In the 19th century, Germany was a world leader in chemicals and dyes. This was due to a superbly rigorous higher educational system that produced highly skilled chemists.[22] It was these skilled German chemists who were first able to isolate pure chemical ingredients, also known as the "active ingredient", from herbs and plants. For example, morphine was isolated from opium in 1803 and used as a painkiller while quinine was isolated from the bark of the cinchona tree in 1820 and used to treat fevers, especially those caused by malaria.[23] Isolating the active chemical ingredient had enormous advantages since it meant that it would be possible to standardize doses depending on the severity of the medical problem, the physical characteristics of the patient, and also help devise the means to stabilize the medicine in a manner that allowed for it to be stored for longer periods of time.

More importantly, German scientists began studying chemicals as a source of new medicines. They turned to chemicals as a source of new medicine because during the course of experiments, German scientists noticed that many synthetic chemicals being produced by Germany's booming chemical industry could have potential medical applications. They came to this realization when they noticed that different cells and tissues of the human body had affinities for different chemicals. This technique of visualizing different cells and tissues through the use of chemicals came to be known as "staining" and led to the development of a new field called "histology" which was crucial to developing diagnostic tools in medicine. One of the key figures in the development of "staining" techniques was the future Nobel Laureate Paul Ehrlich who was able to develop staining techniques to visualize red and white blood cells in leukemia and anemia. He also developed the diazo colour reaction to identify the presence of bilirubin in the urine of patients with jaundice.[24]

Ehrlich's understanding of the chemical interactions between chemical dyes and human cells led to future breakthroughs in the search for new medicines.[25] It was correctly hypothesized at the time that if specific chemicals interacted in particular ways with cells and tissues, these chemicals could also be a source of new medicines for various infections and medical conditions by interfering with disease-causing bacteria. Proving this hypothesis meant testing hundreds of chemicals to identify the ones with potential curative properties. This was an expensive proposition because it involved a "trial and error" approach and success was never guaranteed.

Securing funding for such research was not an easy task because of which the latter half of the 19th century was witness to a new funding model for scientists engaged in the search for new drugs. This new model involved German scientists entering into agreements with German chemical corporations, where the latter would fund research and provide their chemical "library" to scientists, in exchange for the intellectual property rights in the resulting inventions. As one commentator put it, "...the most significant innovation of the great German biochemical revolution was neither drugs not vaccines themselves but the creation of a durable funding source for ongoing lab research."[26]

The funding model and the decision to tap into chemicals and dyestuffs proved to be very fruitful. By the end of the 19th century, the biggest German chemical corporations like Hoescht, Bayer, and BASF had introduced to the market the first analgesics and antipyretics such as Aspirin, Kairin, Phenacetin, Antipyrine, Antifebrin, etc.[27] By 1910, Paul Ehrlich had discovered arsphenamine, the first real antibiotic and "miracle cure". Known internally in Ehrlich's laboratory as Compound 606, the drug which was developed with support from Cassella, a German company, was eventually sold under the brand name "Salvasaran" by Hoescht, another German chemical company.[28] It was found to be highly effective against syphilis, a sexually transmitted disease that was highly contagious and deadly. The disease affected millions across Europe. Needless to say, the drug was a huge commercial success. It presumably made Hoechst AG significant profits and laid the foundations for the modern pharmaceutical industry to pour resources into the discovery of new drugs in exchange for patent rights.

In 1932, a different set of German scientists,

led by future Nobel Laurate Gerhard Domagk, and supported by Bayer, followed Ehrlich's approach of testing thousands of chemicals on disease-infected mice before discovering the effectiveness of a specific variant of sulfanilamide. The new drug demonstrated astounding curative effects on laboratory mice that were infected with streptococci, which is a type of bacteria that causes many life-threatening infections in humans. It was soon discovered that this new drug could also cure a number of non-strep infections such as spinal meningitis, gonorrhea, and childbed fever, all of which were caused by different kinds of disease-causing bacteria. This new "wonder drug" was first marketed as Protonsil by Bayer and proved to be a true blockbuster.[29]

Given all these medical breakthroughs, it was no surprise that Germany soon came to be known as the "pharmacy of the world."[30]

This era of medical breakthroughs laid the foundations for the modern pharmaceutical industry and drug innovation. The challenge now for governments across the world was to ensure the consistent supply of quality drugs while keeping in check the fantastical claims being made by the pharmaceutical industry about their new inventions. This was easier said than done given the fact that many of these pharmaceutical corporations grew rapidly to become very profitable and powerful. Older models of self-regulation had to give way to a more direct intervention by the state.

The nation state steps in to regulate the science of drugs

Historically, in most societies, medicine was formulated by individual apothecaries or pharmacists or *vaids* or *hakims* as they were known in different jurisdictions. These solo practitioners would usually prepare various concoctions from mainly herbs, and sometimes alcohol, which was the common solvent available to extract the "active ingredients" from the herbs. The ingredients of these concoctions would only rarely be disclosed to the public. State regulation of these drugs was limited in the 19th century. For example, in the UK, the state did not directly regulate the quality of drugs. Rather it enacted legislation such as the Apothecaries Act 1815, or the Pharmacy Act 1868, which vested the right to manufacture certain specific drugs in apothecaries and pharmacies, who in turn would regulate themselves through their professional guilds or societies.[31] The other form of regulation was via penal laws, which prohibited the adulteration of drugs. For example, the Indian Penal Code 1860, which was enacted by the British after the Crown took over the administration of India from the East India Company had a specific clause penalizing the adulteration of food and drugs.[32]

These prevalent models of regulation evolved with the discovery of new and effective therapies. Once mass manufacture of these new drugs began, it was necessary to create a new regulatory model especially since biologicals like vaccines and anti-sera were injected directly into the bodies of human beings. Even slight contamination during the manufacturing process could be fatal for the patient. Germany led the way in creating a new regulatory model. A key inspiration for the proactiveness of the German government was the "tuberculin" scandal in the preceding decade where Robert Koch's much anticipated new treatment—tuberculin—for treating tuberculosis failed to prove effective in curing the disease.[33] Eager to ensure the availability of high-quality anti-diphtheria serum, imperial Germany proactively put in place a new regulatory system in 1895 to ensure quality control of serum.

There were two components to the new German regulatory model created specifically for anti-diphtheria serum. The first was the creation of legally binding standards to ensure the potency and purity of the serums meant for use as treatments on humans. This was the first-time standards were being created for serums and it was a complex task. It had to begin with the very basic task of creating units to measure serum. Once standards were created and included in the legally recognized pharmacopeia, they were made binding on all future manufacturers. The ultimate aim of creating standards was to ensure consistency in the purity and potency of anti-diphtheria serum across the industry.

Adherence to these standards by manufacturers was then monitored at two sites. The first was at the site of production where an officer appointed by the state monitored the production process, and the second was at the state-run Institute for Serological Research and Serological Survey (ISRSS), which functioned under the leadership of Paul Ehlrich, where each batch would be tested by a team of experts for adherence to quality standards.[34] This would include testing the serum on infected guinea pigs. If the serum was potent, it would only show a mild reaction at the spot where it was injected. If not, the guinea pig would die in four days.[35] By the standards of the day, this was a remarkably rigorous regulatory set-up.

Like the Germans, the French took a proactive approach to regulating these new anti-sera. The French enacted a legislation in 1895, covering a whole range of biologicals including any "...attenuated viruses, therapeutic sera, modified toxins and analogous products that can serve as prophylaxis against or therapy for contagious diseases..." All such products would require prior authorization from the Ministry of Interior, which relied on inputs from members of the Academy of Sciences and a Consultative Committee on Public Health.[36]

Both the German and French regulatory models were pathbreaking because they ensured perhaps for the first time in history, an assurance from the state regarding the quality of a drug that was being supplied to patients. Not only did this relieve pharmacists of their traditional job of guaranteeing quality but it also acted to boost public confidence in these new therapies.[37]

Not all countries were as proactive as the Germans

and the French when it came to regulating these exciting new drugs. An interesting contrast to the proactive regulatory approach of the German and French, is the American approach to regulation. Till 1962, the American attempt to regulate the pharmaceutical industry has generally been on the heels of death and scandal. The first mass deaths due to contaminated vaccines and anti-sera occurred in the USA in the year 1901. In the first case, anti-diphtheria serum, which was unknowingly contaminated with tetanus, caused the death of 13 children in St Louis, Missouri. The horse that had been bled for the serum had a tetanus infection and was killed on discovery of the infection but the vials of serum drawn from the infected horse had not been destroyed or tested on guinea pigs. When administered on children, the anti-diphtheria serum infected them with tetanus causing their deaths. These deaths received a lot of publicity in the national press. As a result, there was a drop in confidence in this new treatment leading to an increase in deaths due to diphtheria in some cities. In that same year, there were 11 deaths in Camden, New Jersey, of people who recently received small pox vaccinations. They had died of tetanus infections and it was suspected that some of the vaccines were contaminated.[38]

These deaths in St Louis and Camden were the first instances of mass deaths from mass manufactured drugs and served as a reminder that these new life-saving and disease-preventing biologicals could be dangerous if not manufactured and tested properly in completely sterilized premises. The USA at the time did not regulate biologicals. These deaths, along with other cases of bacterial contamination of biological products, led to American doctors and the press demanding some form of regulation of biological products. The very next year, in 1902, the American Congress enacted into law the Biologics Control Act 1902, with an intent to guarantee the safety and efficacy of new biologics.

While most commentators view the Biologics Control Act as a reaction to the deaths in St Louis and Camden, there are academics who argue otherwise, stating that it was the biologics industry that pushed for the legislation. As per this theory, the privately owned pharmaceutical industry was worried that any more incidents of contaminations and death would cause various state and municipal governments in America to expand their existing manufacturing facilities for biologicals in order to better control quality of the biologicals available in their jurisdictions. Unlike today, America in the early 19th century had a public sector manufacturing biologicals. If that manufacturing process expanded further, it would reduce the private sector's market share. Better regulation was thus in the interest of the private sector, since it would check the "bad players" in the private sector and protect the reputation of the private sector.[39]

While the enactment of the Biologics Control Act 1902, brought regulation to the American pharmaceutical industry, it was limited to only "biologicals" i.e., viruses, therapeutic serums, toxins etc. This law did not cover other drugs, such as the newly available anti-pyretic drugs or even the first antibiotics, which were derived from industrial chemicals and dyestuff. The rest of these drugs came to be regulated by another American law called the Pure Food and Drugs Act 1906. This legislation was enacted after being kept pending for 27 years and after muck-raking journalists like Samuel Hopkins Adam and Upton Sinclair shone light on the fraudulent claims by the "patent medicine" industry and the meat-packing industry.[40] This new law focused on issues such as mandating proper disclosure of ingredients on labelling of drugs (in order to combat the secrecy of 'patent medicine'), as well as prohibiting the adulteration and misbranding of drugs with "false claims". The Pure Food and Drugs Act did not focus on either "safety" or "efficacy" of new drugs.

The shortcomings of the model of regulation under the Pure Food and Drugs Act 1906 for non-biological drugs made itself obvious in 1937 when an American drug manufacturer sold Sulfanilamide in a liquid form after dissolving it in DEG, without realizing the dangerous side-effects of DEG on humans. This mistake caused the deaths of more than 100 Americans when they drank the poisoned syrup. The tragedy invited a swift legislative response from the American Congress in the form of the Food, Drug and Cosmetic Act 1938, which amended the existing drug regulatory law to make it mandatory for manufacturers to submit safety data to the United States Food and Drug Administration (USFDA) before they could sell new drugs in America.[41]

Four years after the Sulfanilamide disaster in 1941, tragedy struck once again, this time due to poor manufacturing practices within the American pharmaceutical industry. A batch of Sulfathiazole tablets had been contaminated with a sedative called Phenobarbital at a manufacturing plant owned by Winthrop, leading to over 300 deaths in the United States.[42] The episode led to the birth of modern Good Manufacturing Practices (GMPs) in the USA. As therapies and the pharmaceutical supply chain got more complex, the formulation and enforcement of GMPs by the state became even more crucial. For example, a key concern across the board, especially with injectables has been the challenge of maintaining sterility of all ingredients, including water. Even minor microbiological contamination can lead to serious infections. Given these challenges, GMP regulations have become progressively more detailed with almost every aspect of manufacturing and record-keeping covered by these regulations.

Across the Atlantic, European countries who did not learn from the American reforms of 1938 were about to face one of the most shocking tragedies in the history of the pharmaceutical industry because of a new drug called Thalidomide. Initially marketed as a tranquilizer, Thalidomide was also being prescribed to pregnant women in Europe as a remedy for morning sickness. Unknown to doctors at the time, the drug was teratogenic that is, it had an adverse effect on the fetus, resulting in the birth of thousands of disabled babies in Europe in the late 50s and early 60s. In most cases, the limbs of the baby failed to develop properly while in some other cases, the eyes and ears were not developed properly. While the global toll of Thalidomide is unknown, it is estimated Germany alone saw the birth of 10,000 babies affected by Thalidomide.[43] There were also countless miscarriages across countries where pregnant women had been prescribed Thalidomide. The United States on the other hand saw the birth of only 17 babies affected by Thalidomide and even those births were because of the distribution of samples to doctors who had passed them on to their patients. This was because a heroic and diligent USFDA inspector, Frances Oldam Kelsey, had persistently rejected the marketing application filed by the manufacturers of Thalidomide due to their failure to submit the safety data required by the amendments in 1938.[44]

Kelsey would go on to receive the President's Award for Distinguished Federal Civilian Service from American President J.F. Kennedy. She is considered to be one of the most significant personalities in the history of the USFDA, where she worked until the age of 91 years. On her passing at the age of 101 years, the *New York Times* in an obituary for her described her as a, "...20th-century American heroine for her role in the thalidomide case, celebrated not only for her vigilance, which spared the USA from widespread birth deformities, but also for giving rise to modern laws regulating pharmaceuticals."[45]

The silent heroes of the Thalidomide episode were the policy makers who had amended American regulatory law in 1938 to mandate the submission of safety data as one of the conditions for approving new drugs in the United States. The episode was a stark reminder of the dangers of new medicines and the need to scientifically vet new drugs prior to their introduction in the market.

A new law and the demand for proof of "efficacy"

The timing of the Thalidomide tragedy coincided with a scathing American Congressional inquiry into the workings of the American pharmaceutical industry. This inquiry which was held by the Senate Subcommittee on Anti-trust & Monopoly, from the years 1957 to 1961, was presided by Senator Estes Kefauver.[46]

By the time of this inquiry, the pharmaceutical industry had been transformed by a series of brilliant scientific discoveries. This included the discovery of a range of broad-spectrum antibiotics such as Penicillin, Ampicillin, Streptomycin, Neomycin, Aureomycin, and Erythromycin, all of which revolutionized medicine and slashed mortality rates from bacterial infections in less than a decade.[47] Apart from these antibiotics, scientists also discovered painkillers, anti-psychotropic drugs, hormonal therapies, and cardio-vascular drugs. Most of these discoveries were by private pharmaceutical corporations who were able to ringfence their inventions with patents and then market them under exclusive brand names. The resulting patent monopolies and the fantastical marketing claims quickly resulted in these pharmaceutical corporations becoming the most profitable businesses in America. The monopolistic nature of the pharmaceutical industry, the pricing of these drugs, and the manner in which they were marketed became the focus of the Senate anti-trust committee.

While investigating marketing practices of the pharmaceutical industry, the committee was particularly concerned with the issue of "efficacy" of new drugs given the wildly exaggerated claims being made by their manufacturers and their salesmen, often without scientific basis. The blitzkrieg of advertisements and marketing efforts assumed the form of visits to doctors by "detail men" (the terminology for sales persons employed by the pharmaceutical industry), mailing of brochures and samples, advertisements in medical journals, and exhibits at marketing conference.[48] The challenge for American doctors at the receiving end of these advertisements was to determine for themselves the claims of efficacy of these advertisements. As explained by a Dr Weinstein who deposed before the Committee:

> ...a number of drugs have been put on the market with efficacy claims based on extremely meager and unobjective observations by people not truly qualified to make such observations. Also, there is absolutely nothing in the law to prevent the manufacturer from completely ignoring unfavourable reports. One company in its advertising for one of its products

> blithely states that there have been over 200 reports in the literature about this particular drug. They neglect to say that 60 per cent are not entirely favourable or pertinent.[49]

At that point in time, as explained earlier, American law did not require manufacturers to submit evidence of therapeutic efficacy. It only prohibited companies from making false therapeutic claims. This prohibition could be effectively circumvented by referencing vague scientific and experimental studies, the veracity of which was never verified by the state. As a result, many of the doctors deposing before Kefauver's committee suggested that independent agencies like the USFDA or the National Institute of Health (NIH) play a role in determining the efficacy of each new drug. A Dr Dowling testified as follows before the Committee:

> First, the Food and Drug Administration should be empowered to examine the efficacy as well as the toxic effects of all new drugs. It should be obvious to everyone that insufficient knowledge on the part of the doctor regarding the efficacy of a drug can react to the detriment of a patient just as much as toxic action by the drug, which the Food and Drug Administration now has the power to regulate.[50]

This point was belaboured by other doctors who warned the committee that questions of efficacy had a direct bearing on safety and that it made no sense for the FDA to evaluate only safety without also examining efficacy of the drugs in question.

The hearings of the Senate anti-trust committee were widely publicized in the press with several newspapers providing daily updates to the public on Kefauver's confrontations with the heads of the biggest pharmaceutical corporations, as he hauled them over coals over their astonishing profit margins. By the time the final report was tabled, there was support for a new law to regulate the pharmaceutical industry.

Initially, political differences between the Kennedy administration and Kefauver almost gutted the law that was meant to reform many of the issues that came to the fore during the committee hearings, including the issue of regulatory reform. The thalidomide tragedy however brought them together to enable the enactment of far-reaching reforms on 10 October 1962. Known as the Kefauver-Harris Amendments, after the senators who sponsored the bill to amend the Federal Food, Drug and Cosmetic Act, these amendments empowered the FDA to seek efficacy data in addition to safety data before approving a new drug for marketing in the USA. This data would have to be collected through "controlled" clinical trials.[51]

The enactment of this law was widely welcomed by the press. The *New York Times* declared it a "Victory on Drug Regulation", calling Senator Kefauver the "hero of this victory" for doggedly pushing the "... legislation despite widespread public apathy, lack of Administration interest and bitter opposition from some industry and Congressional sources."[52] As correctly noted by the *New York Times*, Kefauver's efforts would have been in vain if it was not for the unfortunate Thalidomide tragedy that awoke the public, the government, and the legislature to the dangers of this new era of medical innovation. Commenting on the indifference of the elected representatives on such an important issue until the precipitation of a crisis, the editorial remarked on how it did "...not speak too well for Congressional responsiveness to a public need that it took such an unpredictable and chance occurrence as the thalidomide tragedy to secure passage of this law so clearly related to the general welfare." This lack of responsiveness by politicians to the demands of drug regulation is unfortunately a feature in democracies around the world. Nevertheless, given the Thalidomide tragedy, the Kefauver-Harris amendments enacted in the USA were eventually replicated in Europe and other developed countries in the following decades. This new model of regulation was extraordinary for its time because the state for the first time was playing a role in guaranteeing efficacy of all new drugs on the basis of scientific data and expert opinion.

Lessons from history

There are four important takeaways from this discussion on the evolution of medicine and drug regulation in the democracies of the USA and Europe.

The first is that much of drug regulatory law has been written with the blood of citizens who died in hundreds, many of them, children. This tells us that if a country is governed by a poorly designed and enforced drug regulatory system, people will die. The pharmaceutical industry cannot be trusted to regulate itself.

The second takeaway is that even robust democracies with a free press have not always taken proactive steps to ensure efficient drug regulation. The major drug regulatory milestones in the USA and Europe over the last century were triggered mostly by mass deaths or scandals caused by experimental or poorly manufactured medicines. The Germans wanted to regulate the anti-diphtheria serum because of their past experience with Koch's failed tuberculin. The Americans were forced to act in 1902, 1938, and 1941 only because of mass deaths of their citizens due to contaminated drugs. Again in 1962, the Thalidomide disaster forced sweeping reforms in both the USA and Europe because of the deaths and deformities caused by the new drug. There are few other areas of regulatory law where reforms have been catalyzed primarily due to the mass death of citizens.

The third takeaway is that debates around drug regulation have progressively become more scientifically complex. The 1901 scandal in St Louis was because the contaminated sera was due to an infected horse from which the serum was extracted. The Thalidomide tragedy however was because the drug in one particular isomeric form was dangerous to the unborn fetus. The complexity of these issues has increased progressively over the decades. Any regulatory system meant to deal with cutting edge pharmaceutical innovation needs to be upgraded regularly, both in terms of qualified personnel and regulations every time technology makes a leap ahead. Given the lethargy and red-tape of most bureaucracies, the regulator is likely to remain one step behind the industry unless elected representatives crack the whip.

The fourth takeaway is that it is in the interest of the pharmaceutical industry as a whole to welcome better regulatory standards. A major fallout of the above scandals, apart from deaths and lawsuits, is the loss of consumer confidence and this can be a setback for both public health and profitability of the pharmaceutical sector. There are examples from the early 20th century where big players in the American and German pharmaceutical industries welcomed regulation because they were worried that unregulated players may lead to more public sector involvement in manufacturing of new drugs. They expected consumer confidence in their medicines to improve significantly if state regulators played an active role in guaranteeing the safety and efficacy of all drugs in the market. This enthusiasm amongst the pharmaceutical industry towards regulation has fluctuated over the decades but the core sentiment likely remains the same.

The point of discussing the regulatory history of Europe and the USA is to demonstrate, through the course of this book, how little India has learnt from the history of these other countries. The price of this ignorance is often paid by not just Indian citizens but also the citizens of India's trading partners who import copious amounts of medicine from the "pharmacy of the developing world."

Notes

1. William Bynum, *The History of Medicine: A Very Short Introduction* (OUP 2008), 5.
2. ibid 10.
3. ibid 12–13.
4. ibid 11.
5. ibid 53–55.
6. ibid 75–76.
7. Marianna Karamanou and others, "From Miasmas to Germs: A Historical Approach to Theories of Infectious Disease Transmission" (2012) 1 *Le Infezioni in Medicina*, 58, 59.
8. Priya Vrat Sharma, *History of Medicine in India, from Antiquity to 1000 A.D.* (Indian National Science Academy 1992), 382.
9. M.R. Raghava Varier, *A Brief History of Ayurveda* (OUP 2020), 61.
10. Sharma, (n 8), 383.
11. Varier, (n 9), 52.
12. Bynum, (n 1), 93.
13. Paolo Mazzarello, "A Unifying Concept: The History of Cell Theory" (1999) 1 *Nature Cell Biology*, E13.
14. Bynum, (n 1), 99.
15. William Rosen, *Miracle Cure: The Creation of Antibiotics and the Birth of Modern* (Penguin 2017), 23.
16. Bynum, (n 1), 103–104.
17. Les Iversen, *Drugs: A Very Short Introduction* (OUP 2016), 2–3.
18. Syal Kumar, Gustav J. Dobos and Thomas Rampp, "The Significance of Ayurvedic Medicinal Plants" (2017) 22 *Journal of Evidence-based Complementary & Alternative Medicine*, 494.
19. Stefan Riedel, "Edward Jenner and the History of Smallpox and Vaccination" (2005), 18 *Baylor University Medical Centre Proceedings*, 21.
20. ibid.

21. Stefan H.E. Kaufmann, “Remembering Emil von Behring: From Tetanus Treatment to Antibody Cooperation with Phagocytes” 8 mBio e00117.
22. Rosen, (n 15), 40.
23. Iversen, (n 17), 5.
24. Michael Titford, “Paul Ehrlich: Histological Staining, Immunology, Chemotherapy” (2010) 41 *Laboratory Medicine*, 497.
25. ibid.
26. Rosen, (n 15), 57.
27. Kay Brune and Burkhard Hinz, “The Discovery and Development of Antiinflammatory Drugs” (2004) 50 *Arthritis & Rheumatism*, 2391.
28. Rosen, (n 15), 57.
29. Rosen, (n 15), 67.
30. Tobias Cramer, “Building the “World’s Pharmacy’: The Rise of the German Pharmaceutical Industry, 1871–1914” (2015) 89 *Business History Review*, 43.
31. Jon Merrills, *Pharmacy Law and Practice* (Elsevier 2013), 363.
32. Indian Penal Code 1860, s. 272.
33. Axel C. Hüntelmann, “Evaluation as a Practical Technique of Administration: The Regulation and Standardization of Diphtheria Serum” in Jonathan Simon and Christoph Gradmann (eds), *Evaluating and Standardizing Therapeutic Agents, 1890–1950* (Palgrave Macmillan 2010) ch 2, 44.
34. ibid 35.
35. ibid.
36. Jonathan Simon, “The Politics of Serum Production in France”, in Jonathan Simon and Christoph Gradmann (eds), *Evaluating and Standardizing Therapeutic Agents, 1890–1950* (Palgrave Macmillan 2010) ch 5, 96.
37. ibid.
38. Ross E. DeHovitz, “The 1901 St Louis Incident: The First Modern Medical Disaster” (2014) 133 *Paediatrics*, 964.
39. Terry S. Coleman, “Early Developments in the Regulation

of Biologics" (2016) 71 *FOOD AND DRUG LAW JOURNAL*, 544.

40. Bryan Denham, "Magazine Journalism in the Golden Age of Muckraking: Patent-Medicine Exposures Before and After the Pure Food and Drug Act of 1906" (2020) 22(2) *Journalism & Communication Monographs*, 100; James H. Cassedy, "Muckraking and Medicine: Samuel Hopkins Adams" (1964) 16 *American Quarterly*, 85.
41. Suzanne White Junod, "FDA and Clinical Drug Trials: A Short History" (US Food & Drug Administration 2008) 5 <https://www. fda.gov/media/110437/download> accessed 28 June 2021.
42. John P. Swann, "The 1941 Sulfathiazole Disaster and the Birth of Good Manufacturing Practices" (1999) 41 *American Institute of the History of Pharmacy*, 16.
43. "What's Happened to Thalidomide Babies?—BBC News" (3 November 2011) <https://www.bbc.com/news/magazine-15536544> accessed 28 June 2021.
44. Katie Thomas, "Pursuing an Untold Story of Thalidomide", *The New York Times* (23 March 2020) <https://www.nytimes.com/2020/03/23/ reader-center/insider-thalidomide-fda.html> accessed 27 June 2021.
45. Robert D. McFadden, "Frances Oldham Kelsey, Who Saved U.S. Babies From Thalidomide, Dies at 101", *The New York Times* (7 August 2015) <https://www.nytimes.com/2015/08/08/science/frances-oldham-kelsey-fda-doctor-who-exposed-danger-of- thalidomide-dies-at-101.html> accessed 28 June 2021.
46. United States Senate (Sub-committee on Antitrust and Monopoly), *Study of Administered Prices in the Drug Industry* (Rep No 448, 1961).
47. Rosen (n 15).
48. United States Senate (Sub-committee on Antitrust and Monopoly) (n 46), 156.
49. ibid 187.
50. ibid.

51. Jeremy A. Greene and Scott H. Podolsky, "Reform, Regulation, and Pharmaceuticals—The Kefauver—Harris Amendments at 50" (2012) 367 *The New England Journal of Medicine*, 1481.
52. "Victory on Drug Regulation", *The New York Times* (5 October 1962) <https://www.nytimes.com/1962/10/05/archives/victory-on- drug-regulation.html> accessed 28 June 2021.

CHAPTER TWO

Controlling the Craze for Medicinal Drugs in Colonial India

One of the earliest public debates in India on the need for regulating the manufacture and sale of pharmaceutical drugs took place in 1927 in the Council of States of the bi-cameral Indian Legislature when India was still under British rule. A legislator from the Bombay Presidency, Sir Haroon Jaffer, had moved a resolution on the 9 March 1927, before the Council of States, titled "control of the craze for medicinal drugs." The short text of the resolution was as follows:

> This Council recommends to the Governor General in Council to urge all Provincial Governments to take immediate measures to control the craze for medicinal drugs by legislation for the standardisation of the preparation and sale of such drugs.[1]

In his address to the Council, Sir Jaffer took aim at four issues pertaining to medicinal drugs.

The first was the indiscriminate availability of all kinds of medicines of doubtful efficacy. In his words, several of the new drugs made "claims that were never properly demonstrated and which are prepared merely to put money into the pockets of the manufacturers."[2]

The second issue was "the indiscriminate use of drugs by doctors in their prescriptions."[3] These included the so called "patent & proprietary drugs" whose ingredients were kept confidential and not disclosed to the public. This problem was greatly magnified in India, according to Sir Jaffer, by the number of "unqualified or only partly qualified and very inexperienced doctors" practising in India.

The third issue was the growing demand from the public for all kinds of powders, tonics, serums, vaccines, and injections, regardless of the absurd claims made by the manufacturers of such medicines. Sir Jaffer jokingly remarked:

> I have not yet heard of any case in India where the monkey gland has been grafted on to an old person to make him as frisky as a full-blooded boy, but I presume it is possible that many enthusiasts getting on in years have atleast made inquiries about it based on what they have read of so called successful graftings in the West.[4]

The fourth issue was the problem of adulteration and substandard drugs. He explained how there were many cases where a local drug was "absolutely useless" and "inactive, if not adulterated" and boosted by the "unsolicited testimonials" from "non-existent individuals".[5]

The bleak picture painted by Sir Jaffer was not surprising since at the time there was no uniform law in British India regulating the manufacturing standards and sale of medicinal drugs. Although some provinces like Bengal, the Central Provinces, Assam, Ajmer-Merwar, and United Provinces had provincial legislations to regulate the sale of adulterated drugs, none of them dealt with standardization of drug quality or efficacy of drugs. These were presumably very basic laws, since it is almost impossible to guarantee quality without the creation of binding legal standards. Some of the remaining provinces, like Madras, had enacted legislation only on the issue of food adulteration.[6]

Of the four speakers that followed Sir Jaffer, two supported the resolution with amendments and two others opposed it. One of the supporters was Major General T.H. Symons who was then the Director General of the Indian Medical Service (IMS), which although primarily a military service, played an important role in influencing public health policies in British India until 1947 when it was disbanded.[7] General Symons described to the Council an inspection of dispensaries and mofussil hospitals in the Madras Presidency by experts which had revealed certain dispensaries to contain expensive drugs that he had never heard of during his career as a doctor. Supporting the urgent need for standardization of drugs in India, General Symons pointed out how both the USA and the UK had already enacted legislation to regulate the manufacture and sale of pharmaceutical drugs.[8] The USA had enacted two laws to regulate the manufacture and sale of medicinal drugs: the Biologics Control Act

1902, and the Pure Foods and Drugs Act 1906.[9] The British had enacted The Sale of Food and Drugs Act 1875, which was limited in its scope, and the more thorough Therapeutic Substances Act 1925, which regulated only biologics.[10]

Opposing the motion was Dr U. Rama Rau, a legislator from Madras who was outraged by Sir Jaffer's criticism of doctors, describing the speech as "nonsense and libel".[11] Dr Rau blamed the "craze" for medicines not on doctors but unregulated advertisements in the press. Addressing the Council, he said:

> Sir, the craze for patent medicines is not because of doctors. It is because of numerous advertisements appear in the papers, not only the Indian papers but also the English and other papers, in which the patent medicines are advertised to cure every illness on the face of the earth. If my Honourable friend had moved a Resolution to prevent these patent medicines from being advertised in India I could understand it, or if he had said that advertisements must not appear in the papers regarding patent medicines, I would have entirely supported him. Or if he had moved that there should be no importation of patent medicines from foreign countries to India, I would have entirely supported him.[12]

The second speaker opposing the motion was Mr P.C. Desi Chakra, a representative from Burma. His opposition was borne from the fact that such regulation would lean in favour of Western medicine and against Ayurvedic medicine.[13] According to him, doctors trained in Western medicine had a "natural bias" that would tend to put out of the market all Unani and Ayurvedic preparations which at the time were popular choice of medicine in British India.[14] This concern is not entirely surprising because there was always some tension between Western medicine and traditional Indian medicine in the pre-independence era not only for commercial reasons but also because of cultural conflicts over practices such as dissection of the human body.[15]

Notwithstanding the opposition, the motion ultimately was adopted by the Council of States after some amendments, notably to drop the word "craze for medicinal drugs" which was replaced with "indiscriminate use of medicinal drugs".[16] It was a momentous occasion for British-ruled India because until this motion was adopted, the interest of India's British rulers in the issue of drug quality was motivated by their desire to control the trade in narcotics and taxation. The government laboratories that existed at the time were primarily affiliated to tax authorities because they were meant to check the amount of opium or alcohol in food and drug products so as to determine the excise duty payable. The issue of adulteration or drug quality from a safety perspective was not on the radar of India's colonial rulers until this motion by Sir Jaffer forced the British Government to take note.[17]

The debate preceding the vote on the resolution is fascinating because of the many parallels it has to the debate on drug regulation in India of the 21st century.

This includes the perception of a problematic nexus between doctors and pharmaceutical companies, the issue of misleading advertisements by an assorted group of charlatans selling all kinds of concoctions as medicines, the tension between traditional medicine and modern evidence-based medicine, and lastly, the continuing problem of adulterated and sub-standard medicine.

The colonial government drags its feet on the issue

Despite Sir Jaffer's resolution being adopted by the Council of States, the British administrators of India continued dragging their feet on the issue. In 1928, yet another motion was moved in the Legislative Assembly of the Indian Legislature; this time asking for an adjournment of the proceedings of the House to discuss the urgent issue of "quinine fraud".[18] The legislator behind that motion was Lt Colonel H.A.J. Gidney. A prominent member of the Anglo-Indian community and formerly a member of the IMS, he was a nominated member to the Legislative Assembly.[19] He was no stranger to the debate on regulating medicinal drugs. Many years before his motion to discuss the "quinine fraud", in 1921, when Gidney was a member of the Legislative Assembly, he had attempted to convince the government during a discussion on the budget that the customs duty on import of patent medicines from the UK. And other countries should be increased to 20% from 7.5% because many of these drugs (whose composition was secret at the time) were perpetuating false claims through their "cure-all" advertisements. That amendment to the budget failed because the government did not think that customs tariffs were the best solution to the problem described by Gidney.[20]

But returning to his address to the House, on 4 September 1928 demanding an adjournment, Gidney warned the government that the mortality due to malaria in India was a staggering four million patients a year and that "spurious" quinine was likely one of the reasons for the large number of avoidable malarial deaths in India. At the time, quinine, which was first isolated in 1920 from the bark of the cinchona tree found originally in Peru, was the most effective treatments for malaria. In Gidney's words, the quinine fraud was "the most terrible fraud that has ever been perpetrated on this country and the unrestricted sale of this spurious drug has, I submit, been largely responsible for the steady high mortality from malaria."[21]

Illustrating with an example, Gidney described the results of an examination of Quinine by a Chemical Examiner of the Punjab Government who certified that a sample advertised to have five grains of Quinine Bisulphate actually had only one grain or less of Quinine and three and a half grains of chalk, along with one grain of alum or some other substance to lend taste! He also made the sensational claim that "most of the quinine offered in the bazaars for sale to the public...is not quinine but chalk."[22] This was no exaggeration. Earlier that year, the *Indian Medical Gazette* had published a small survey documenting the quality of quinine sold in India by J.W.D Megaw, an officer in the IMS along with Sudhamoy Ghosh and N.R. Chatterjee who were both professors at the Calcutta School of Tropical Medicine. They drew 90 samples of quinine tablets from the market and tested them for the quantity of quinine in each sample.They discovered that 23 samples were 25% weaker than the stated strength. More than 40% of the samples had a deficiency of more than 10%. Some 11 samples had more quinine content than advertised. Although the survey was quite small, it was the first empirical evidence of the quinine fraud in India at the time.[23]

According to Gidney, the problem was not limited to quinine since India was "par excellence the dumping ground for every variety of quack medicine and adulterated drug manufactured in all parts of the world."[24] The sole responsibility for the sale of such spurious medicine according to Gidney, was thc failure of the government to take steps to regulate the sale of medicinal drugs at a time when even countries like Egypt, Palestine, and Mesopotamia had drug regulatory laws in place.[25]

Reminding the government of Sir Jaffer's motion that was adopted by the Council of States, on 9 March 1927, Gidney upbraided the government for dragging its feet on the issue despite the widespread support for such a law from both the medical profession and the industry. He rattled off the following names of eminent personalities who supported the enactment of such a law:

> The Tropical School of Medicine in Calcutta has also pronounced its opinion about the danger of this drug adulteration and pressed for legislation. The Senior Trade Commissioner has also exposed these dangers and advised a Food and Drugs Act. Mr. J.C. Ghosh of Calcutta has also exposed these dangers and pressed for legislation. The Indian Chambers of Commerce in Bombay have also written to the Government of India, Education, Health and Lands Department, and asked for a Food & Drugs Act and standardisation of all drugs manufacturers or imported into India. Representatives of well-known drug manufacturers and the public Press have also widely ventilated the fraud and dangers. I ask the Government, what has it done? Nothing! When it was clearly its duty to act at once and save India. Why has it failed to do its duty? Why has it not introduced a Food and Drugs Act, a Pharmacy and Poisons Bill and other remedial measures?[26]

There indeed appeared to have been a groundswell of support at that time in the Indian press across the industry and the medical profession on the issue of legislation to improve the quality of drug supply. It was a topic of discussion at the recent Indian Science Congress held at Lahore, where in Sir Jaffer's words "...the drug craze in India and the tendency for it to reach dangerous proportions were...fully discussed and...it was unanimously agreed that some control was urgently needed."[27] Similarly, the Secretary of Indian Merchants Chamber of Bombay complained to the government that the uncontrolled sale of inferior quality drugs was creating a bad name for the pharmaceutical industry and that the Chambers was of the view that "the introduction of a Food and Drugs Act in this country would be desirable from the point of view of both dealers and consumers, as some continental and English firms are known to make a practice of wilfully adulterating their goods for shipment into India in response to trade demands for such goods."[28]

Similarly, medical journals like the *Indian Medical Gazette*, the *Indian and Eastern Druggist*, and the *Pharmaceutical Journal of England*, as also newspapers like the *Statesman* and the *Civil and Military Gazette* had voiced their support for governmental regulation of the sale of drugs.[29]

Despite this popular support for the government to regulate the manufacture and sale of medicinal drugs, the British administrators of India appeared to be indifferent to the issue. In its response to Gidney's motion for adjournment, the British India Government speaking through Mr G.S. Bajpai, the Secretary of the Department of Education, Health and Lands and a bureaucrat belonging to the Indian Civil Service (ICS), managed to successfully convince the President of the Council of States to dismiss Gidney's motion for adjournment because it dealt with a vintage issue rather than a recent event as required by the rules of the house.[30] In other words, the issue was not urgent enough because it had been raised in India repeatedly and for a long time.

Regardless of Gidney's failed, yet heroic, effort

to pin the government into a corner, it is worth reflecting on the possible reasons for the delay in the government's lethargic response to unregulated sale of medicinal drugs.

The first and most likely reason is that the British colonial project in India was focused on extracting economic resources from India rather than governance for the well-being and improvement of lives of the average Indian citizen. In the eloquent (and famous) words of John Sullivan, an Englishman who had headed the Board of Revenue, "Our system acts very much like a sponge, drawing up all the good things from the banks of the Ganges, and squeezing them down on the banks of the Thames." Not only did India serve as a base for raw materials like cotton required by the textile mills of Manchester, England, it also served as a market for finished goods from England and this included medicinal drugs such as the quinine sample referenced by Gidney during his address to the Legislative Assembly. The British, therefore, had very little incentive to create a regulatory framework in India to regulate the import of medicinal drugs from their very own country in order to protect their colonial subjects. For their own citizens in Great Britain, the British Parliament had enacted the Sale of Food and Drugs Act 1875, and the Therapeutics Substances Act 1925. In India however, the extent of the British interest in drug quality was guided by its desire to regulate the narcotics trade and levy excise duties. Protecting Indians from the detrimental effect of substandard and adulterated drugs did not feature on the British agenda.

The second likely reason for the delay in enacting a new drug regulatory law was the federal scheme brought in by the Government of India Act 1919. This law devolved legislative powers regarding medicine from the Indian Legislature to the various provincial legislatures. Gidney had referred to this aspect in his speech, saying, "I know that medicine is a transferred subject and that the Devolution Rules state that food adulteration is also a provincial matter."[31] However, as Gidney pointed out, the "Government [could not] evade direct responsibility in this quinine fraud because this spurious drug is imported into India at various seaports" and the regulation of imports fell within the purview of the Government of India and the Indian Legislature.[32] Regulation of imports could have had a substantive impact on the quality of drugs available in India because it was clear from government records in 1931 that most of these medicinal drugs were imported rather than domestically manufactured.[33] While it is likely that convincing provincial legislatures to act on this issue with haste may have been a difficult exercise, there is little doubt that the British could have moved swiftly to curb imports of adulterated medicine from the UK and the other countries if the Governor General appointed by the British Government had the political will to do so.

The Chopra Committee—The Report of the Drugs Enquiry Committee, 1930–31

Although slow to react, the Government of India finally did take note of the resolution moved by Sir Jaffer in 1927 and after consultations with the provincial governments issued an order on 11 August 1930, appointing an expert committee to study the magnitude of manufacture and sale of "impure or defective" medicine in India and to make recommendations to improve the situation as well as to enquire into the necessity of legislation to restrict the profession of pharmacy to only "duly qualified persons".[34]

This committee was headed by Lt Col R.N. Chopra who was a member of the IMS and a Professor of Pharmacology, School of Tropical Medicine and Hygiene, Calcutta. Educated at Cambridge, Chopra is often referred to as the "Father of Pharmacology" in India because of his contributions and illustrious scientific career in the field of Pharmacology at the Calcutta School of Tropical Medicine.[35] The other members were Rev. Fr. J.F. Caius, a pharmacologist at the Haffekine Institute, Bombay, Mr H. Cooper of Messrs Smith, Stanistreet & Co. Ltd., Manufacturing Chemists, Calcutta, and Maulvi Abdul Matin Chaudhury.

The Committee conducted extensive consultations, issuing over 2,180 questionnaires to the medical profession, pharmacists, medical universities, medical journals, industry experts, government analysts responsible for testing medicine, and other assorted experts, soliciting both opinions and recommendations on the quality of medicinal drugs being sold in India. It received 638 replies, 392 from official sources and 246 from non-official sources, making it an incredible consultative exercise even when compared to most contemporary law-making exercises in independent India.[36]

Much of the testimony to the Committee painted a terrifying picture of the situation on the ground, especially with regard to the quality of quinine that was much required to combat malaria. It appeared that the legislators in the Council of State and Legislative Assembly had been correct about the extent of the problem. Prof P.S. MacMahon, a public analyst to the Government of the United Provinces, explained to the committee that "...it is not surprising to find 'quinine' pills sold with impunity on the market composed of clay and chalk, and containing less than half per cent of quinine."[37]

A Mr W.J. Campbell of Smith & Campbell, Pharmaceutical Chemists, who was a chemist from Lahore with 24 years of experience, was of the opinion that: "The Indian market is flooded with spurious drugs and chemicals which are certainly cheap, but worthless as medicinal agents." He then proceeded to give a list of examples of drugs that had failed testing due to either adulteration or lack of the advertised active ingredient.[38]

Another pharmacy from Lahore, by the name Beli Ram & Brothers, described to the committee how "locally" made quinine tablets often contained chalk with a bitter taste of quassia or burnt alum and were sold in considerably large quantities throughout Sindh. Imported drugs were no better according to them, as they cited examples of German-made drugs failing quality testing after import because these drugs were only one-fourth of the advertised strength on the labels.[39]

Yet another testimony from Punjab came from Major G.C. Maitra, of the IMS. He presented particularly worrying examples from the quality testing performed by the army on drugs that it purchased. According to Major Maitra:

> In the last 18 months, 39 samples of Sulfarsenol and 3 of Neosalvarsan were tested. About 40 per cent of the former and 100 percent of the latter were found to have become toxic on injection into the experimental animal—a specially bred strain of English white mice.

A second problem according to Major Maitra, were the "very extravagant claims" being made in advertisements. One remedy, titled "Conquest of death", was accompanied by literature which claimed that, "In case the medicine has reached the patient too late and he has breathed his last, he may be revived if made to inhale this remedy within three hours of death by artificial respiration."[40]

The committee heard similar complaints from across the country. From down south in Madras, it heard from Mr D.R. Mawnay, a wholesale chemist who supplied to several southern pharmacies and who was of the opinion that "legislation must be enacted to put an immediate stop" to adulteration of medicines and that "central laboratories must be established where all drugs must be tested before they are allowed to enter the market."[41]

Another voice from Madras was Dr Lakshmanaswami Mudaliar, who was a physician at the Government Hospital for Women and Children. He informed the committee that:

> ...it may be stated from clinical experience of the therapeutic value of certain well-known drugs, that at present the market is flooded with a large number of preparations of inferior quality and doubtful purity, which must necessarily be deleterious to the patients. There are certain preparations, such as Extract Ergot Liquidum, preparations of Digitalis and certain preparations of Quinine, which have been found defective from clinical experience. Even in regard to well-known British Pharmacopial preparations, the clinical results of drugs obtained from different firms, vary. It is also a fact that there are certain drugs sold in the market at rates which are so widely different that it is but reasonable to infer that the cheaper drugs are probably of doubtful quality.[42]

Similarly, from Bangalore, Dr C.V. Natarajan, who was the Superintendent of the Health Institute, Bangalore, stated in his testimony to the Committee that:

> The necessity for controlling drug traffic and drug adulteration is a long desired want. Locally

> manufactured indigenous preparations as well as imported preparations fall very often very low regarding their potency...Another unknown factor is the period of maintenance of the full potency of such extracts and tinctures during transportation and storage at the existing temperature of tropical climate.[43]

From Bombay, Colonel B. Higham, IMS, who was a Chemical Analyser at the Government Laboratory in Byculla, Bombay, and tested drugs for the Collector of Customs and others, also narrated instances of several drugs failing testing. Expanding on one particular episode he informed the committee that:

> In 1928, I was sent several samples of quinine tablets and the amounts of quinine present were found to be very much less than those shown on the labels...I regarded this as so important that I addressed the Surgeon General in the matter and suggested that an *ad interim* Quinine Act should be introduced in the legislature pending the introduction of the General Drugs Act that I considered must eventually be required.[44]

The testimony from an academic in Calcutta, Mr P. Neogi, Professor of Chemistry, Presidency College, Calcutta, spoke out against "secret remedies". Many patent and proprietary medicines at the time were "secret" with no obligation under the law to disclose their ingredients. In his words:

> I am of opinion that secret remedies should be banned. The approximate composition of each patent medicine

> must be disclosed to the public. A legislation should be passed requiring manufacturers of patent medicines to disclose on the labels of the phials containing those medicines their approximate composition.[45]

Also, from Calcutta was the Editor of the *Indian Medical Gazette*—Lt Col E. Knowles. The *Indian Medical Gazette* had been reporting about the crisis of counterfeit and adulterated drugs in India and the need in India for a legislation like the Therapeutic Substances Act that was enacted in the UK in 1925. Like the others, Knowles rattled off a long list of examples of how Santonin, Quinine, and Cinchona Febrifuge were being heavily adulterated in the Indian market. In no uncertain terms, Knowles told the committee that, "There can be no question as to the imperative necessity of legislation to deal with this situation."[46]

The Drug Inquiry Committee thus received testimony from literally all four corners of the country and there appeared to be a near consensus that the drugs being supplied to the Indian market were of poor quality and marketed through grossly exaggerated advertisements. There were, however, some contrary views from Indians who were worried that the attempt to impose regulation was nothing but a strategy to stifle the nascent but growing pharmaceutical sector in India. The key proponent of this argument was the Indian Medical Association (IMA), which continues to be the pre-eminent association of medical doctors in India.

In its testimony to the Committee, the IMA claimed

that its members had "considerable misgivings" about the enquiry being conducted by the committee and that they apprehended that that the committee's findings would be "...used with the ulterior purpose of prejudicing the position of the infant drug industry in this country" so as to benefit the British drug industry at a time when there were "...manifestations of a strong national desire for using indigenous preparations and drugs." The IMA also claimed that "...though the Food and Drugs Act in the United Kingdom makes it compulsory to examine all drugs and food substances consumed in the United Kingdom, the products for export to India are beyond the provisions of this Act."[47] Regarding the specific allegation contained in the Committee's questionnaire that there was widespread sale of inferior quality drugs in India, the IMA stated that it could not "...accept this statement in the absence of accurate and proper evidence."[48]

It most certainly did not help the Government's case, as the IMA pointed out in its testimony, that although the membership of the Committee consisted of a representative of a British firm, no Indian firm was given similar representation on the Committee. This, according to the IMA, lent credence to its claim that the enquiry was a pretext to stifle the growth of the Indian pharmaceutical industry.[49]

It must be remembered that this was the era of the independence struggle and the Swadeshi movement, which had been initiated in 1905 by Indian nationalists. This movement called upon Indians to boycott

British goods in favour of swadeshi or domestically manufactured products, was meant to protest the British plan to divide the province of Bengal on communal lines. The simple strategy behind the call to purchase only swadeshi goods was to hurt British economic interests and thus undermine one of the main motivations of its colonizing mission in India. It should also be noted that the year 1930 was also witness to the famous Dandi March, which involved Gandhi leading a march of satyagrahis from Sabarmati Ashram in Ahmedabad to Dandi in order to "produce" salt and sell it without paying the salt tax imposed by the British. The Dandi March is considered to be one of the most iconic civil disobedience moments of the Indian freedom struggle and is today considered to be a pivotal moment in the struggle for Indian independence from the British Empire. It is thus no surprise that nationalist sentiment was making an appearance in the debate regarding the regulation of the pharmaceutical industry.

On the other hand, it should also be remembered, as pointed by Sir Jaffer's speech in the Council of States in 1927, that doctors of that era were likely playing a major role in prescribing dubious medicines to their patients. It is possible that the IMA had financial incentives to resist any new law or authority that would interfere with the authority of their members to prescribe drugs of their choice to their patients.

The IMA's view on the topic was, however, the minority opinion. A majority of the testimony received by the Committee weighed overwhelmingly in favour of a legislation to control the sale of drugs, with several terming it as an "urgent" requirement in the Indian context.

After reviewing all the testimony and drug control legislation in other countries, the Committee recommended in its final report dated 29 March 1931, that a drug control legislation be enacted for India. Although the Committee did not submit a draft bill, it did recommend that any future law should ensure standardization of medicine through the creation of an Indian Pharmacopeia, prohibit misleading advertisements of drugs, regulate the sale of patent and proprietary remedies (whose ingredients were secret at the time), ensure better regulation of the profession of pharmacists, the licensing of manufacturers, importers and retailers of medicinal drugs, the setting up of laboratories at the central and provincial level to undertake testing of quality of drugs, the creation of an advisory council, and most importantly, criminalizing the sale of adulterated or misbranded drugs.[50]

In a move that appeared to be designed to pre-empt any criticism that the Committee was attempting to throttle the rise of the local drug industry, the Committee also made recommendations for "fostering" the growth of the Indian drug industry.[51]

On the most important issue of whether there should be one central law or a multitude of provincial legislations addressing drug regulation, the Committee recommended the route of a single central law to ensure uniformity across British-India. It made this recommendation despite the fact that as per the Devolution Rules framed under Section 45-A of the Government of India Act 1919, the subjects of medical administration, public health, and administration of justice would fall within the purview of the provincial legislatures. The Committee argued that it was possible under Section 67(2) of the Government of India Act 1919, for the Indian Legislature to pass legislation on subjects devolved to the provincial legislature with the prior sanction of the Governor General.[52]

In its concluding remarks, the Committee acknowledged that some of its proposals would "... strike at vested interests and are sure to arouse vigorous opposition" but that it was "...impressed with the sincerity, force and earnestness of the general demand for reform." It signed off by asking for "energetic action on the part of the Government."[53]

The wait for a new law continues

Despite the thorough investigation by the Drugs Inquiry Committee and the near unanimous consensus that the issue of drug control urgently required legislative action, the government of the day continued to drag its feet while Indian legislators grew increasingly impatient. On 18 September 1935, an Indian legislator in the Council of State, Sir Nasarvanji Choksy, frustrated with the slow pace of reforms, moved a resolution before the Council calling upon the Governor General in Council to initiate "early measures" to implement the recommendations made by the Drugs Inquiry Committee. While moving the motion, Sir Choksy informed his peers that the matter of poor quality or adulterated medicine had become far worse since the submission of the report of the Drugs Inquiry Committee, providing several recent examples where spurious or adulterated medicine had been detected in India.[54]

The Government representative tasked with resisting Choksy's resolution was Mr Ram Chandra who tried placating the Council by explaining the reasons for the delay. Chandra explained to the House that the problem was not a lack of a law since several provinces or in some cases municipalities had local laws to deal with drug adulteration. In addition, he pointed out that the Indian Penal Code (IPC) had provisions penalizing the sale of adulterated drugs. The challenge according to Chandra, was the lack of standardization of drugs and the lack of laboratories and experts to test the quality of drugs and the funding these laboratories and experts would require to enforce a new legislation. Apparently, many of the provinces like Bombay, Bengal, United Provinces, and Madras had told the Government of India that they lacked the funds to run drug testing laboratories. This lack of co-operation from the provinces was a key problem in enacting any legislation for the entire country, according to Chandra. He said that the Government of India itself, although "unable to incur any substantial expenditure", would try to provide an effective solution to this problem if the provincial governments were more co-operative on this issue.[55] In other words, the Government of India simply passed along the blame to the provincial governments, ignoring the fact that the Drugs Inquiry Committee had actually recommended that a central law be enacted for this purpose.

The Government of India's defence before the Council of State did not win it much support. The suggestion that the lack of funds was stalling the creation of an effective drug control system rankled some of the legislators. Mr Hossain Imam, a legislator from Bihar and Orissa, was one such legislator who sought to remind the Government of India that there existed a "Silver Jubilee Fund", which had sufficient funds to create the necessary infrastructure under a new drug control legislation.[56] The "Silver Jubilee Fund" was likely a reference to a fund created by the British to celebrate King George V's 25th coronation ceremony on 6 May 1935. Many other legislators spoke in favour of Choksy's resolution and a majority of the Council of State voted in favour of the following, slightly amended resolution:

> This Council recommends to the Governor General in Council to initiate early measures to implement the conclusions of the Report of the Drugs Inquiry Committee, or, if for financial or other reasons he has to delay giving effect to all the conclusions of the Committee, to take early steps to pass legislation which would effectively prevent the sale of spurious drugs.[57]

A failed legislative attempt

Perhaps due to the above resolution, the Government of India finally introduced, on 7 October 1937, the Import of Drugs Bill, in the Legislative Assembly. As obvious from the title, the legislation dealt with only the import of drugs and kept away from regulating domestically manufactured drugs. The reason for limiting the scope of the bill to only imported drugs, as pointed out by Secretary Girja Shankar Bajpai who introduced the bill in the Legislative Assembly, was apparently a legal limitation in the new Government of India Act 1935 (which had replaced the old Government of India Act 1919). Under the old Government of India Act 1919, as pointed out by the Drugs Inquiry Committee (1931), the Indian Legislature could override the provincial legislature with the prior approval of the Governor General. However, the Government of India Act 1935 envisaged a stricter separation of legislative powers between the Federal Legislature and the provincial legislatures. Under the new scheme, the legislative powers were identified in three lists under Schedule VII to the Act. List I contained subjects for the Federal Legislature, List II contained subjects for provincial legislatures and List III contained subjects on which both the federal and provincial legislatures could enact laws.

As per the government of the day, the issue of legislation to control the quality of drugs manufactured and sold within India fell within the powers of the provincial legislature and thus the Federal Legislature could not enact a new law in this regard. As a result, the Government of India passed the buck on regulation of domestically manufactured drugs to the provinces, hoping that the Bill under consideration would "serve as a stimulus" for the provinces to enact their own legislation.[58] This strategy however did not pan out. Ultimately the Import of Drugs Bill 1937, was referred to a Select Committee of the Legislative Assembly for further examination, which predictably ended with the recommendation that the Bill be reworked to regulate even the domestic manufacture and distribution of drugs.[59] This was not a surprising ask given that this issue of a uniform law across India had been raised repeatedly in the legislature in previous years.

Finally, a new comprehensive drug law

After the rejection of the Import of Drugs Bill 1937 by the Select Committee, the Government of India adopted a new strategy for creating a uniform legislation across British India. This strategy involved a request to all the provincial legislatures to pass a resolution under Section 103 of the Government of India Act 1935 empowering the Federal Legislature to pass a drug control law to regulate the domestic manufacture and sale of drugs, including those in their provinces. Once all the provincial legislatures passed such resolutions under Section 103, the Federal Legislature could enact a legislation even on those legislative subjects that fell within List II.[60]

The new law, which came to be known as the Drugs

Act 1940, separated the powers and responsibilities of the federal and provincial governments, allowing both provinces and the federal government to set their own pharmacopeial standards. In simple English, "pharmacopeial standards" are standardized methods of testing the identity, purity, and quality of drugs. Drugs that fail to pass these standards are considered to be substandard drugs. Imports would be regulated only by the Federal Government. The domestic manufacture and sale of drugs were to be regulated by provincial governments who were required to appoint their own drug inspectors and government analysts to staff their laboratories.[61] Similarly, rule-making powers were distributed between the federal and provincial governments to correlate with the distribution of powers under the legislation. For example, the provincial governments were at liberty to make their own rules regarding qualifications for hiring their own drug inspectors and government analysts and prescribing the format of manufacturing licences, regulating the mode of labelling of drugs etc.[62] The federal government could make similar rules with respect to imported drugs.[63] In order to ensure some coordination and expertise on the issue of standards and the various rules drafted by different governments, the law also created two bodies—the Drugs Technical Advisory Board (DTAB), which had a mix of interdisciplinary expert members to advise on technical issues, and the Drugs Consultative Committee (DCC), which had as its members representatives from the various provincial governments.[64]

This new version of the Bill was largely welcomed by weary legislators who had been seeking legislative action on this issue for more than a decade. There was the inevitable criticism about the significant delay in enacting such law during the legislative debates. Sir Gidney, who had repeatedly raised the need for legislative action against adulterated and counterfeit medicine since 1921 was thankful to the government and effusive in his praise of Colonel Chopra who had headed the Drugs Inquiry Committee.[65] However, like many of his colleagues, he called upon the government to take similar actions and regulate the profession of pharmacists since they played a crucial role in providing medicine to consumers. That was an era where pharmacists actually "manufactured" or "compounded" some of the medicines meant for patients.

Others like Mr J.D. Boyle, a legislator from Bombay, were critical of the fact that manufacturers and importers of drugs were being given representation on the DTAB. In his opinion, it was "...to a certain degree improper that those who will be bought within the mischief of this Act should find a seat on the technical board which will formulate the policy."[66] This was an important articulation of the possible "conflict of interest" between the DTAB's role in protecting public health and the pharmaceutical industry's goal of increased profits. Other legislators like Pandit Lakshmi Kant Maitra had the polar opposite view. He argued that there should be more representation of persons from the Indian pharmaceutical industry on the board, as was the case in other countries and that it could not be presumed that they would "pollute" the atmosphere of the advisory board.[67] This line of argument was not entirely out of place in that era where the most prevalent form of regulation was "self-regulation". In those times, most professions and trades were regulated by self-representative bodies such as guilds and councils. The idea of regulation of a trade or profession by the state was still in its infancy.

Notwithstanding the criticism posed by some legislators, the government's bill was passed in both chambers of the Federal Legislature, thereby giving India its first ever Drugs Act 1940, more than 13 years after Sir Jaffer's resolution in the Legislative Assembly had called upon the government to pass such a law.

Many of the issues raised during the debate on Sir Jaffer's motion in 1927 were not addressed by the new law. These include issues such as the lack of requirement for the pharmaceutical industry to provide any clinical proof of safety and efficacy of new drugs, lack of regulation of traditional medicinal industries like Ayurveda and Unani, exaggerated and misleading advertisements by the pharmaceutical industry, and finally, the unhealthy nexus between the pharmaceutical industry and the medical profession. Some of these issues continue to plague India almost a century after being raised in the legislative debate of 1927.

During the course of the 20th century, the global pharmaceutical industry has seen an explosion of innovation as well as tremendous growth. The Indian pharmaceutical industry has grown exponentially earning itself the moniker of being the "pharmacy of the developing world" because of its ability to manufacture low-cost generic drugs. Despite leaps in medical innovation and the dramatic growth of the industry, India's drug regulatory infrastructure has evolved at snail's pace because of the reluctance of successive governments to improve the quality of regulation, lest it muzzles the growth of the pharmaceutical industry. The cost of this inaction is felt by not just India but by all countries importing drugs from India, especially those countries with weak domestic regulatory systems.

Notes

1. At the time though India was still a colony of the British Empire, the Government of India Act 1919, which was enacted by the British Parliament, provided for a small measure of self-government in India wherein Indians could elect their own representatives to a bicameral central legislature as well as provincial assemblies. The Council of States was the upper house of the Indian Legislature. Council of State Debates, 9 March 1927, vol I, 515.
2. ibid 516.
3. ibid 515.
4. ibid 516.
5. ibid 517.
6. Government of India, *Report of The Drugs Enquiry Committee* (1930–31) 24–31.
7. Donald McDonald, "The Indian Medical Service. A Short Account of its Achievements 1600–1947" (1955) 49 *Proceedings of the Royal Society of Medicine* 13, 17.
8. Council of State Debates (n 1) 522.
9. Peter Barton Hutt, "Drug Regulation in The United States"

(1986) 2 *International Journal of Technology Assessment in Health Care* 619.

10. R.G. Penn, "The State Control of Medicines: The First 3000 Years" (1979) 8 *British Journal of Clinical Pharmacology*, 293.
11. Council of State Debates (n 1) 519.
12. ibid 520.
13. ibid 523.
14. ibid 524.
15. David Arnold, *Colonizing the Body: State Medicine and Epidemic Disease in Nineteenth-Century India* (University of California Press 1993) 5–6.
16. Council of State Debates (n 1) 543–44.
17. Patricia Barton, "'The Great Quinine Fraud': Legality Issues in the 'Non-Narcotic' Drug Trade in British India" (2007) 22 *The Social History of Alcohol and Drugs*, 1, 11.
18. Legislative Assembly Debates, 4 September 1928, vol III, 154.
19. Esther Mary Lyons, "THE TWO GREAT ANGLO-INDIANS" (2000) 5 *International Journal of Anglo-Indian Studies*, 37.
20. Legislative Assembly Debates, 19 March 1921, 1364–65.
21. Legislative Assembly Debates, (n 18).
22. ibid 155.
23. J.W.D. Megaw, Sudhamoy Ghosh and N.R. Chatterjee, "Stock Solutions of Quinine" (1928) 63 *The Indian Medical Gazette*, 244.
24. Legislative Assembly Debates, (n 18).
25. ibid.
26. ibid 156.
27. Sir Jaffer, Council of State Debates, (n 1) 515.
28. *Report of The Drugs Enquiry Committee*, (n 6) 2.
29. ibid 2–3.
30. Legislative Assembly Debates, (n 18) 157.
31. ibid 156.
32. ibid.
33. *Report of The Drugs Enquiry Committee*, (n 6) [para 29] 14.

34. ibid 3, 4.
35. Harkishan Singh, "Ram Nath Chopra (1882-1973)—A Visionary in Pharmaceutical Science." (2008) 43 *Indian Journal of History of Science*, 231.
36. *Report of The Drugs Enquiry Committee*, (n 6) 16.
37. ibid 247.
38. ibid 251–52.
39. ibid 254–56.
40. ibid 285.
41. ibid 256, 279.
42. ibid 286.
43. ibid 289.
44. ibid 279.
45. ibid 280.
46. ibid 267.
47. ibid 262.
48. ibid 263.
49. ibid.
50. ibid 158–70.
51. ibid 173.
52. ibid 172.
53. ibid 173.
54. Council of State Debates, 18 September 1935, vol II, 128.
55. ibid 134–35.
56. ibid 139.
57. ibid 143.
58. Legislative Assembly Debates, 7 October 1937, vol VII, 3213–4.
59. J.D. Tyson (Education, Health and Lands Secretary), Council of State Debates, 10 April 1940, vol I, 558.
60. ibid.
61. The Drugs and Cosmetics Act 1940, ch III and IV.
62. ibid, s 33.
63. ibid, s 12.
64. ibid, ch II.
65. Legislative Assembly Debates, 4 April 1940, vol III, 2171.
66. ibid 2181.
67. Legislative Assembly Debates, 5 April 1940, vol III, 2208.

CHAPTER THREE

Of Botched Investigations, Dodgy Prosecution Guidelines and Lenient Judges

In August 2013, government analysts working at the Drug Testing Laboratory in Chennai under the Tamil Nadu Drug Control Administration received as a matter of routine, drug samples from the Drug Inspectors in Gudiyattam, Vellore. The samples in question were supposedly of Glipizide, a drug used to treat Type 2 diabetes. Drug inspectors routinely purchase such samples and send them to government laboratories for testing as prescribed in the Drugs and Cosmetics Act, 1940. These particular tablets were allegedly manufactured by the Tamil Nadu based Alfred Berg & Co. Pvt. Ltd. and had been purchased in bulk by the Tamil Nadu Medical Services Corporation, a government company responsible for purchasing and distributing drugs to government-run hospitals across the state of Tamil Nadu.[1]

The usual adverse outcome during the testing process by government analysts is for the drug to be declared as "Not of Standard Quality" (NSQ) because of its failure to comply with the standards laid down in the Indian Pharmacopoeia. Except in this case, the government analysts made the shocking allegation that the tablets in question contained not Glipizide as mentioned on the labelling of the samples sent to them but instead another drug called Glibenclamide! While Glibenclamide is also used to treat Type 2 diabetes, it should not be used as a substitute for Glipizide without the advice of a doctor. It takes the human body three to four times longer to metabolize Glibenclamide when compared to Glipizide, thereby increasing the possibility of hypoglycemia in patients who unwittingly take one drug instead of the other.[2]

The allegations in question were so scandalous that the drug inspectors from the Tamil Nadu Drug Control Administration, instead of merely summoning manufacturing records as is the usual practice during such investigations in India, visited the manufacturing premises of Alfred Berg & Co. to inspect the manufacturing facility for regulatory compliance. The inspection allegedly revealed shocking lapses at the facility. Not only did the drug inspectors accuse the facility of lacking a "separate quality assurance department" as mandated by the GMP code laid down in Schedule M, but also alleged that the staff were unable to produce quality control records that they were mandated to retain under the law.[3] The staff had apparently claimed to the drug inspectors that they had sent their quality control records to their headquarters and did not maintain records at the manufacturing facility. Similarly, when the raw materials register and packing material register were sought by the inspectors, the director of the company produced a compact disk that was supposed to contain these records but which allegedly did not open on the computer.[4] In other words, the most critical records about the manufacturing process were not accessible to the drug inspectors and in the records that were accessible, the inspectors alleged several discrepancies.

Subsequently, a criminal complaint filed before the Judicial Magistrate at Gudiyattam on 8 December 2014 by the Drug Inspector Mrs S.L. Dheivanar alleged that Alfred Berg's manufacturing facility did not follow "good manufacturing practices"; that the premises were congested with raw material that was not properly labelled and that required records were not being maintained by the company. The complaint filed in court also "observed" that Alfred Berg & Co. was "simply manufacturing the drugs first and then creating records thereafter" and that the investigating team was of the opinion that "the manufacturer did not produce the proper and genuine records."[5]

The drug inspector also accused Alfred Berg & Co. of substituting Glipizide with Glibenclamide for purely profit motives; the cost of Glipizide was ₹9,000 per kilogram, while the cost of Glibenclamide was only ₹1,900 per kilogram. If these allegations against the company were in fact true, Alfred Berg & Co. presumably profited enormously from this substitution (regardless of whether it was a mistake) because as per the complaint filed in court, it had sold a whopping total of 567,000 Glipizide tablets to the Tamil Nadu Medical Services Corporation![6]

Given the seriousness of the allegations, it was no surprise that the drug inspectors sought to prosecute Alfred Berg & Co. under a provision of the Drugs & Cosmetics Act that carries a maximum punishment of life in prison and a fine that could go up to three times the value of the consignment seized.[7] In an ideal world, this was exactly the kind of case that should have been swiftly prosecuted. The Indian legal system, however, has its own logic. As we discovered to our utter astonishment, this case which was filed in December 2014, had not proceeded to trial as of December 2024! According to the e-courts record for this case, the court was unable to serve summons on the company despite the fact that Alfred Berg & Co. is headquartered in Chennai, merely 167 kilometers away from Gudiyattam. At some point in 2016, the Judicial Magistrate finally issued non-bailable warrants against the company, thereby clearing the path for the police to arrest the accused management personnel in charge of the company. Yet as of 2024, according to the e-courts record, these warrants had not been executed.[8]

During this very time period, we discovered that Alfred Berg & Co. has been actively litigating other cases before other courts and tax tribunals across the country, including several appeals before the Madras High Court. It is thus a mystery to us as to why the state has not been able to secure the presence of the management personnel of Alfred Berg & Co. in the prosecution before the court at Gudiyattam.

The allegations against Alfred Berg & Co. are extraordinary even by Indian standards. Typical allegations made by Indian drug inspectors against the members of the Indian pharmaceutical industry are better captured in the criminal complaint filed before the Chief Judicial Magistrate, Pune, in August 2009, by drug inspectors from Maharashtra against Olcare Laboratories, a Gujarat-based pharmaceutical firm. In this case, the drug inspectors alleged that Azithromycin tablets manufactured by the firm sent to a government laboratory for testing were declared to be NSQ by a government analyst after it was found to contain only 25.69 mg of Azithromycin instead of the 200 mg advertised on the label i.e., 12.85% of the advertised amount.[9]

After the case bounced around in the judicial system for a period of seven years, the proprietor of Olcare Laboratories, along with the manufacturing chemist and analytical chemist who oversaw the manufacturing process at the manufacturing facility of the firm, finally pled guilty before the Chief Judicial Magistrate to the charge of manufacturing NSQ drugs. The judge now had to decide an appropriate punishment for the guilty parties in this case. The punishment prescribed by the Drugs & Cosmetics Act for the manufacture and sale of NSQ drugs is a minimum of one year imprisonment and a maximum imprisonment of two years, with a small monetary fine of ₹20,000. The law allows the judge to impose a prison term of less than one year for "adequate and special reasons to be recorded in the judgment". In the circumstances of this case, the Chief Judicial Magistrate hearing the case decided that it would be adequate punishment to sentence the guilty, to "simple imprisonment till the rising of the court" along with a paltry fine of ₹70,000.[10]

A sentence of "simple imprisonment till the rising of the court" is exactly as it sounds. It basically allows the convicted persons to go free once the judge "rises" from the court for the day. Technically, if the judge rises 15 minutes after passing the sentence, the guilty can leave court in 15 minutes. This is the most lenient form of sentencing. The reason offered by the Chief Judicial Magistrate for this lenient punishment in this case was that at most a prospective patient consuming the NSQ drug would not have received immediate relief and would simply have had to consume more of the medicine. Thus, as per the court's logic, it was okay to let the accused off with a lenient fine since, "They have undertaken that they will take proper care in future."[11] A key factor in the court arriving at this conclusion was a statement by the prosecuting drug inspector before the judge that the NSQ drug would not be injurious to health and that a "heavy fine" would be sufficient in the facts of the case.[12]

The above reasoning is deeply problematic for two reasons. First, the provisions of the Drugs & Cosmetics Act, 1940, invoked in this case do not require such an assessment of the possible adverse impact of a NSQ drug on patients. Second, the judge and drug inspector were completely wrong in concluding that the drug with only 12.85% of the active ingredient would not pose any harm to patient. The fact of the matter is that Azithromycin is a broad-spectrum antibiotic that is used to treat a wide range of life-threatening infections. If a patient battling a serious life-threatening infection was administered the defendant's NSQ tablets that contained only 12.85% of the active ingredient advertised on the labeling of the drug, there is a high possibility of the patient dying. Dosage of antibiotics is usually decided by doctors based the weight of the patient. If a doctor prescribed a 200 mg tablet keeping in mind specific body weight and metabolism, the infection will not be cured if the tablet has only 25.69 mg of the antibiotic. Apart from the issue of the possible death of patients administered such NSQ drugs, it should be noted that substandard antibiotics contribute to a rise in antimicrobial resistance, which is one of the biggest public health issues facing the world today.[13] Yet the manufacturing firm in this case escaped with a slap on the wrist from the judge. Such judicial outcomes are unfortunately quite routine in prosecutions under the Drugs & Cosmetics Act, 1940.

Even in cases where it is obvious that a NSQ drug poses a danger to public health, Indian courts have been very lenient. Take for example the case filed by drug inspectors of the Tamil Nadu Drug Control Department in 2019 against Tamman Titoe Pharma Pvt.

Ltd. after vials of a drug manufactured by the company allegedly failed both the assay test and the bacterial endotoxin test (BET). The presence of endotoxins in a drug can have dangerous consequences for patients, ranging from aseptic shock to death. After a relatively speedy trial that concluded in April 2021, the XV Metropolitan Magistrate, Georgetown, Chennai found the company guilty of manufacturing the NSQ drug in question. However, as a punishment, the judge merely sentenced the management of the company to "simple imprisonment till the rising of the court along with a paltry fine of ₹50,000."[14] The court also ordered the company to pay the charges for an advertisement in the paper publishing details of the conviction in the newspaper. The court justified this leniency on the grounds that the prosecution did not argue that the drug caused any "injury or harm" to the public.[15]

In a similar case in neighbouring Kerala, when the Chief Judicial Magistrate of Thalassery found the Madhya Pradesh based Modern Laboratories guilty of manufacturing an Ampicillin injection that failed the tests for bacterial endotoxin, sterility and assay, it sentenced the management to simple imprisonment for three months and a fine of ₹10,000 each.[16] (This sentence was stayed by the Sessions Court pending the outcome of an appeal.[17]) The reason for the leniency offered by the judge to avoid the minimum sentencing requirement of one year in the Drugs & Cosmetics Act, 1940, was the fact that the accused had been appearing before the court over a period of 13 long years![18]

It is not unknown for such prosecutions to take more than a decade to conclude. Take for example in Maharashtra, we were able to collect from the e-courts database, a set of 95 judgments in prosecutions against pharmaceutical manufacturers under the Drugs & Cosmetics Act, 1940 that were filed between 1993 and 2015. For this dataset, the median time to disposal was 10.5 years with the average being 11.35 years! These figures would have actually been much higher if it was not for one particular judicial magistrate in whose courtroom, pharmaceutical companies suddenly began pleading guilty to manufacturing NSQ drugs after having contested their cases for several years. In all these cases, the manufacturers received, as punishment, only a light fine without having to serve any jail time.

In cases where the pharmaceutical manufacturers decide to slog it out through an entire trial, a typical case can take up to 20 years only to result in an acquittal. Take for example the criminal complaint filed by a Drug Inspector of the Maharashtra FDA on 1 September 1994, against Macleods Pharmaceuticals and its management personnel before the Judicial Magistrate First Class at Palghar district in Maharashtra. The drug inspector accused the company of manufacturing and selling Ampicillin, an antibiotic that had been declared to be NSQ by a government analyst in a government laboratory on the grounds that it contained only 47.50% of the active ingredient advertised on the label of the drug. After a trial and arguments that dragged on for 23 years, 5 months and 25 days, the Judicial

Magistrate on 26 February 2018, acquitted all the accused on a host of procedural grounds, including the fact that the drug inspectors were not able to establish whether the drug was properly stored in the dispensary, from where it was drawn by the Drug Inspector, in a "cool place" as required on its labelling in order to prevent the drug from degrading.[19]

But the situation is not the same across all states. In Karnataka for example, the situation is very different. We discovered that the Special Court for Economic Offences, Bangalore, Karnataka was concluding similar prosecutions in a matter of months in judgments spanning three pages without even a mention of the nature of the defect that led to the drug being declared NSQ. This appears to have been possible because this court was content with handing out paltry fines and "simple imprisonment till the rising of the court". By way of illustration, this particular court took cognizance of a criminal complaint filed by a Drug Inspector on 6 November 2012, against BRD Medilabs, accusing it of manufacturing NSQ drugs. The management of the company pled guilty to all charges on 15 December 2012, and on the same day was "sentenced till the rising of the court" along with a fine of ₹20,000! The judgement does not even mention the name of the drug that was declared NSQ or the nature of the defect.[20] There are several such judgments where the same court dealt with such cases in the same manner as it would deal with prosecution of traffic offences.

Of the various types of cases discussed above, the

case against Macleods Pharmaceuticals which involved NSQ drugs is the most representative of the typical case filed by a Drug Inspector in India, both in terms of facts and outcomes.

Subverting parliamentary will through prosecution guidelines

While the acquittals and lenient sentencing discussed in the cases above is worrying, what worries us more is the fact that only a very small percentage of cases where the system detects NSQ drugs are actually prosecuted by the drug inspectors. This is not due to the corruption or negligence of individual drug inspectors but due to the dubious prosecution guidelines laid down by the Drugs Consultative Committee (DCC); a committee consisting of representatives from all the state drug control administrations, the Drug Controller General of India (DCGI) who heads the Central Drug Standard Control Organization (CDSCO) and the top brass of the Ministry of Health.[21] These guidelines are only meant to offer guidance to drug inspectors on the type of cases under the Drugs & Cosmetics Act, 1940 that they must prosecute and lack any binding legal value. Except, these guidelines are not in tune with the letter or spirit of the law. In fact, it can be argued that the DCC guidelines actively undermine the parliamentary will expressed in the bare reading of the Drugs & Cosmetics Act, 1940, by advising drug inspectors to consider administrative measures such as licence suspensions in lieu of criminal prosecutions for certain offences. What follows is an explanation of how the prosecution guidelines drafted by the bureaucracy have subverted the Drugs & Cosmetics Act, 1940.

Under the Drugs & Cosmetics Act, 1940, any drug sample tested in a government laboratory that fails quality parameters prescribed in the officially recognized Pharmacopoeias can be prosecuted for one of the following offences: misbranding, adulteration, being declared spurious or being "not of standard quality" (NSQ).

The actual legal definitions of these offences are complicated, but here is a simple explainer of each term. Adulterated drugs usually involve cases where the drug is contaminated with foreign substances that are harmful or reduce its quality or when the drug is manufactured in unsanitary conditions.[22] Spurious drugs generally mean counterfeit drugs where a drug is an imitation of another company's drug and is meant to deceive customers of the true source of manufacture.[23] This includes using a name or a packaging that belongs to another drug. Misbranded drugs are those which make false claims on the labelling of the drug or which fail to follow the law on labelling.[24] A drug which fails quality testing prescribed in the recognized pharmacopoeia but does not fall in any of the previous categories is declared as "Not of Standard Quality" or "NSQ".[25] Majority of the quality problems with Indian drugs fall in this last category where drugs manufactured by licensed manufacturers fail quality testing due to poor manufacturing practices. These drugs tend to have too little of the active ingredient to be effective or fail dissolution tests thereby indicating their inability to dissolve in bloodstream of patients. In some cases, where government laboratories in fact do test for contamination (which is relatively rare), there have been instances where drugs fail tests for microbial contamination as well.

The punishment for each offence listed above differs. In 2008, the punishment under this law was increased dramatically by Parliament to extend to life in prison with a minimum punishment of ten years, if such adulterated, spurious or not of standard quality drug caused or was likely to cause "grievous hurt" or death.[26] The same provision also allows for the imposition of a fine of ₹10 lakhs or three times the value of the drugs confiscated, whichever is higher.

The manufacture of spurious or adulterated drugs unlikely to cause death or "grievous hurt" is punishable with a minimum punishment of seven years and a maximum punishment of life in prison, along with a fine that is not less than Rs 3 lakhs or three times the value of the drugs confiscated, whichever is higher.[27]

On the other hand, manufacturers of NSQ drugs that do not cause death or "grievous hurt" is punishable by a minimum imprisonment of one year and a maximum imprisonment of two years, along with a fine of up to a maximum of ₹20,000.[28]

In each of the provisions mentioned above, the law allows the court the discretion to impose a lesser sentence for special reasons which are to be recorded in writing,

For most of the offences mentioned above, such as the manufacture of NSQ drugs, the state is not required to establish either "criminal negligence" or "criminal intent" in order to secure convictions. The mere fact that the drug has failed testing is sufficient to secure a conviction. Such provisions reflect Parliament's zero-tolerance policy towards the issue of drug quality. This is quite an imposing standard for the pharmaceutical industry since it mandates imprisonment of the responsible personnel and the management of the pharmaceutical company even if a single drug it manufactured is found to be NSQ when it is procured by a drug inspector from the market. While it is always open to the pharmaceutical industry to lobby the Parliament asking it to reform the law and lower punishments, it is not open for a body of bureaucrats like the DCC to ignore the law laid down by the Parliament by directing drug inspectors to wink at the law enacted by Parliament. Yet, this is exactly what has happened with the DCC's prosecution guidelines. Two different versions of these prosecution guidelines, one in 1993 and another in 2008, basically dissuade drug inspectors from prosecuting every case where a drug has failed to meet quality standards laid down in the pharmacopeia. For example, even if a drug has failed quality norms because it was found to be contaminated or due to failing dissolution tests or if it contains less than 70% of the active ingredient, the "guidelines" advise the drug inspectors to prosecute only if there is evidence of "criminal intent" or "gross negligence".

This despite the law enacted by Parliament not requiring such a determination of "intent" or "negligence". Such leniency in the guidelines is surprising, since these quality failures which have been exempted from prosecution, can lead to serious treatment failures for patients, which at times can also result in the death of patients. Instead of criminal prosecution, these guidelines recommend "administrative measures" such as suspension or cancellation of manufacturing licenses.

Further, the guidelines also create another category called "minor defects", in which only administrative measures are recommended. Including the definition of "minor defects" are quality issues such as "broken or chipped tablets", "presence of spot/dis-colouration/uneven coating", "clear liquid preparations showing sedimentation" etc.[29] These kinds of defects are generally a result of poor manufacturing processes but it is misleading to classify them as "minor defects". For example, a tablet could be discolored, due to contaminants in raw materials or poor formulation of the drug. The chemical composition of a poorly formulated product reacts with surrounding air and light if not stored under the conditions specified on the label, resulting in molecular conversion and possible changes in coloration. Similarly, liquid formulations may degrade over time, resulting in visible sedimentation. Such degradation may be linked to potential adverse events. Thus, classifying such degradation as "minor defects" is unscientific to say the least and to propose only administrative measures like license suspension and not criminal prosecutions for these categories of defects, is morally reprehensible.

Despite the DCC guidelines lacking the force of law (since the DCC has no rule-making powers) there is conclusive evidence that drug inspectors follow the guidelines and avoid criminal prosecution of pharmaceutical manufacturers. We were able to access via the RTI Act, consolidated state level data on the frequency of prosecutions in cases where NSQ drugs were detected during varying time periods, for five states: Karnataka, Maharashtra, Uttarakhand, Delhi and Gujarat. Scrutiny of this data revealed that criminal prosecutions were ordered only in a small fraction of the cases where NSQ drugs were discovered.

In Maharashtra, between 2010 and 2015, of the 2,176 drugs found to be NSQ by the state laboratories, only 293 prosecutions were ordered by the department. (Prosecution data for 18 months was unavailable in the registers.)[30] Similarly in Karnataka, between the years 2009 and 2013, of the 755 drugs that were found to be NSQ by the state laboratories, the department ordered prosecutions in only 81 cases.[31] In Uttarakhand, during the period of January 2010 to May 2015 of the merely 68 drugs found to be NSQ by the state laboratory, only four prosecutions were ordered.[32]

For the city of Delhi, publicly available data on the website of the Delhi Drugs Control Department, indicates that of the 130 drugs declared NSQ by the state laboratory between 2012 and 2018, prosecutions were ordered in merely 29 cases.[33]

Lastly, the Commissioner for FDCA, Gujarat, in response to a request we made under the RTI Act revealed that between 1 January 2016, and December 2021, a mere 65 prosecutions were ordered.[34] During the same time period, as per the XLN website, the state laboratories in Gujarat declared a total of 1,617 drugs as NSQ. This would mean that Gujarat is prosecuting approximately 4% of the NSQ cases that it detects.

In the remaining cases, where the state drug controllers do not prosecute the erring manufacturer, they fall back on "administrative measures" such as suspension or cancellation of licences. Gujarat, for example suspended a total of 1,318 licences in the same time period that it ordered only 65 prosecutions. In cases where the manufacturer of the NSQ drug is located outside the jurisdiction of the state drug inspector who has detected the NSQ drug, the general practice is for the drug inspector to refer the report to the state drug controller who has issued the manufacturing licence for further action. The Karnataka NSQ Register provided more details in this regard, since it also recorded the response from other states after they were informed by the Karnataka Drug Control Department that a drug manufactured in a facility under their jurisdiction tested NSQ. For example, drug inspectors from Himachal Pradesh, which is the primary source of NSQ drugs in Karnataka, typically informed the Karnataka Drug Control Department that they punished the company in question by "suspending" their manufacturing licence for the drug in question for a time period ranging between 10 days and 180 days.

Technically speaking, if a manufacturing licence has been suspended, the pharmaceutical company cannot manufacture the drug for the duration of the "suspension" but we have serious doubts as to whether these licence "suspensions" amount to a punishment at all. A typical pharmaceutical manufacturer likely holds multiple manufacturing licences for different drugs at the same facility. It is perfectly profitable for these companies to stop a manufacturing line for one drug temporarily while continuing to manufacture other drugs during the suspension period. A better indicator of the extent to which such licence suspensions actually punish or hurt erring pharmaceutical manufacturers is whether they litigate these licence suspensions before a court of law. A search of all High Court judgments across India over a period of 75 years threw up only two judgments dealing with the issue of suspension of manufacturing licences under the Drugs & Cosmetics Act, 1940.[35] The most likely reason there is no substantial litigation on the issue of licence suspension is because such suspensions are either not enforced or even if enforced, are not materially hurtful to the business interests of these erring pharmaceutical companies.

It is more likely that only a cancellation of a manufacturing licence will hurt their business interests. These cancellations however appear to be rarer than suspension of a manufacturing license. In any event, there is no bar under the law against reissuance of the suspended manufacturing licence on payment of the required licence fee and fulfilment of required conditions.

From the data presented above, it is very clear that the DCC guidelines are being followed by drug inspectors despite these guidelines having effectively subverted the Drugs & Cosmetics Act, 1940 to create a parallel framework which lacks any legal basis and which is exceptionally lenient towards errant pharmaceutical companies manufacturing NSQ drugs. In no other country in the world is the business of manufacturing pharmaceutical drugs such a low-risk enterprise.

Of faulty investigations and prosecutorial errors

In the relatively few instances where a drug inspector proceeds to prosecute a manufacturer of a NSQ drug, it is the responsibility of the drug inspector to conduct an investigation and file a criminal complaint before a court of law.

For successful prosecutions of a case involving a NSQ drug, the law does not really require a very detailed investigation. A conviction can be procured solely on the basis of the government analyst's report declaring the drug to be NSQ, provided the drug inspector complies with all procedural safeguards. As a result, most drug inspectors conduct a limited investigation, generally aimed at establishing the chain-of-custody between the manufacturing facility where the drug was manufactured and the pharmacy from where it was purchased by the drug inspector. This is usually done by sourcing the trail of invoices from the wholesaler, retailer etc.

Once the journey of the drug through the supply chain is established, the focus of the criminal investigation shifts to the manufacturer of the drug. In an ideal world, this aspect of the investigation should begin by reviewing past inspection reports of the manufacturing facility along with any information on past investigations or prosecutions against the same drug manufacturer. Unfortunately, such information is not available in consolidated public databases, which is a big problem since India has 38 different drug regulators in each state, union territory and at the centre. None of them publish their inspection reports online; only a few have searchable databases of drugs failing quality testing. In effect, this means that a regulator in Karnataka cannot access inspection reports of a pharmaceutical facility in Himachal Pradesh unless the latter agrees to provide a copy.

An ideal investigation into the manufacture of a NSQ drug should also include a surprise inspection of the manufacturing facility in order to inspect for GMP compliance and conduct a "root-cause analysis" for the failure, which is industry lingo for identifying the specific reasons for failure in the manufacturing controls that caused the drug to be NSQ. This is very important from a public health perspective because only once the manufacturer is forced to identify the cause of the defect, will it rectify the same, thereby ensuring that future batches of the drug meet quality specifications or can be mandated by the regulator to put procedures in place to avoid such failures in the future. Surprisingly however, Indian drug inspectors rarely, if ever, conduct inspections of facilities as part of their investigations. In an overwhelming number of the approximately 225 criminal complaints, investigation reports and judgments that we researched upon, the drug inspector in charge would simply write to the pharmaceutical company that manufactured the NSQ drug, asking for a copy of the manufacturing records of the batch in question. Only a few enterprising drug inspectors turn up at the manufacturing facility to ask for a copy of the records and conduct an inspection in person.

Only in a small minority of cases, like the Alfred Berg case discussed in the beginning of this chapter, do drug inspectors actually carry out a "surprise inspection" or "raid" of facilities suspected of flouting quality norms. Even in these small number of cases, drug inspectors can run into jurisdictional issues because of the federal nature of India's drug regulatory framework wherein each state appoints its own drug inspectors to carry out licensing and enforcement. Due to this distribution of powers which dates back to 1940, the Drugs & Cosmetics Act, 1940, limits the search and seizure powers of drug inspectors to the jurisdiction of the area for which they have been appointed by the state government. Most states usually appoint a drug inspector for a district or to oversee a couple of districts. For the drug inspector to enter and search facilities outside her jurisdiction, she will have to coordinate with the drug inspector who has jurisdiction over the facility that manufactured the NSQ drug. This may be relatively easy in case the manufacturer is located within the same state, since both drug inspectors work for the same regulator. However, if it turns out that the manufacturing facility is located in a different state, matters can get severely complicated since it involves coordination between two different regulators working under different state governments and with different political aims. For example, a state like Himachal Pradesh which has consciously worked to turn into a hub for pharmaceutical manufacturing may not be interested in permitting inspections of its facilities by drug inspectors from other states where drugs manufactured in its facilities are sold. In his book on the functioning of the India drug regulatory system, K.L. Sharma who was a former joint secretary in the drug regulation section of the Ministry of Health, documents the extreme resistance of states like Himachal Pradesh and Tamil Nadu in allowing drug inspectors from the CDSCO to conduct joint inspections of manufacturing facilities along with the respective state drug inspectors.[36] In his words, "...it particularly proved to be a Heculean task to convince the Government of Himachal Pradesh who agreed to the state participating in inspections after detailed discussions on the condition that the modalities of inspection were to be first discussed by the inspecting team with the State Drug Controller." Similarly, he notes, "The Tamil Nadu Government also refused to cooperate initially; however on persuasion, the state government reluctantly agreed."[37]

Perhaps for the above reasons, most Indian drug inspectors limit themselves to asking for the manufacturing records to be sent to them by mail. There are two problems with this approach. First, asking pharmaceutical manufacturers to send the records via postal mail gives them ample time to manipulate the manufacturing records to paper over any wrongdoing on their part. There is great incentive for them to do so in the face of a possible criminal prosecution. In her book *Bottle of Lies*, Katherine Eban documents in detail the scale of data fabrication discovered by the USFDA during its surprise inspections at manufacturing facilities owned by Indian pharmaceutical companies. Indian companies have even had to cough up fines for destroying documents. Take for example Fresenius Kabi, an Indian manufacturer of cancer drugs which pled guilty to concealing and destroying records prior to an inspection conducted by the USFDA in 2013. It agreed to pay $50 million in fines to the United States government.[38]

The second problem with this approach of asking for manufacturing records via mail is that merely perusing manufacturing records does not give the drug inspector a reasonable idea of the physical conditions at the manufacturing facility. Take for example the allegations against Alfred Berg; of congested premises without proper labeling and the lack of a separate quality assurance department or the allegations regarding the lack of sterile manufacturing conditions. These issues go to the heart of compliance with GMP and can be discovered only through a physical inspection of the facilities.

In any event, under the Drugs & Cosmetics Act, 1940, even without a physical inspection of the premises or an in-depth scrutiny of the manufacturing records, it is possible for the drug inspector to secure a conviction of the manufacturer solely on the basis of the government analyst's test report *unless* the accused company is able to establish a failure of the drug inspector to comply with all the procedural safeguards laid down in the law. If and when pharmaceutical companies decide to contest the charges and take the case to trial, their chances of getting acquitted are very high. For example, in Maharashtra, of the 95 judgments that we were able to access through the e-courts database, in cases against pharmaceutical companies between 1993 and 2016 on the charges of manufacturing NSQ drugs, drug inspectors of the Maharashtra FDA were able to secure convictions only in five cases where the accused contested charges. In another 54 judgments where the accused contested the charges, the trials ended in acquittals. In another 28 of these 95 cases, the pharmaceutical companies pled guilty in exchange for no jail time and a small monetary fine. The remaining cases ended in discharge of the accused since the evidence was not adequate to conduct a trial.

In Andhra Pradesh, of the 54 judgments delivered (between 1999 and 2017) in cases filed against pharmaceutical companies on the charges of manufacturing NSQ drugs, drug inspectors were able to secure convictions in only eight cases. In another 38 cases, the courts acquitted the pharmaceutical manufacturers after the trial and in the remaining cases there was no trial because the accused were discharged due to lack of sufficient evidence.

In Telangana, of the 24 judgments that we were able to access through the e-courts database in cases filed against pharmaceutical companies between 2002 and 2015 on the charges of manufacturing NSQ drugs, drug inspectors of the Telangana Drug Control Department managed to secure zero convictions!

Based on an analysis of the above judgments from Maharashtra, Andhra Pradesh and Telangana, we were able to identify eight common errors that were committed by drug inspectors during the investigation and prosecution of the cases under the Drugs & Cosmetics Act which eventually led to the acquittal of the accused pharmaceutical company.

To begin with, a drug inspector is required to file a copy of the Gazette notification establishing her appointment and jurisdiction to investigate and prosecute the case. Failure to provide such evidence, especially the notification outlining the drug inspector's jurisdiction, can be fatal to the case. Despite being such a basic requirement, we have seen a few judgments where the courts acquitted pharmaceutical companies because they were not convinced that the drug inspector had the jurisdiction to investigate or prosecute the case.

Second, the drug inspector must absolutely file as evidence, a receipt showing purchase of the drug samples of the impugned drug from a pharmacy as well as documentation demonstrating that the pharmacy purchased the drug from the manufacturer, even if it is through wholesale dealers. This is necessary to establish that the sample was in fact manufactured by the manufacturer. Failure to file this paperwork will lead to the case falling apart.

Third, when a sample of a drug is purchased by the drug inspector, she is required under Rule 4 of the Drugs & Cosmetics Rules, 1945, to send the drug sample in a sealed packet via registered post to the government analyst in the government laboratory for testing. Rule 4 also requires that the "specimen impression" of the "seal" affixed on the packet containing the drug, be sent separately to the government analyst. This is to reduce scope for manipulation of the sealed package in transit. A failure to comply with this requirement can lead to the case falling apart. On receipt of the sample, the Director of the government laboratory, or a person authorized by the Director is supposed to match the specimen of the seal impression to the seal on the sealed packet containing the drug sample in order to compare and check for any signs of tampering and record the same in the test report. When a prosecution is filed before a court, during the course of the trial, the drug inspectors need to lead evidence before the court proving that all of these procedural requirements have been met. For example, the receipt from the post office acknowledging that the sample was sent by registered post to the laboratory needs to be filed before the court to prove that the sample was sent to the laboratory in the prescribed mode. If the drug inspector fails to provide evidence on these issues, the entire prosecution case can fall apart.

A fourth set of errors typically made by drug inspectors is the failure to record the condition of the storage of the drug sample being purchased, both at the pharmacy from where it is purchased and during the process of transit of the sample to the government laboratory. Recording the conditions of storage is very important because many pharmaceutical companies will try to argue in their defense that the sample degraded during transit or at the pharmacy because it was not stored properly. For example, if the drug in question is known to be sensitive to temperature, the drug inspector must produce documentation to show that the drug was properly stored during transit to the government laboratory. Yet, many drug inspectors fail to address this issue while leading evidence during the course of a prosecution. Failure to do so can lead to the prosecution's case collapsing because in a criminal trial, the court will give the accused pharmaceutical company the benefit of the doubt.

A fifth set of errors which is the predominant reason for acquittals in most states we studied, is the failure of the drug inspectors and government analysts working in the government laboratory to complete the testing process of the drug sample before the expiry date printed on the label of the drug. In fact, the first round of testing, usually in the state government laboratory, needs to be completed with enough time left to facilitate an "appeal" by the accused manufacturer before the Central Drug Laboratory (CDL), Kolkata. This "appeal" is the statutory right of the manufacturer under the Drugs & Cosmetics Act, 1940 and it allows the manufacturer to request the court to send the sample stored with it to CDL for a second round of testing. The appeal process before CDL must conclude before the expiry date printed on the drug packaging. If the accused pharmaceutical company is denied this right to have the sample tested at CDL prior to the expiry date of the drug, the court will dismiss the prosecution because a statutory right granted to the accused pharmaceutical company has been frustrated by the government.

A sixth set of errors, which are quite rare, are attributable to government analysts who conduct the testing. Rule 6 of the Drugs & Cosmetics Rules, 1945, requires government analysts to disclose in the form sent back to the drug inspector, the complete protocols used to test the drug sample along with test results. A failure to disclose the test protocols can lead to a dismissal of the case.

The seventh set of errors, although relatively rare, is the failure to serve a copy of the report of the government analyst on the pharmaceutical company in order to enable them to prepare for their defense.

The eighth set of errors that are made generally at the stage of trial, involves "panch witness". These "public witnesses" are supposed to be independent citizens who can verify that the sample has been seized and sealed properly by the drug inspector. This is not a procedural requirement in the Drugs & Cosmetics Act, 1940, but a general practice during criminal investigations in India. The aim is to have someone outside of the investigating agency verify seizures and sign the "panchanamma" or "seizure memorandum"'. These "panch witnesses" are then supposed to turn up during the course of the trial and corroborate their signature, the items seized, the placement of the seals etc. Very often, these "panch witnesses" do not turn up or do not "remember" crucial facts—this could be attributed to the long gaps between the sampling/ seizure and the trial.

It is obvious from the above analysis that there is a lot of scope for errors during the course of a criminal prosecution against a pharmaceutical company charged with manufacturing NSQ drugs. These lapses by drug inspectors during investigations and prosecutions have not missed the attention of judges in the High Courts, who are often asked to quash criminal prosecutions under the Drugs and Cosmetics Act, 1940, due to the failure of drug inspectors to comply with procedure under the law. Some judges have blamed the lapses on corruption, an allegation that is entirely believable given the number of drug inspectors arrested on charges of accepting bribes.[39]

Of easy convictions and lenient sentencing

The only aspect of the enforcement mechanism which is more astonishing than the high percentage of acquittals is the rate at which pharmaceutical companies plead guilty in some states to charges of manufacturing NSQ drugs. The incentive for such guilty pleas lies in the fact that many judges are only too eager to ignore the minimum mandatory punishment of one year prescribed in the Drugs & Cosmetics Act, 1940, by invoking a special exception in the law, to sentence the management of these companies to "simple imprisonment till the rising of the court" along with a paltry fine which is usually ₹20,000 as prescribed in the law.[40] In some cases, the fines may be higher but rarely above ₹1 lakh.

As mentioned earlier, "simple imprisonment till the rising of the court" is literally how it sounds—the accused has to be in court till the judge rises, after which the accused is deemed to have served the sentence and is free to go, provided the fine has been paid. The wide prevalence of this sentencing practice across the Indian states that we surveyed was astonishing.

In Maharashtra, of the total 95 judgments in our dataset, accused pharmaceutical companies pled guilty in 28 cases! In every one of these cases, the courts handed out sentences of "simple imprisonment till the rising of the court" along with paltry fines in the range of ₹5,000 to ₹80,000. This includes the case discussed earlier against Olcare Laboratories where the

Azithromycin tablets manufactured by the company tested for only 12.85% of the content advertised on the labelling.

In Maharashtra, in almost all the cases, the Judicial Magistrates justified these lenient sentences on one (or a combination) of the following grounds: *first,* that the accused had pled guilty voluntarily; *second,* since the case had languished in court for several years, the accused had already spent much time and money in court[41]; and *third,* that the defective drug in question was not "dangerous to life" since it was not adulterated or spurious but "only the required ingredient is found to be less than the standard prescribed". Judges in Maharashtra made such statements in cases where Azithromycin tablets tested for only 12.85% and 13.05% of the quantity advertised on the label and where Glimepiride tablets for diabetic patients had less than 33.85% of the quantity advertised on the label.[42] In all three cases, patients could have been seriously harmed if the drugs failed to perform as expected.

For the state of Karnataka, we managed to get access to some interesting data for a period of seven years from 2015 to 2021. We got this information in the form of a photocopy of an untitled handwritten register from the Karnataka Drug Control Department that was given to us under the Right to Information Act, 2005 when we sought information from it on the number of NSQ drugs etc. in the state. On perusing the contents of the register, it became clear to us that it contained the details of all prosecutions filed by the Drug Inspectors of the Karnataka Drug Control Department over a period of seven years across the entire state of Karnataka.[43] These included prosecutions filed against manufacturers of NSQ drugs, pharmacists and a tiny number of cases pertaining to the violation of price control laws.

The conviction-related data from the registers revealed some stunning information. Of the 285 cases in which the accused were convicted, the courts in Karnataka sentenced the guilty to "simple imprisonment till the rising of the court" in a total of 248 cases! In the remaining cases, fines were imposed just in 23 cases and prison terms were awarded only in 14 cases. We were also able to access 13 judgments delivered by a court in Bangalore between 2010 to 2018 in cases against pharmaceutical manufacturers under the Drugs & Cosmetics Act, 1940, for manufacturing NSQ drugs. In these 13 judgments, the pharmaceutical companies pled guilty and were merely sentenced to "simple imprisonment till the rising of the court" with fines ranging from ₹5,000 to ₹35,000. In almost all the judgments, the judges justified going below the minimum prescribed punishment of one year on grounds that the accused either had a family that they had to support or alternatively that the NSQ drugs were not spurious or adulterated or the fact that the accused employ a large number of employees who will go unemployed in case of his imprisonment.

Similarly, we were able to access 30 judgments from Tamil Nadu in prosecutions against pharmaceutical companies on the charges of manufacturing NSQ drugs. In 27 of these cases, the accused pled guilty either before trial or during the trial after the prosecution led its evidence. In the remaining three cases, the pharmaceutical companies were found guilty of manufacturing NSQ drugs (in one case the company only failed to maintain records) after a trial. In all 30 cases, the courts in Tamil Nadu passed sentences of "simple imprisonment till the rising of the court" accompanied with fines that were significantly higher than those imposed in Maharashtra or Karnataka. This is because the courts in Tamil Nadu imposed the statutory fines of ₹20,000 on each of the accused charged in the case. Depending on the number of accused, the cumulative fines could go up to ₹1,20,000. As with the courts in Karnataka and Maharashtra, the courts in Tamil Nadu justified awarding sentences lesser than the one-year mandatory prison term prescribed in the Drugs & Cosmetics Act, 1940 on the grounds that the accused had families to support or that the case had taken years to resolve itself or more misleadingly, that there was no harm caused to anyone by the NSQ drugs. In many cases the Judicial Magistrates appear to have not been accurately informed on the nature of the defect in the drug. For example, as discussed earlier in one case, the vials of a drug had tested positive for bacterial endotoxins, which can be dangerous for humans. Yet, the court justified the lesser sentence on the grounds that the drug in question did not harm anyone.[44]

The manner in which the courts in these states routinely circumvent the minimum mandatory imprisonment terms in the law runs against precedents of the Supreme Court on the scope of "special reason" exceptions in criminal law. In the words of the Supreme Court, "'Special reasons' have to be distinguished from 'good' or 'other reasons'."[45] It has also ruled that "pendency of a criminal case for over a period of time cannot be treated as a special reason" since "Prolonged litigation in the country is admittedly a general reason in criminal cases."[46]

Lenient sentencing, combined with a statutory cap on monetary fines at a mere ₹20,000 means that pharmaceutical companies found guilty of manufacturing NSQ drugs seldom face any significant punishment for a crime that could seriously hurt or kill patients.

So, why is it that judges are so lenient towards pharmaceutical manufacturers? The leniency is likely reflective of a larger structural flaw in the Indian justice system wherein judges tend to take a very lenient view of white-collar crime committed by the rich and the middle class. As far back as in 1978, the Supreme Court lamented upon this very issue in a case where a professor found guilty of forging university degrees was sentenced to "simple imprisonment till the rising of the court". In that case the Supreme Court had condemned such lenient sentencing practices in the following words:

> We are scandalized by this soft justice syndrome vis-a-vis white collar offenders. It stultifies social

> justice and camouflages needed severity with naive leniency... It is surprising that the Public Prosecutor has consented, on behalf of the State, to this unsocial softness to an anti-social offender on conviction for grave charges. Does the Administration sternly view white-collar offenders, or abet them by agreeing to award of token punishment, making elaborate trials mere tremendous trifles?[47]

Reversing this trend of lenient sentencing in prosecutions under the Drugs & Cosmetics Act, 1940, will require public prosecutors to push back against such sentencing practices by judicial magistrates and if required, appealing such decisions to higher courts. Except, as explained in the next section, India has decriminalized the manufacture of substandard drugs in 2023.

Diluting the law further

We had hoped that the publication of the first edition of this book in October of 2022, would spur a broader discussion on the leniency being shown towards pharmaceutical manufacturers under the Drugs & Cosmetics Act, 1940. Instead, approximately two months after the first edition of this book was published and on the heels of the two cough-syrup scandals in The Gambia and Uzbekistan, the government introduced a law in Parliament called the Jan Vishwas Bill to decriminalize "minor offences" across 42 legislations. One of the offences sought to be decriminalized by this law was the offence of manufacturing substandard drugs under the Drugs & Cosmetics Act, 1940.

The Jan Vishwas Bill proposed converting the offence of manufacturing substandard drugs into a compoundable offence. A "compoundable offence" is one where a prosecution is dropped in exchange for paying a monetary fine. We flagged the issue in the national press, writing opinion editorials explaining how the government was decriminalizing the manufacture of substandard drugs (such as antibiotics with only 12% of active ingredient or a contaminated injection) that could lead to deaths and treatment failures. At one point after some of our arguments went viral on social media, the Ministry of Health was forced to publish a press release countering our argument—it chose to obfuscate the issue in the press by confusing journalists on the different categories of offences under the Drugs & Cosmetics Act, 1940. The Ministry seemed to imply that only adulterated and spurious drugs were dangerous, without admitting at any point that substandard drugs, where the active ingredient was lacking or where there was contamination were as dangerous.

The bill eventually sailed through Parliament in August of 2023 with no debate, since the Opposition had staged a walkout in protest on an unrelated issue. As a result, the manufacture of substandard drugs was effectively decriminalized in India. The fine print in this law states that only the first offence can be compounded but we suspect that due to the lack of searchable databases, judges will never know whether a particular offence was the first offence. Moreover, by declaring the manufacture of substandard drugs a compoundable offence, Parliament has signaled to the judges that it is a minor offence, thereby furthering lenient sentencing practices.

Much after the law was enacted, when we accessed under the RTI Act, the "Cabinet Note", which is a document prepared for the Union Cabinet informing it about the policy objectives behind the Jan Vishwas Bill as a precursor to its introduction in Parliament, we realized that the note never really explained to the Cabinet the dangers posed to public health by sub-standard drugs. Similarly, when we reviewed the report of the Joint Parliamentary Committee (JPC), which examined the legislation before it was voted upon, we noticed that the public health implications of decriminalizing the manufacture of substandard drugs were never examined.[48] Since the JPC invited only bureaucrats, it was not possible for us to present our views to the committee. In effect, neither Cabinet nor Parliament were informed by the bureaucracy of the public health implications of the law that they were enacting.

This amendment, via the Jan Vishwas Act, was a massive win for the pharmaceutical industry which had been lobbying for complete decriminalizing the manufacture of substandard drugs. Instead of tightening the law, India has moved backwards by treating the manufacturing of substandard drugs as a compoundable offence.

Notes

1. Criminal Complaint filed by the Drug Inspector, Vellore under the Drugs and Cosmetics Act 1940 before the Judicial Magistrate, Gudiyattam on 8 December 2014.
2. World Health Organization, "Should elderly patients with type 2 diabetes be treated with Glibenclamide or different sulfonylurea?" <https://www.who.int/selection_medicines/committees/expert/19/applications/Sulfonylurea_18_5_A_R.pdf> last accessed 5 May 2022.
3. The Drugs and Cosmetics Rules 1945, sch M: para 6.2 (Independent QA) and para 12 (Documentation); Criminal Complaint (n 1) 4.
4. Criminal Complaint (n 1) 4.
5. Criminal Complaint (n 1) 5.
6. ibid.
7. The Drugs and Cosmetics Act 1940, s 17B read with s 27(c) (amongst other provisions).
8. *Drug Inspector, Gudiyatham vs Alfred Berg and Co Pvt Ltd & Ors* PRC/4/2016 before the Judicial Magistrate, Gudiyatham, Tamil Nadu (CNR No.: TNVL11-000414-2016).
9. *State of Maharashtra represented by Drug Inspector vs Jayesh Chandulal Mehta, proprietor of Olcare Laboratories* RCC No. 3771 of 2009 before the Chief Judicial Magistrate, Pune decided on 28 September 2016.
10. ibid 5.
11. ibid 4, para 10.
12. ibid 3, para 7.
13. Theodoros Kelesidis and Matthew E. Falagas, "Substandard/Counterfeit Antimicrobial Drugs" (2015) 28 *Clinical Microbiology Reviews* 443; Atholl Johnston and David W. Holt, "Substandard Drugs: A Potential Crisis for Public Health" (2014) 78 *British Journal of Clinical Pharmacology* 218.
14. *State represented by the Drugs Inspector vs Tamman Titoe Pharma Pvt Ltd* & Ors C.C. No. 1348 of 2020 before the

Court of XV Metropolitan Magistrate, Georgetown Chennai decided on 17 April 2021 at 5.

15. ibid 5, para 10.
16. *Drug Inspector vs Modern Laboratories & Ors* STC No. 107/2018 before the Chief Judicial Magistrate, Thalassery, Kerala decided on 21 January 2020.
17. *Modern Laboratories & Ors vs Drug Inspector* Crl.A/038/2020 before the Principal District & Sessions Judge, Thalassery, Kerala decided on 4 February 2020.
18. *Modern Laboratories* (n 16) 22.
19. *State of Maharashtra vs Dr Rajendra Agarwal, Director Macleods Pharmaceuticals & Ors* R.C.C. No. 230 of 1004 before the Court of Judicial Magistrate First Class, II Court, Palghar decided on 26 February 2018.
20. *Drug Inspector, Bangalore Circle-VI vs M/s BRD Medilabs & Anr* C.C. No. 134 of 2012 before the Special Court (Economic Offences), Bangalore decided on15 December 2012.
21. Central Drugs Standard Control Organization, Drugs Consultative Committee (DCC), "Guidelines for Taking Action on Sample of Drugs declared spurious or not of Standard Quality in the light of Enhanced Penalties under the Drugs & Cosmetics (Amendment) Act, 2008" (DCC Guidelines) <https://cdsco.gov.in/opencms/export/sites/CDSCO_WEB/Pdf-documents/Consumer_Section_PDFs/DCC_Guidelines_Spurious_Drugs.pdf> last accessed 5 May 2022.
22. The Drugs and Cosmetics Act 1940, s 17A.
23. ibid, s 17B.
24. ibid, s 17.
25. ibid, s 16.
26. ibid, s 27.
27. ibid, s 27(c).
28. ibid, s 27(d).
29. ibid 3.
30. Reply to RTI application dated 25 August 2015, Office of Commissioner Food & Drug Administration, Maharashtra

(Application No D&C/MaAdhi./352/126-15/15, 17 July 2015).

31. Reply to RTI application dated 27 June 2015, Drugs Control Department, Karnataka (Application No DCD/20/RTI/2015-16, 2 June 2015).
32. Reply to RTI application dated 28 October 2015, Drug Licensing & Controlling Authority, Uttarakhand (Application No 17/P/8/216/2015/26098 dated 29 September 2015).
33. Government of NCT of Delhi, Drugs Control Department, "Not of Standard Quality Sample 2012 to 2018" <http://drugscontrol.delhigovt.nic.in/wps/wcm/connect/doit_drug/DoIT_Drug/Home/Not+of+Standard+Quality+Sample/> last accessed 23 March 2022.
34. Reply to RTI application dated 14 March 2022, Commissioner, Food and Drugs Control Administration, Gujarat (Application No RTI/ID-117-2021/2022, 14 February 2022).
35. *Digital Vision vs State of Himachal Pradesh & Anr* CWP No. 2572 of 2020 before the High Court of Himachal Pradesh decided on 14 August 2020; *Dr Louis Biotech vs State of Bihar* CWP No. 9487 of 2016 before the Patna High Court decided on 12 July 2016.
36. K.L. Sharma, *Healing the Pharmacy of the World: An Inside Story of Medical Products Manufacturing and Regulation in India* (Notion Press 2021) 102.
37. ibid 103.
38. The United States Department of Justice, Office of Public Affairs, *Indian Cancer Drug Manufacturer Agrees to Plead Guilty and Pay $50 Million for Concealing and Destroying Records in Advance of FDA Inspection* (Press Release No 21-137, 9 February 2021).
39. *Albert David & Ors vs State of Rajasthan & Anr* S.B. Criminal Misc. Petition No. 411 of 2008 before the Rajasthan High Court at Jodhpur decided on 13 April 2012; *State of Maharashtra vs Jethmal Himatmal Jain & Anr* 1994 Cri. L.J. 2613 before the Bombay High Court decided on 22 March

1994; *Shivkumar & Ors vs State of Maharashtra & Anrs* Criminal Application No. 3439 of 2006 & Ors before the Bombay High Court decided on 21 June 2010).

40. The Drugs and Cosmetics Act 1940, s 27(d).
41. *P.P. Mhanvar vs Ram Gulwady MD of Sanmour Pharma Pvt Ltd* R.C.C. No. 109/2009 before the Chief Judicial Magistrate, Thane decided on 16 January 2019.
42. *State of Maharashtra vs Vinod Ratilal Shah MD of Iatros Pharmaceutical Pvt Ltd & Ors* R.C.C. No. 1831 of 2006 before the Chief Judicial Magistrate, Pune decided on 21 November 2016; *State of Maharashtra represented by Drug Inspector vs Jayesh Chandulal Mehta proprietor of Olcare Laboratories* RCC No. 3771 of 2009 before the Chief Judicial Magistrate, Pune decided on 28 September 2016; *State of Maharashtra vs Harpreet Singh Kalra* R.C.C. No. 349 of 2007 before the Chief Judicial Magistrate, Satara decided on 11 February 2019.
43. Reply to RTI application dated 26 May 2022, Karnataka Drug Control Department (Application No DCD/RTI/114/2021-2022 dated 10 February, 2022).
44. *Tamman Titoe Pharma* (n 14).
45. *State of Jammu & Kashmir vs Vinay Nanda* AIR 2001 SC 611. <https://indiankanoon.org/doc/492051/> last accessed 5 May 2022.
46. ibid.
47. *Madhav Hayawadanrao Hoskot vs State of Maharashtra* 1978 AIR 1548. <https://indiankanoon.org/doc/513169/> last accessed 5 May 2022.
48. Prashant Reddy T., "Jan Vishwas Act, 2023: Symbol of a Broken Legislative Process", *India Forum* (20 October, 2023) <https://www.theindiaforum.in/public-policy/jan-vishwas-act-2023-symbol-broken-legislative-process>

CHAPTER FOUR

Of Glass Particles and Bacterial Endotoxins in Drugs

In the decades following the enactment of the Drugs Act in 1940, as the Indian pharmaceutical industry grew by leaps and bounds, nobody in government paid much attention to the functioning of its drug regulators. At best, individual Members of Parliament would raise questions during "Question Hour" about the questionable approval and sale of certain drugs not authorized for sale in any developed countries.

The only expert committee constituted by the Government of India since independence to exclusively study the functioning of the drug regulatory framework was the Mashelkar Committee in 2003.[1] While this Committee made useful recommendations to improve the existing system, it failed to conduct an empirical evaluation of the various components of India's complex regulatory system partly because it was chasing the red herring of spurious or counterfeit drugs. Given that nobody in India was really paying attention to the quality issues in the pharmaceutical industry, it was not surprising that the Indian pharmaceutical industry faced its first major scandal with Ranbaxy at the hands of a foreign drug regulator like the United States Food & Drug Administration (USFDA).

In June 2013, a few weeks after Ranbaxy Laboratories finally pled guilty to the offence of selling adulterated drugs in the USA after a seven-year long investigation by their government, the Ministry of Commerce of the Indian Government put out a boisterous press release claiming that the Indian pharmaceutical sector is a "highly regulated one" and that "vested interests are raking up isolated issues" to attack the reputation of the country's pharmaceutical industry.[2] In the following years, most senior government officials and even some public health activists adopted this position as foreign regulators began to discover a horrifying number of quality-related violations at manufacturing facilities of major pharmaceutical companies located in India.

Far away from the politics of trade and faux nationalism, the mostly ignored records of Indian drug inspectors and government drug laboratories narrated a completely different story about the quality woes of the Indian pharmaceutical industry. The records of just three of India's 28 state governments and eight union territories (each of which has its own drug controller to regulate manufacturing of drugs), which are available on XLN website reveal that between 2007 and December 2020, a total of 7,525 drugs sampled from the market in these states had been declared NSQ after failing quality testing in the state government laboratories run by Gujarat, Karnataka and Kerala.[3] Similarly, the drug alerts announced by the national regulator—the CDSCO—based on random testing conducted by central drug laboratories, reported 2,668 NSQ drugs between 2013 and 2021.[4] Tamil Nadu, which shared information with us under the RTI Act reported that its laboratories detected a total of 2,355 NSQ drugs between 2015 and 2021.[5] It is important to remember that each failed drug sample represents an entire batch of medicine; meaning that the entire batch which often runs into hundreds of thousands of tablets, capsules, injections etc., is NSQ; unless of course storage conditions at individual pharmacies have resulted in the degradation of the tested samples. It is thus evident from the official records of the drug regulators that India is staring at a tsunami of NSQ drugs circulating in its market. It is worth remembering here that these statistics do not include data from some of India's most heavily populated states like Uttar Pradesh, Madhya Pradesh and Rajasthan (none of which co-operated with us under the RTI Act).

It is also important to remember that since each of these samples have been drawn by drug inspectors from random pharmacies, these drugs were already in circulation and being consumed by patients when the government laboratories declared them to be NSQ. Yet, if you search the news archives for "drug recalls" being announced by the government, you are unlikely find much information on recalls. As a result, we suspect that the total number of patients affected by these

NSQ drugs possibly runs into hundreds of thousands, perhaps millions over the last decade, given that each NSQ drug represents an entire batch of substandard/contaminated drugs that was most likely not recalled from the market. To truly understand the depth of the problem, it is also important to understand the nature of the defects due to which these drugs are declared NSQ.

In simple terms, a drug is declared to be NSQ when it fails the quality tests prescribed in the legally recognized pharmacopeia. For formulations sold as tablets, these tests usually include an assay test which determines the quantity of the active ingredient in the tablet. It is not uncommon for NSQ drugs in India to test for only 10% or 20% of the active ingredient advertised on the label. Depending on the medicine in question, failure to contain the advertised quantity of active ingredient can lead to a range of poor health outcomes, ranging from death of the patient (in case of life-saving antibiotics) to severe discomfort (in case of drugs like antacids). Then there is the "dissolution" and "disintegration" test which establishes the ability of the tablet to break down and dissolve in the bloodstream. Drugs declared NSQ on this count will fail to dissolve in the bloodstream and hence will therefore have no real therapeutic action on the patient. Once again, depending on the quality of drug, these failures can have implications ranging from death to discomfort. For formulations sold as liquids in vials to be administered as injections, there are other kinds of tests, such as "sterility" testing, that are meant to test the sterility of the drug in order to ensure it is free of any kind of contamination. Since these drugs are injected directly into the body, any contamination can have a severe outcome in the patient. Failure to use sterile water when formulating such injectables will result in contamination with bacteria and other microorganisms which will invariably result in severe illness and/or death of the patient. In many cases, such contaminated injectables will make otherwise healthy patients dangerously ill. An additional problem with injectables is the presence of "glass particles" in vials meant to be administered as injections. Needless to say, since injections deliver the drug directly into the body, it is dangerous for it to contain "glass particles".

For most but not all of these 7,525 drugs, the XLN database (which contains data from Gujarat, Karnataka and Kerala) discloses the reason for the drug samples being declared NSQ by government analysts. Approximately 2,332 of these samples failed to meet standard pharmacopeial tests for "assay" which aims to test for the quantity of active ingredient present in a drug formulation. Another 1,164 tests failed the "dissolution" test which is meant to test the ability of drug formulation to dissolve into the bloodstream and become bioavailable. A smaller set of approximately 463 drugs failed tests for sterility or were found to contain bacterial endotoxins or unidentified particulate matter. Another set of approximately 90 drugs, most of which were meant to be administered through injections (and in one case, eye drops) were found to be contaminated with glass particles. We do not know the number of samples that were actually tested by these labs since the data in the XLN database only reports those that failed testing. From the little data publicly available it is clear that India is facing a systemic crisis from a public health perspective and not mere "isolated issues" as claimed by the Ministry of Commerce or public health activists speaking in support of the Indian pharmaceutical industry.

The question to ask is how exactly did things get so bad in India? Afterall, under current Good Manufacturing Practices (GMPs), including those mandated by Indian law since 1988, a pharmaceutical company is required to conduct quality testing at each stage of manufacture, including before shipping a batch of their drug to the market to guarantee the identity, purity and strength of a drug.[6] In fact, the law requires continued testing of retained samples of batches shipped to the market through its expiry date in order to detect any degradation that may occur over time due to stability issues. Yet, given the sheer quantity of drugs detected as NSQ over the last decade from the open market, it is obvious that a number of Indian pharmaceutical manufacturing facilities are completely flouting quality and process control procedures that form the core of GMPs. The answer we suspect, lies in the design of the Drugs & Cosmetics Act, 1940. As originally enacted in 1940, this law focused on a "market surveillance" approach which requires drug inspectors to randomly sample drugs from the open market and send them for testing. The legal requirement to follow GMPs came in much later, in 1988, and it is possibly the institutional culture of state drug regulators that still concentrates on market surveillance instead of focusing on GMP compliance.

Trying to protect public health through market surveillance, as described above, is less rigorous and efficient than focusing on GMP compliance during the manufacturing process. More importantly though, the market surveillance approach is more difficult to enforce. Right from the stage of sampling drugs to testing the samples for quality and recall process, the Indian system is riddled with loopholes, shortage of infrastructure and other inherent inefficiencies that leaves too much of the regulatory process to the mercy of lady luck. A deep dive into these issues is critical to understanding the severity of the failures of the Indian drug regulatory framework that has led to the flood of NSQ drugs in India.

The random sampling of drugs for market surveillance without any strategy

Since its enactment in 1940, the Drugs & Cosmetics Act has given drug inspectors powers to draw samples of drugs from the market provided they follow a very specific procedure laid down in the law.[7] This procedure requires the drug inspector to intimate the seller of the drugs in writing that the drug was being purchased for the purpose of testing, tender the fair price for the drug and then divide the purchase into four portions in the presence of the seller. All four portions are then sealed and marked, with the seller being permitted to add his own seal. Of these four portions, one is returned to the seller, another is sent to the government analyst, a third is sent to the manufacturer and the fourth is produced before the court before which proceedings may be instituted.

This practice of drawing four samples can be traced back to an old British law called the Sale of Food and Drugs Act, 1875, and continues to exist in Indian law.[8] It is not the most efficient of methods to monitor drug quality in the market. In an ideal world, testing should be conducted on a statistically significant number of samples of a batch in order to determine the quality of the entire batch. Testing just one sample from a commercial batch which typically has hundreds, if not thousands of samples is not scientific or statistically defensible.

The second big problem with this sampling approach is the failure to cover a wide cross-section of the market both in terms of manufacturers and formulations. In an ideal world, the Ministry of Health should lay down a scientifically designed sampling methodology to guide drug inspectors across states on the type of drugs they should be drawing samples from different manufacturers for the purpose of quality testing at a predetermined frequency. The aim of such sampling should be to cover a large cross-section of different drugs sold in the open market and manufactured by different companies for different treatment regimens.

As of today, state drug controllers, who conduct the bulk of testing in India, do not proactively disclose their sampling strategy. We filed applications under the RTI Act with a few state drug controllers as well as CDSCO asking them whether they had specific sampling guidelines in place instructing their drug inspectors on the type of drugs/frequency to be drawn from the market for the purpose of testing. From their responses, we discovered that none of them had any guidelines to ensure either wide or statistically meaningful sampling of drugs. At most, the CDSCO in one of its manuals and one state drug inspector in one district of Tamil Nadu had vague guidelines specifying "locations" from where drugs are to be sampled (i.e., government hospitals and dispensaries).[9] There was, however, nothing in these guidelines about the type of drugs to be sampled. An independent study of the Kerala Drug Control Department also made similar observations, stating in pertinent part that, "The statutory sampling target for drugs seems arbitrary and there was no document to suggest risk-based sampling strategies."[10]

The lack of such guidelines means that drug inspectors in each district of the country are randomly sampling drugs of their choice without a state level strategy; forget a national strategy. The most likely outcome of such an approach is that certain categories of drugs are either under-represented or over-represented. We further suspect that limited budgets to purchase drugs (drug inspectors have to tender a fair price under the law to the seller while drawing samples from the market) may be further skewing the type of drugs that are bought by drug inspectors for the purpose of testing. Drug inspectors may be buying a larger number of cheaper drugs instead of a smaller number of more expensive drugs. An independent study conducted on the functioning of the Kerala Drug Control Department discovered that there was a state-wide ceiling of ₹400,000 in the year 2018 for purchase of drugs from private sellers, thereby making it difficult for the drug inspectors to buy the more expensive drugs.[11] Modern cancer medication can cost a few thousand rupees for a single dose.

As a result of the factors described above, in our opinion, the starting point of the "market surveillance" model of regulation under the Drugs & Cosmetics Act, 1940, is deeply flawed. We had pointed this out in a report to the Ministry of Health in 2016. One of us, Dinesh Thakur, even petitioned the Minister of Health in July 2020, on the urgent need to put in place sampling guidelines.[12] As usual, the Health Ministry failed to even acknowledge receipt of the petition, much less act on it.

Dysfunctional state laboratories

The second limb of the "market surveillance" approach to drug regulation are the laboratories operated by both central and state governments. These laboratories are tasked with testing samples of drugs purchased from the market by drug inspectors. Samples that fail testing can lead to an investigation and prosecution of the manufacturer by the drug inspector. Thus, if these laboratories are dysfunctional or not fully functional, there is little hope of actually enforcing the quality standards prescribed in the Drugs & Cosmetics Act, 1940.

In order to understand the functioning of these laboratories, we filed applications under the RTI Act with 15 state laboratories. Only a handful of them responded but those responses revealed worrying information.

The first point of worry is the almost negligible number of drugs tested in most states when compared to Tamil Nadu, a better governed state in the Union. For example the state of West Bengal, which has a population of 90 million people, tested just 2,637 samples for the six years between 1 January 2016 and February 2022.[13] In the same time period, in the state of Delhi, with a population of 19 million people, drug inspectors sent merely 3,433 samples for testing and of these, the laboratory operated by the Drugs Control Department of Delhi claimed to have tested only 2,610 samples.[14] Bihar on the other hand, with a population of 128.3 million people tested merely 14,103 samples during the same time period.[15] These are paltry figures when compared to the 57,567 samples tested during the same time period in Tamil Nadu, a state with a population of 67.9 million people.[16]

The second problem, and the reason that the above numbers do not tell us the complete story, is that many of these laboratories do not have the equipment required to conduct all the tests required to establish whether a drug is actually of standard quality. We asked all the laboratories whether they had testing equipment like High Performance Liquid Chromatography (HPLC) machines which are essential to separate, identify and quantify each ingredient in a drug sample and a dissolution apparatus that is required to test whether the drug dissolves as intended. The answers provided by many of these laboratories are simply shocking.

For example, the Combined Food & Drug Laboratory in Patna which is responsible for testing drugs for the entire state of Bihar informed us that it had only one HPLC machine which was 20 years old and non-functional and that it was instead using an outdated method involving a spectrophotometer for the assay test.[17] This despite it being well known that spectrophotometers are far less accurate than HPLC machines when it comes to identifying individual ingredients in the drug sample.

Two other states had HPLC machines which were ancient. The Composite Testing Laboratory located in Solan, Himachal Pradesh, which is responsible for testing drugs in the pharmaceutical hub of the country reportedly had just one HPLC machine which was 16 years old.[18] Similarly, in Delhi, the laboratory under the Drugs Control Department reported having only one HPLC machine, which was bought 18 years ago in 2004.[19] Only the state laboratories in Tamil Nadu and West Bengal were well equipped with 16 and 8 HPLC machines.[20]

A second quality test required to be carried out in these laboratories is "dissolution testing"; this is a critical test because drugs formulated as tablets will not have any therapeutic effect if they do not dissolve as per specifications. Unless such testing is carried out, a drug cannot be declared to be of standard quality. We asked all the laboratories whether they had the necessary equipment to carry out dissolution testing for tablets. Once again, the answers from some of these laboratories were shocking. The Combined Food and Drug Laboratory in Bihar informed us that, "No Instruments is available for dissolution test."[21] Similarly, the Composite Testing Laboratory in Himachal Pradesh informed us that, "Dissolution testing not carried out in this Laboratory".[22] That the one state laboratory in the pharmaceutical manufacturing hub of India does not conduct such testing should worry us all. Only the laboratory in Tamil Nadu reported having nine such dissolution-testing apparatus.[23] West Bengal was close, with four dissolution-testing apparatus.[24]

Apart from conducting assay and dissolution tests, state laboratories are also required to conduct a critical test called "impurity testing". Impurities in drugs can be organic or inorganic and are usually a result of problems with the manufacturing process. These impurities can be dangerous for patients. For example, a protein impurity in the antibiotic ampicillin was linked to a severe skin rash in some patients. There are several more examples where impurities in drugs were found to be causing anaphylaxis or injuries to specific organs.[25]

Many of these impurities are known and classified and can be tested against "impurity standards" sold by the Indian Pharmacopeia Commission (IPC) which is the main standard-setting body in India. This is a critical test from a quality perspective but is not always conducted in India. In response to our query about whether it conducted impurity testing, the Combined Food and Drug Laboratory in Bihar informed us that it could not carry out impurity testing because it did not have HPLC machines.[26] Similarly, the Composite Testing Laboratory in Himachal Pradesh replied with a one line answer informing us that, "Impurity testing is not carried out in this Laboratory."[27] This is a shocking state of affairs, especially considering the fact Himachal Pradesh is the hub of pharmaceutical manufacturing in India.

It is thus clear that even when Bihar and Himachal Pradesh claim that they are testing 14,103 and 11,103 drug samples respectively, they are not actually performing all the tests that are legally required under the Indian Pharmacopeia to certify a drug as being of standard quality.

Given that testing is the basis of the entire regulatory framework under the Drugs & Cosmetics Act, 1940 it is worth questioning the extent to which this Act is enforced across different states in India. We suspect the situation to be far worse in many states, a fact that we were not able to confirm because of their refusal to reply to our queries under the RTI Act. Only a few states like Tamil Nadu and Gujarat appear to have well-equipped laboratories capable of testing even complex formulations like injectables. Similarly, the six central and regional laboratories setup by the Ministry of Health, were equipped with far better testing facilities, most likely because of the Ministry's deeper pockets and also because these facilities are relatively new.

The shaky foundations of the Indian Pharmacopoeia Commission and its impact on testing laboratories

One of the crucial elements of any regulatory framework is the issue of standards laid down in the pharmacopeia. A typical pharmacopeia will comprise different monographs detailing standardized testing protocol for each new drug formulation that enters the market. These include the testing protocols for identity, purity, dissolution, disintegration and sterility. Only a drug that complies with all these tests, and also passes a visual inspection, is considered to be of standard quality.

In India, the pharmacopoeia being followed by a pharmaceutical company is generally printed on the packaging of its drugs. IP indicates that the company is following standards laid down in the Indian Pharmacopoeia which is published by the Indian Pharmacopoeia Commission. Similarly, the abbreviations such as BP and USP, expand into the British Pharmacopoeia and the United States Pharmacopoeia, respectively.

In addition to publishing a monograph, a

pharmacopoeia will also manufacture and sell "reference standards" and "impurity standards" to both the pharmaceutical industry and government drug laboratories. A "reference standard" is essentially a small sample of the pure active ingredient of a particular drug. A useful analogy to understand the role of reference standards are the designated weights that were once used in grocery stores to weigh fruits or vegetables that were being bought. These weights, which were basically iron blocks of 250 gm, 500 gm and 1 kg were used to weigh produce and confirm to the consumer the quantity being purchased. The reason consumers trust these weights is because they are calibrated against a standard that is guaranteed under the law. A similar process applies to the reference standards produced by the pharmacopeia. When a lab conducts drug testing, it compares the sample of the drug drawn from the market with the "reference standard". These tests are conducted using a HPCL system. The results of this test tell the analyst tasked with certifying the drug whether the test sample has the same "chemical" as the reference standard and the quantity of the "chemical" when measured against the reference standard.

Similarly, a pharmacopoeia is also required to supply "impurity standards". As the name suggests, these are critical to test for the presence of impurities in a drug sample that are known to be generated during the process of manufacturing a drug or while storing it, as a by-product of degradation.

A well-functioning pharmacopeia that understands the science of standards and guarantees the supply of high-quality standards is critical for both the pharmaceutical industry and regulator. Prior to independence, the Drugs Act, 1940 and the Drug Rules, 1945 recognized only foreign pharmacopoeias, some of which like the USP continue to exist as non-governmental, non-profit organizations. After independence, India setup the Indian Pharmacopoeia Committee in 1948 to act as India's standard-setting body for the pharmaceutical industry.[28] It published the first Indian Pharmacopoeia, as a collection of all its monographs in 1955. In 2008, the Ministry of Health, acting on a proposal first put forward by the Drugs Technical Advisory Board (DTAB) in 1984,[29] converted the Indian Pharmacopoeia Committee into the supposedly more autonomous Indian Pharmacopoeia Commission (IPC) but for all practical purposes the IPC operates under the administrative control of the Ministry of Health and the Secretary of the Ministry of Health & Family Welfare remains the Chairperson of the IPC.[30]

The IPC is the most important standard-setting body in India not due to its scientific acumen but because an amendment in 1977 to Rule 124 of the Drugs & Cosmetics Rules, 1945 ensured that the standards in the Indian Pharmacopoeia are legally binding in India.[31] Only if a drug is not listed in Indian Pharmacopoeia, can a manufacturer adopt the standards laid down in other official pharmacopoeias such as the USP, BP etc.

Making the standards prescribed by the IPC mandatory would have been fine if it were not for one major problem. As per the government's own records, the IPC has been found to be lacking in its ability to ensure the timely availability of reference and impurity standards. We documented multiple instances of complaints by state drug controllers against the Indian Pharmacopoeia Commission starting in 2004 at the 35th meeting of the statutory Drugs Consultative Committee (DCC). At this meeting, some of the state drug controllers complained that a shortage of both reference standards and impurity standards was making it difficult for government analysts in the state laboratories to conduct all the prescribed tests in the pharmacopoeia.[32] The minutes of the meeting also state that this shortage rendered the entire exercise of drug inspectors drawing the samples from the market as "an exercise in futility". Instead of demanding more efficiency from the IPC, the committee resolved that in case of shortage of reference standards or chemicals, the government analyst should insert a disclaimer in the test report, mentioning the shortage as the cause for not conducting all the mandated tests in a monograph.[33] From a public health perspective, this was a disastrous decision because it meant that an otherwise NSQ drug would get a clean chit. Strangely, there was no discussion at that DCC meeting on how exactly to solve the issue of shortage of reference standards.

Since that meeting in 2004, the inability of the IPC to supply sufficient reference standards has been raised by drug controllers from Karnataka and Goa amongst others at the 43rd meeting (2011), the 45th meeting (2013), the 48th meeting (2015) and the 56th meeting (2019).

Reporting in 2021 confirms that state testing laboratories continue to face difficulties in procuring reference standards as a result of which they are unable to conduct several types of testing, including for the presence of impurities.[34]

One of the possible reasons that the minutes of the DCC do not record a strong condemnation of the inefficient workings of the IPC is the simple fact that the DCC meetings are chaired by the Drug Controller General of India who in rank, is subordinate to the Secretary of the Ministry of Health & Family Welfare who is the Chairperson of the Governing Council of the IPC. To criticize the functioning of the IPC is in effect to criticize the Secretary of Health & Family Welfare and that is not how the Government of India functions.

In 2022, when we asked the IPC, through an application under the RTI Act, whether it had received complaints from drug testing laboratories about delays in supplying reference standards, it stated, quite incredibly, in no uncertain terms that it had not received any complaints from state drug controllers or government analysts about delays in the supply of standards![35]

The shortage of standards is not the only problem with the functioning of the IPC. A second significant problem identified by experts is the absence of monographs for many drugs approved for sale in India. Each monograph contains the scientific methodology by which the quality of a drug can be assessed on different parameters. A drug that fails to meet the parameters laid down in the monograph is considered to be NSQ. As per one estimate, the Indian Pharmacopeia has published only 2,030 monographs, despite 5,868 drugs being approved for sale in India. This means that only an estimated 34.5% of all formulations approved in India have a monograph in the official pharmacopeia.[36] As a result of this shortage, both government testing laboratories and the industry have to continue relying on the far more expensive monographs published by the USP or BP. There are no answers forthcoming from the IPC on its failure to prepare the remaining monographs.

A third problem, after the shortage of reference standards and monographs, is the quality of the monographs. This is a far more serious problem because if a monograph does not lay down accurate and up-to-date standards, it follows that poorly formulated drugs will be sold in the market. An example in this regard is Albendazole, a drug used in the prevention and treatment of a range of parasitic diseases such as roundworms, hookworms and mosquito-borne lymphatic filariasis. Although this drug has been used since 1975, the IPC introduced a key dissolution test in the monograph for Albendazole only in 2019, despite the fact that such a testing requirement for dissolution existed in the USP from many years earlier. This new requirement was introduced only when the World Health Organisation (WHO) raised the issue with India, after the WHO's own testing indicated that most versions of Albendazole failed to dissolve as a result of which the drug was not having the expected effect on patients. When the new dissolution test was introduced in the Indian Pharmacopeia, many Indian manufacturers reportedly struggled to meet the new requirement causing delays in government-sponsored deworming programs.[37] The episode raises the question of why the IPC did not introduce the dissolution testing earlier and the human cost of this delay for children treated with Albendazole. This example hopefully drives home the importance of the role played by the IPC and the urgent need to reform the workings of this body. At the very least, the IPC should prioritize producing quality monographs for those medicines that are listed on the National List of Essential Medicines and publish these monographs without any further delay.

Given its importance to public health in India, there is no denying that the IPC is in need of urgent reforms. This is easier said than done. Running a standard-setting body like the IPC is the equivalent of running a rather complex business enterprise involved in precision manufacturing. It is well known that the Government of India has a terrible record of running business. Hopefully the Ministry of Health will conduct transparent and open deliberations with stakeholders to identify the failings of the IPC and embark on reforms that improve the efficiency of this very crucial cog in the Indian regulatory system.

The murderous apathy of the Indian state in enacting a recall law

Presuming that a government analyst in a government laboratory is able to overcome all of the aforementioned obstacles to actually test the drug sample and determine that it is NSQ, the next logical step from a public-health perspective should be to recall the entire batch of the drug from the market before it is consumed by any more patients and also inform patients who have already consumed the NSQ drug. This is especially true in cases like the one discussed in the prologue where a cough syrup adulterated with DEG caused deaths of at least 11 children from Jammu. A less-discussed aspect of that case is the death of a two-year-old toddler in August 2020, approximately eight months after the deaths of the 11 children from Jammu. The toddler was admitted at PGIMER, Chandigarh with renal failure and the doctors at the hospital discovered that the child's parents had given her a different brand of cough syrup manufactured by Digital Vision, the same company whose cough syrup was allegedly responsible for the deaths of the 11 children from Jammu. The doctors at PGIMER then sent the cough syrup for testing to a laboratory which alleged that the sample was found to be adulterated with DEG. It is very possible that the same batch of adulterated ingredients was used to manufacture different brands of cough syrups at Digital

Vision but the other brands were not recalled after the tragedy in Jammu. The doctors at PGIMER reported the adulteration to CDSCO asking it to take urgent steps.[38] The manufacturer for its part has denied these second set of allegations in interviews to the press.[39]

The CDSCO's response in this case was to simply write to different state drug regulators informing them of the brand name and asking them to take steps to withdraw the drug from the market.[40] This was the same modus operandi followed by the CDSCO after the first tragedy in Jammu. There was no attempt by the national drug regulator to co-ordinate a public communications strategy to inform the public, trace other potential victims or supply other state drug controllers with sales records so as to enable them to identify distributors and enable a swift recall of the entire batch of adulterated medicine from the market.

Contrast the above approach of the CDSCO with the following two incidents where doctors or regulators discovered adulterated cough syrup: the American government's response in 1937 after discovering that the DEG-adulterated cough syrup was killing patients and the response of Indian doctors in Chennai in 1972 who discovered the adulterated Pipmol cough syrup. In the first incident, the USFDA deployed its entire field force of drug inspectors to trace every bottle of the DEG-adulterated syrup that had been manufactured and sold by the manufacturer. The USFDA made active efforts to track down all the salespersons involved in selling the adulterated formulations and contact all of their customers. In addition, shipping records and sales receipts of the company that manufactured the adulterated syrup were individually checked to trace the sales. Doctors and pharmacists joined the effort in large numbers. This effort was combined with public service announcements on the radio and television. The FDA inspectors did not stop until they traced each and every bottle of the syrup that had been sold in the market.[41]

In the second incident, the doctors in Chennai who discovered the DEG-adulterated Pipmol C took matters into their own hands by coordinating with All India Radio to make public announcements and holding a press conference to publicize the poisoned batch before the media. They made sure that news of the adulterated Pipmol C was broadcast loud and clear to the general public.[42]

Left to their own devices, pharmaceutical companies lack the incentive to communicate clearly with doctors and patients on potentially dangerous quality issues. For example, in 1941 in the USA, a company called Winthrop had sold an entire batch of Sulfathiazole tablets contaminated with Phenobarbital, a sedative. After hearing of adverse reactions from doctors who had prescribed its drug, the company tested the batch in its labs and discovered the contamination. Its recall process was, however, too slow and ineffective, resulting in the loss of 64 lives and another 134 adverse reactions after the company discovered the contamination! A post mortem of the recall process noted that the company was not transparent with its own branch offices. Instead of informing them that the drug was contaminated, the company headquarters misled them by telling them that the batch had to be recalled because the tablets were not disintegrating properly. Further, the company had focused on recalling the drug at only primary distribution points and not the end consumers or hospitals. It was only when the USFDA stepped in that Winthrop was compelled to be transparent and notify all the stakeholders of the actual reason for the withdrawal. The USFDA also issued a press release to inform the general public and involved a range of stakeholders from state health boards to pharmacy organizations to conduct an efficient recall of the contaminated medicine.[43]

The example above is a reminder of why countries like India need a law providing for supervision by the drug regulator of recall of drugs that have failed quality testing. Yet, India does not have a law on recall and the reason as to why it lacks such a law is a story of epic bureaucratic procrastination.

This is a story that begins with a meeting, in 1976, of the DCC, consisting of all state drug controllers, the DCGI and representatives from the Ministry of Health & Family Welfare.[44] Item No. 11 on the agenda of that meeting was "To review the existing procedure of recall by manufacturers of drugs found deficient". The minutes of that meeting recorded the Chair's observation that, "...when a drug is found deficient and is required to be withdrawn from the market, the instructions sent to manufacturers in this regard in many cases are not carried out with the result that the stocks of the defective drugs continue to move in the market."[45] Another participant at the meeting narrated an instance of how a drug declared NSQ because it contained phenol was found to be on sale in Rajasthan 18 months after the manufacturer had been ordered to withdraw it from the market.[46] For this reason, the Chair of the DCC warned against leaving the issue of withdrawals solely to the manufacturer and recommended drug inspectors verify whether withdrawals of NSQ drugs were actually taking place from the market.

At that meeting in 1976, it was also resolved that for future recalls, the state drug controller where the manufacturer was located would be responsible for gathering the names and addresses of all the distributors to whom the NSQ drug had been sold by the erring manufacturer and then transmitting those details to the state drug controllers in whose jurisdiction the distributor was located. It was then supposed to be the duty of those state drug controllers to communicate to dealers in writing to withdraw the stocks and destroy them in the presence of the state drug inspector.[47] All of this was fine except for the fact that this decision was never translated into law via an amendment to either the Drugs and Cosmetics Act, 1940 or the Drugs & Cosmetics Rules, 1945. In effect, the issue of recall was left entirely to the individual discretion of state drug controllers.

The issue of recalls came up once again in 1989 at the 26th meeting of the DCC. This time, it was the Secretary of Health & Family Welfare who expressed his concern about the recall of drugs found to be toxic and hazardous to public health. He wanted in place a mechanism to ensure complete recalls of such drugs in a span of 72 hours. The minutes of the same meeting record the fact that a high-powered group under the Chairmanship of the Health Minister of Maharashtra had already been constituted by the Central Council of Health to make recommendations on a number of issues including "strengthening of procedure for quick recalls of drugs in emergency situations".[48] We do not know what became of these recommendations.

The issue then came up again in 1996, this time at a meeting of the DTAB which is another statutory body under the Drugs and Cosmetics Act, 1940 with a mandate to advise the government on technical issues arising under this Act. Item No. 12 on the agenda was a proposal to ensure the swift recall of spurious, sub-standard or adulterated drugs, within a time span of 48 hours. The minutes specifically mention that this was an issue of concern that had been "expressed in various fora" and yet settled on a proposal to put in place only non-binding guidelines, which also never happened.

Two years later, in 1998, the DCC once again discussed a proposal for amending the Drugs & Cosmetics Rules, 1945 to ensure the expeditious recall of NSQ drugs. Like their counterparts in the DTAB, the members of the DCC decided that, "...it is very difficult to incorporate any statutory provisions in the Drugs and Cosmetics Rules relating to the time-bound recall of the drugs at the present moment."[49] Instead like the DTAB, the DCC resolved that uniform non-binding guidelines by the DCGI would suffice.

Six years later, in 2004, the issue of amending the law to guarantee effective recalls came up once again before the DCC at its 35th meeting and the matter was sent to a sub-committee for a more detailed discussion.[50] We were unable to access the report of the sub-committee.

Three years later in 2007, the DCC once again flagged the issue of recall guidelines at its annual meeting. This time the issue acquired some urgency, most likely because WHO had conducted a National Regulatory Assessment (NRA) of the Indian regulatory framework and had possibly flagged the lack of recall and destruction guidelines as an issue to be remedied.[51] Yet, when the issue of time sensitive recalls of NSQ drugs came up once again four years later at its 43rd meeting in 2011, the DCC recommended creating yet another subcommittee to examine the issue.[52]

And so, yet another sub-committee was setup to look into the issue. Its recommendations were never discussed in future meetings of the DCC, possibly because it never submitted a report.

The very next year, in 2012, the Parliamentary Standing Committee on Health & Welfare examined the issue of recalls while reviewing the functioning of the CDSCO in its now-famous 59th report. The report noted the lack of any effective system to recall NSQ drugs, noting that "this cannot be allowed to go on". It recommended a system of widespread publicity to inform the public of NSQ drugs.[53]

One would have expected the government to respond to a demand by the highest law-making body with the utmost urgency and sincerity. Regretfully, this was not the case. Rather than put together a swift policy response, the bureaucracy of the Ministry of Health engaged in a lethargic game of passing the buck. The Ministry of Health in its Action Taken Report (ATR) assured Parliament that the "CDSCO had also formulated guidelines on recall and rapid alert for drugs and that the same was uploaded on its website".[54] While a document called "Guidelines on Recall and Rapid Alert System for Drugs" was made available on the CDSCO's website on 23 November 2012, the Ministry simply omitted mentioning to Parliament the crucial detail that those recall guidelines lacked the force of law and were hence not binding on any governmental authority.[55] A separate issue was the fact that the guidelines were very poorly drafted and lacking in detail on who in government would be responsible for overseeing the recall of drugs across the country.

At around the same time, the then DCGI, Dr G.N. Singh was quoted in the press claiming that after the public comments were received, the guidelines would now be forwarded to the Ministry of Health and Ministry of Law to translate the same into binding law in 3 to 4 months.[56] This never happened, even after the issue was discussed in 2013 at a meeting of the DCC.[57]

A few years later, in 2015, we filed requests under the RTI Act, 2005 with several state drug controllers asking them whether they followed any specific guidelines to effect drug recalls. We received six different answers from six different state drug controllers—not a single one of those responses referred to the CDSCO's recall guidelines![58] Clearly these state drug controllers did not even know that the CDSCO's recall guidelines even existed.

While this policy paralysis continued at the level of the Ministry of Health, some of the state drug controllers rang the alarm bells about the lack of an adequate recall law in India. In 2015, Ravi S. Menon, a Deputy Drugs Controller from Kerala made a public appeal in the media on the need for a more efficient recall system in India. In pertinent part, he stated:

> There is gigantic quantity of NSQ drugs in the Indian pharma market. They are marketed in several places by separate marketing companies. Most of these drugs are manufactured in the excise free zone areas in Uttarakhand and Himachal Pradesh. Those manufacturers should be accountable for withdrawing the batches immediately from the market. The state and central law enforcing agencies are helpless in weeding out these batches from circulation or imposing any fine on the manufacturers due to lack of adequate provisions in the law.[59]

In July 2016, exactly 40 years after the issue of recalls was first flagged at the meeting of the DCC in 1976, the issue was taken up once again at a meeting of the DTAB. Noting the importance of recall guidelines, the minutes referenced the version of recall guidelines drafted by the CDSCO and recorded the fact that, "...concerns about lack of proper implementation of recall and alert system in the country still exist." As a solution, the DTAB proposed translating the guidelines into the law by incorporating them into the Drugs & Cosmetics Rules, 1945 and recommended that a group be setup to study the issue.[60]

The matter then went back to the DCC which took it up at its 50th meeting in November 2016. The minutes of this meeting record the standard spiel on the lack of an effective drug recall system and the need to put one in place.[61] A two-pronged strategy was thus proposed to the members of the DCC. The first step was to amend the rules to create a legal binding framework for recall and second was for all states to display information about their NSQ drugs on the e-governance platform developed for drug controllers. These were both sensible recommendations, yet what followed was an example of not just bureaucratic apathy but pure malice. Instead of fixing the responsibility to monitor recalls on state or central drug controllers, the DCC sought an amendment to the Drugs & Cosmetics Rules, 1945 to basically impose upon manufacturers the responsibility for withdrawing NSQ drugs from the market if their drugs failed quality testing. This was an utterly daft recommendation because Schedule M to the Drugs & Cosmetics Rules, 1945 already placed such a duty on the manufacturers which was not being followed by manufacturers and hence the entire discussion of a government-monitored recall system. As is usually the case when the DCC wants to kick the can down the road, this meeting of the committee wrapped up discussions by creating yet another sub-committee to review and update the existing recall guidelines.

The issue of binding recalls was discussed again at the 54th meeting held in 2018 but the discussions never translated into effective law or policy.

The next year, in 2019, at its 55th meeting, the DCC minutes record that one of the earlier sub-committees set up for the purpose of reviewing the recall guidelines had not submitted its final report and hence another sub-committee was setup under the Chairmanship of the Drug Controller of Andhra Pradesh. Although this report was not proactively published by the Ministry, we managed to get a copy of the final report under the RTI Act in 2021, after some initial resistance from the CDSCO.[62] This report made some useful recommendations on short and long-term reforms to facilitate recalls but skirted the issue of imposing a duty on drug inspectors to monitor drug recalls.

At its 57th meeting, also held in 2019, the DCC agreed to most of the recommendations of the aforementioned sub-committee, including the need for better sharing of information about NSQ drugs, but as usual none of the decisions at the meeting translated into law. In early 2024, the DCGI once again circulated recall guidelines, which lacked the force of law, meaning that state drug controllers were not obliged to follow these guidelines.

As a result, *48 years* after the issue of recalls was first raised at the DCC meeting in 1976, India still lacks a robust law on recalling NSQ drugs, despite thousands of drugs failing quality testing in government laboratories.

The continued lethargy of the government on the issue of robust recall guidelines can be pinned down to the fact that a well-designed and transparent recall system will shine a bright light on the rotten state of drug regulation in India. If the press and the common public were to be informed every other day of a batch of drugs that have to be recalled from the market because of quality concerns, they are bound to demand greater accountability of state drug controllers. Just imagine if you as a citizen heard or read of 12,548 recall notices (combined figures from XLN, the CDSCO's drug alerts and Tamil Nadu) in the press over 10 years publicizing the recall of drugs that were NSQ. Chances are that you would demand accountability from drug regulators. Therein lies the nub of the issue. The average Indian bureaucrat will do anything to escape even an illusion of accountability, which is why India does not have any recall guidelines.

If and when the government does decide to institute binding rules on drug recall, the focus must be on mandatory public notice and fixing accountability for inter-state recalls. When a drug manufactured in Himachal Pradesh makes its way across the country, as far as Mizoram and Tamil Nadu, the responsibility for monitoring and enforcing a recall should be on the central drug regulator, CDSCO. State drug regulators lack the jurisdiction to act beyond their state borders.

For our part, after a failed attempt by one of us, Dinesh Thakur, to raise the issue of recalls before the Supreme Court of India in 2016 via a broader public interest litigation, we sent a report to the Ministry of Health on the failures of the drug regulatory framework in India—one of the issues we discussed in the report was the lack of a law on drug recalls in India.[63] As you can guess, nothing much has happened.

The failure to guarantee GMPs

The reason that thousands of drugs have failed quality testing in government laboratories over the last decade is the simple fact that many Indian pharmaceutical companies regularly flout the GMPs code that they are legally required to follow under Indian law. The history of GMPs can be traced to a tragedy in the USA in 1941, referenced earlier in this chapter, when approximately 300 people died or fell ill because of contamination of a batch of 4,10,000 Sulfathiazole tablets with a powerful sedative called Phenobarbital, at a manufacturing plant owned by a company called Winthrop.[64] That tragedy led to the USFDA bringing in the first "Good Manufacturing Practices" code for the pharmaceutical industry.

Since its inception, GMP codes have evolved to put in place a set of highly sophisticated procedures which when followed, guarantees that only quality drugs are shipped to the market. Under the latest version of the GMP code, pharmaceutical companies are under a duty to maintain highly sanitized premises, to test inputs before these are used in the manufacturing process, to test batches before market release and to also retain samples for future testing. The retained samples are meant to be tested at different timepoints after sale to examine whether the drug has degraded due to stability issues.

Given the manner in which the GMP code is written, and the safeguards envisaged in it, it should be possible to detect most quality issues before the drug is shipped to the market. If NSQ drugs are still making it to the market, it is likely that the manufacturer is not following the GMP code.

From a quality perspective, ensuring GMP compliance is far more thorough and efficient when compared to drawing samples of manufactured drugs from the market for testing. It is logistically possible to conduct at least one surprise inspection every year of every manufacturing facility in the country but it is certainly impossible for the government to sample every manufactured batch of drugs in the country in order to test it for quality.

Like the USA, India too has incorporated GMP standards into the Drugs & Cosmetics Rules in the year 1988, via Schedule M, making it a precondition for issuing a manufacturing licence.[65] In 2001, these regulations were replaced with new regulations that brought Indian law closer to international standards and Rule 52 was amended to require yearly inspections of licensed premises for compliance with the terms of licence.

More worrying though, three years after the new GMP regulations were notified, the government significantly watered them down by amending Schedule M. Many of these "dilutions" were shocking. For example, the original requirement inserted into the law in 2001 required that "all manufacturing premises shall be used exclusively for production of drugs and no other manufacturing activity shall be undertaken therein". Spelling this out in the law was likely required since it is possible that, at the time, many Indian companies that manufactured pharmaceuticals also manufactured chemicals at the same premises and this is never advisable, given the sterility requirements at facilities manufacturing pharmaceutical drugs. In 2004, this clause was amended to create an exception for all manufacturing facilities that were licensed prior to 11 December 2001, meaning that all the older units could continue to manufacture chemicals in the same premises that were manufacturing pharmaceuticals.[66] This was an absurd exception since it makes no rational sense to have different GMP standards based on the year in which the manufacturing facility was licensed by the government. Another amendment introduced in 2004 omitted the limits of microbiological and endotoxin levels in steam systems that were specified in Schedule M as drafted in 2001. These steam systems are absolutely crucial to sterilize manufacturing surfaces used in pharmaceutical manufacturing facilities. It is critical for the steam to not contain bacteria or endotoxins in order to prevent contamination of manufacturing services. Yet, this critical requirement was deleted in 2004.

The reason for these amendments lowering standards can be found in an answer provided by the government to a Parliamentary Question in December 2004. In this response, the government basically admitted to receiving many "representations", including a memorandum from 34 Members of Parliament that the new GMP standards inserted into Schedule M were threatening the closure of thousands of small-scale pharmaceutical manufacturing units and that in response to these concerns, the government was in the process of "rationalizing" GMP standards contained in Schedule M.[67] The survival of the small-scale manufacturing units was clearly more of a priority than ensuring the quality of medicine for the people of India.

The problem however does not stop with the quality of the GMP code followed in India but also the attitude of Indian regulators in enforcing the existing GMP code. Nothing captures their attitude better than the following statement by former DCGI Dr G.N. Singh, who defended the lax standards in India when compared to those followed in the USA on the grounds that, "If I follow US Standards, I will have to shut down almost all drug facilities."[68]

Under Indian law, the state drug controllers who are responsible for issuing manufacturing licences are also required to carry out yearly inspections of the manufacturing facility. But are they actually carrying out these yearly inspections? This is a difficult question to answer because unlike the USFDA which publishes its inspections reports, the Indian state drug controllers who are supposed to carry out scheduled inspections do not make any information publicly available on their findings. However, from insider accounts by those familiar with the functioning of the Indian regulatory mechanism, it is quite clear that most state drug controllers are not inspecting Indian manufacturing plants for GMP compliance. One such account is in the book *Healing the Pharmacy of the World* written by K.L. Sharma, the former Joint-Secretary, Drug & Food Regulation, Government of India, who had the responsibility for setting the course of India's drug regulatory policy for a few years. Sharma narrates the story of how the Ministry of Health ordered the CDSCO to conduct risk-based inspections after a national drug survey report had thrown up shocking results. Of the 170 manufacturing facilities that were jointly inspected (after much resistance by the state drug controller) by the central and state drug inspectors, compliance with GMP standards in 33 facilities was found to be less than 25% with several plants having "critical deficiencies"![69]

A more revealing account of the state affairs in Indian pharmaceutical facilities can be found in

Katherine Eban's *Bottle of Lies: The Inside Story of the Generic Drug Boom*. As Katherine Eban documents in her book, Indian pharmaceutical companies exporting to the USA found ways to rig the entire system by fabricating quality data to paint a false and misleading picture of GMP compliance. One company was found to literally pull the plug on the testing equipment every time a sample failed testing so as to crash the software that would have logged the failed tests.[70] USFDA inspectors accused another large Indian company of having an entire testing laboratory, that was "off the books" and used only for the purpose of fabricating quality data.[71] The incentive for fabricating such data lies in the fact that ensuring strict compliance with GMPs is usually a time-consuming and expensive exercise. For example, if a batch fails accelerated stability testing before it is shipped to the market, it will have to be destroyed. Similarly, if a batch fails stability testing after it has been shipped to the market, the manufacturer will have to publicly announce a recall, account for every unit of that batch and destroy it. All of this entails huge financial losses because of which there is little incentive to comply with GMPs unless there is a strong deterrent under the law.

Separate from the data integrity issues, Eban also casts a spotlight on issues like basic cleanliness and sanitation issues raised by the USFDA in its inspection reports. American inspectors came across bird infestations at a sterile manufacturing plant, bathrooms with pools of urine on the floor, gloves designated for use in sterile areas that were flaking, crushed insects in a shipping box for gloves, failure to maintain records of sterilization and in one instance a snake coiled to laboratory equipment![72] Sharma, in his aforementioned book, mentions how during an inspection in Tamil Nadu, inspectors found the "premises filthy with open drains".[73]

The more shocking observations in our opinion are the ones contained in 29 "stop production orders" issued by the Karnataka Drug Control Department between 2014–2021 and provided to us in response to an application under the RTI Act, 2005.[74] The observations in these inspection reports reveal severe lapses in following GMP standards laid down in Schedule M to the Drugs & Cosmetics Rules, 1945. In all 29 cases the lapses were so serious that the manufacturers were ordered to stop production of the drugs that they had been licensed to manufacture by the Karnataka Drug Control Department. Many of the observations in these reports bear strong similarity to observations in USFDA Form 483 (which lists the observations made during an inspection) of other manufacturing facilities in India.

A common issue that cropped up in several of these inspection reports pertained to the quality of water being used in the manufacture of drugs. Pharmaceutical manufacturing requires the water used in the manufacturing process to be free of any microbiological contamination. But several of the 29 inspections reports found that many facilities lacked the required equipment to generate purified water and those that had equipment were not maintaining it properly.

It is because of such lapses in validating the quality of water being used in the manufacturing process that so many of the drugs (especially the injectables) we discussed earlier, are found to be contaminated with bacterial endotoxins and other assorted particulate matter that could be dangerous to patients.

A second recurring observation in some of the "stop production orders", is with the lack of basic cleanliness and sanitation at facilities manufacturing drugs. GMPs require pharmaceutical manufacturing facilities to be meticulously clean. As important as maintaining actual cleanliness is the need to maintain records and documentation of the frequency at which sanitation procedures are carried out. Yet many of the "stop production orders" reportedly found "open drains", lack of air filtration systems, open windows in manufacturing rooms and the lack of basic hygiene and cleanliness in the facilities that were inspected.

A third series of problems that we observed in these "stop production" orders from Karnataka pertains to the non-compliance with the quality control requirements laid down in the GMP section of Schedule M. As per the law, pharmaceutical companies are supposed to conduct extensive testing throughout the manufacturing process, starting from the input material to the final formulation by qualified personnel in the quality control department which is supposed to be independent from the manufacturing department.

As some of these "stop production orders" reveal, several of the inspected companies did not even have a quality assurance department and even when such a department existed at some facilities, it was often found that they lacked the equipment for testing or that they were not retaining samples for post sales testing or that the authorized personnel meant to supervise manufacturing were not present on the premises at the time of inspection.

These 29 "stop production orders" reveal alarming violations of the GMP code and if more drug controllers made public their inspections reports, we suspect that more such instances will come to light. The more convincing evidence that the lack of GMP compliance is a systemic issue across the industry and not limited to companies like Ranbaxy, are recent revelations by the CDSCO in June 2024 that over 36% of the 400 manufacturing facilities inspected by it were shut down due to lack of compliance with GMP standards. 10% were shuttered permanently. These are staggering numbers, calling into question the actual volume of NSQ drugs moving around in the Indian market.

Conclusion—Transparency and reform

One of the reasons why boisterous press releases like the one referenced at the start of this chapter were never challenged by journalists or even well-meaning public health activists is because there is a complete lack of transparency in the way the law is enforced by drug regulators. As mentioned earlier, only three states took it upon themselves to upload their test results to the XLN database. Even this data on the XLN website is very messy; there is no consistency in the way data is catalogued, making it difficult to perform any meaningful analysis. And asking for this information from the CDSCO and the State Drug Controllers via the RTI Act is an abject lesson in how the bureaucracy lives to frustrate anyone asking for accountability. Requests for information are routinely transferred to "other" office, denied on illegal grounds which then lead to appeals that go on forever.

A simple reform measure that can dramatically alter the present status-quo is to force drug controllers to disclose more information proactively to the general public. This should include proactive publication of all test reports prepared by government laboratories and all inspection reports prepared by drug inspectors. This data should be released in an organized, searchable format in a central database. Such transparency would make it possible for doctors, journalists and regular citizens to understand the levels of efficiency of different state drug controllers and identify the problematic pharmaceutical companies.

The more complicated reforms will require auditing state government laboratories in order to gauge their testing capability, reforming the Indian Pharmacopeia Commission and putting in place a special law on nationwide recalls. None of this is going to happen without sustained public pressure.

Notes

1. Government of India, Ministry of Health and Family Welfare, *Report of The Expert Committee on a Comprehensive Examination of Drug Regulatory Issues, including the problem of Spurious Drugs (Mashelkar Committee Report)* (No Z.28015/112/2002-D/DMS&PFA, 2003). Two other reports which studied the entire pharmaceutical industry merely touched upon the workings of the regulator.
2. Government of India, Ministry of Commerce & Industry, "*Clarifications on Reports of Malpractices of Pharma Manufacturing in India*" (Press Information Bureau, 3 June 2013).
3. The Gujarat Food & Drug Control Administration which pioneered the XLN website in 2007, The Maharashtra Food & Drug Administration which joined in 2011 and the Kerala Drugs Control Department which joined in 2013. "XLN-Xtended Licensing, Laboratory & Legal Node" <https://xlnindia.gov.in/> accessed 23 Jan 2022.
4. CDSCO Drug Alerts: https://cdsco.gov.in/opencms/opencms/en/Notifications/Alerts/.
5. Reply to RTI application dated 23 March 2022, Drug Testing Laboratory, Chennai, Government of Tamil Nadu (Application No 379/A1/2022, 17 February 2022).
6. Reply by the Minister of State (Ministry of Health & Family Welfare) Kumari Saroj Khaparde to question raised by Shri Dharanidhar Basumatari, Rajya Sabha Deb 2 May 1989, Question No 737, 140-141.
7. The Drugs Act 1940, s 23.
8. The Sale of Food and Drugs Act 1875, s 14.
9. Central Drugs Standard Control Organization (CDSCO), "Guidelines for the Zonal, Sub-zonal and Port Offices of the Central Drugs Standard Control Organization" (2011) 15-16; Reply to RTI application dated 30 November 2011, Office of the Director of Drugs Control, Tamil Nadu (Application No 17436/E1/2011).

10. Dr Ravi Prasad Varma P., "Effectiveness of Drugs Control and Regulating Mechanism of the Drugs Control Department in Kerala State" (Kerala State Planning Board 2021).
11. Ibid at 29.
12. Dinesh Thakur to the Union Minister for Health, "Petition to setup Expert Committee to examine the sampling and testing protocols of drugs withdrawn under Section 23 & Section 25 of the Drugs & Cosmetics Act, 1940" (3 July 2020) <https://casemindia.org/wp-content/uploads/2020/07/Samplying-Testing-Petition-Unsgned.pdf> accessed 12 January 2021.
13. Reply to RTI application dated 7 March 2022, State Drugs Control & Research Laboratory, Government of West Bengal (Application No SDCRL/29, 17 February 2022).
14. Reply to RTI application dated 25 March 2022, Drugs Control Laboratory, Government of NCT, Delhi (Application No (0019)/2022/RTI/DC/6700, 17 February 2022).
15. Reply to RTI application dated 17 March 2022, Joint Food and Drugs Laboratory, Government of Bihar (Application No 709, 17 February 2022).
16. Reply to RTI application dated 23 March 2022, Drug Testing Laboratory, Chennai, Government of Tamil Nadu (n 5).
17. Reply to RTI application dated 17 March 2022, Joint Food and Drugs Laboratory, Government of Bihar (n 15).
18. Reply to RTI application dated 16 March 2022, Composite Testing Laboratory, Khandagat, District Solan, Directorate of Health Safety & Regulation, Government of Himachal Pradesh (Application No HSR-H (RTI) 2022-IX-9528, 17 February 2022).
19. Reply to RTI application dated 25 March 2022, Drugs Control Laboratory, Government of NCT, Delhi (n 14).
20. Reply to RTI application dated 7 March 2022, State Drugs Control & Research Laboratory, Government of West Bengal (n 13); Reply to RTI application dated 23 March 2022, Drug Testing Laboratory, Chennai, Government of Tamil Nadu (n 5).

21. Reply to RTI application dated 17 March 2022, Joint Food and Drugs Laboratory, Government of Bihar (n 15).
22. Reply to RTI application dated 16 March 2022, Composite Testing Laboratory, Khandagat, District Solan, Directorate of Health Safety & Regulation, Government of Himachal Pradesh (n 18).
23. Reply to RTI application dated 23 March 2022, Drug Testing Laboratory, Chennai, Government of Tamil Nadu (n 5).
24. Reply to RTI application dated 7 March 2022, State Drugs Control & Research Laboratory, Government of West Bengal (n 13).
25. U.S. Department of Health and Human Services, Food and Drug Administration, Center for Drug Evaluation and Research (CDER), *Guidance for Industry—ANDAs: Impurities in Drug Substances* (November 1999); Priyanka Pulla, "Inside the Fight to Decide How Pure India's Drugs Need To Be", *The Wire Science* (25 June 2022) available at https://science.thewire.in/india-drug-impurities-fight accessed 16 July 2022; Alexander Cartwright, "Toxicology of Impurities in Organic Synthetic Drugs" (1990), *International Journal of Pharmacy*.
26. Reply to RTI application dated 17 March 2022, Joint Food and Drugs Laboratory, Government of Bihar (n 15).
27. Reply to RTI application dated 16 March 2022, Composite Testing Laboratory, Khandagat, District Solan, Directorate of Health Safety & Regulation, Government of Himachal Pradesh (n 18).
28. Indian Pharmacopoeia Commission, "Annual Report 2010-11" (Ministry of Health & Family Welfare, Government of India 2011) 1.
29. Drugs Technical Advisory Board (DTAB), "*MINUTES OF THE THIRTYNINTH DRUGS TECHNICAL ADVISORY BOARD MEETING HELD ON DECEMBER 19, 1984 AT NEW DELHI*" (1984). <https://cdsco.gov.in/opencms/opencms/system/modules/CDSCO.WEB/elements/common_download.jsp?num_id_pk=NTcz> accessed 13 January 2022.

30. Vide resolution: Resolution (F.No.X.11035/2/06-DFQC, 8 May 2008); Indian Pharmacopoeia Commission, "Annual Report 2019-20" (Ministry of Health & Family Welfare, Government of India 2020) 16.
31. The Drugs & Cosmetics Rules 1945, Rule 124.
32. Drugs Consultative Committee (DCC), "*MINUTES OF THE 35TH MEETING OF THE DRUGS CONSULTATIVE COMMITTEE HELD ON 29TH & 30TH APRIL, 2004*" (2004) 483. <https://cdsco.gov.in/opencms/opencms/system/modules/CDSCO.WEB/elements/common_download.jsp?num_id_pk=Nzk3> accessed 13 January 2022.
33. ibid 484.
34. Priyanka Pulla, "India's Drug Testing Has a Big Blind Spot: Officials Rarely Check for Impurities", *The Wire Science* (3 November 2021) <https://science.thewire.in/health/india-drug-testing-blind-spot-imprity-test-rare-pharmacopoeia-commission/> accessed 13 January 2022.
35. Reply to RTI application dated 22 March 2022, Indian Pharmacopeia Commission (Application No CIPGZ/R/E/22/00017 dated 9 March, 2022).
36. Priyanka Pulla, "A study on the Indian Pharmacopoeia and how it impacts drug quality", Thakur Family Foundation accessed at <https://www.thakur-foundation.org/upload/public-health/1670345698_Indian%20Pharmacopiea%20and%20Drug%20Quality.pdf>
37. *Ibid* at p. 50.
38. Email from Bhavneet Bharti to Chandigarh CDSCO titled "Regarding child with Renal failure at PGI Chandigarh & Contamination of Syp Cofset-At with Diethylene Glycol", provided under the RTI Act in response to RTI application no. APC/2021/550 (On file with authors); Priyanka Pulla, "How weak drug laws are costing lives" (*Mint*, 27 September 2021) <https://www.livemint.com/politics/policy/how-weak-drug-laws-are-costing-lives-11632761831130.html> accessed 13 January 2022.
39. Savita V. Jayaram, "Digital Vision under DGCI Scanner:

Renaming Coldbest to Cofset AT Cough Syrup Didn't Help Manufacturer" *IB Times* (10 August 2020) <https://www.ibtimes.co.in/digital-vision-under-dgci-scanner-renaming-coldbest-cofset-cough-syrup-didnt-help-manufacturer-826143> accessed 28 March 2022.

40. Usha Sharma, "DCGI asks drug controllers to prevent sale, distribution of DEG contaminated cough syrup, Cofset" *Express Pharma* (7 August 2020) <https://www.expresspharma.in/latest-updates/dcgi-asks-drug-controllers-to-prevent-sale-distribution-of-deg-contaminated-cough-syrup-cofset/> accessed 30 May 2021.
41. Carol Ballentine, "Sulfanilamide Disaster" [1981] *FDA Consumer Magazine* 144.
42. V.R. Ravi Kumar, "When a Drug Turned Killer" *The Hindu* (9 February 2020) <https://www.thehindu.com/opinion/open-page/when-a-drug-turned-killer/article30770710.ece> accessed 13 January 2022.
43. J.P. Swann, "The 1941 Sulfathiazole Disaster and the Birth of Good Manufacturing Practices" (1999) 53 *PDA Journal of Pharmaceutical Science and Technology* 148.
44. Drugs Consultative Committee (DCC), *"REPORT OF THE 19TH MEETING OF THE DRUGS CONSULTATIVE COMMITTEE HELD ON 12TH & 13TH APRIL, 1976 AT NEW DELHI-110001"* (1976) Item No. 11 <https://cdsco.gov.in/opencms/opencms/system/modules/CDSCO.WEB/elements/common_download.jsp?num_id_pk=ODUy> accessed 13 January 2022.
45. ibid 20.
46. ibid 21.
47. ibid.
48. Drugs Consultative Committee (DCC), *"MINUTES OF THE 26TH MEETING OF THE DRUGS CONSULTATIVE COMMITTEE HELD ON 14TH & 15TH SEPTEMBER 1989"* (1989). <https://cdsco.gov.in/opencms/opencms/system/modules/CDSCO.WEB/elements/common_download.jsp?num_id_pk=Nzg4> accessed 13 January 2022.

49. Drugs Consultative Committee (DCC), "*MINUTES OF THE 32ND MEETING OF THE DRUGS CONSULTATIVE COMMITTEE HELD ON 22ND & 23RD SEPTEMBER, 1998*" (1998) <https://cdsco.gov.in/opencms/opencms/system/modules/CDSCO.WEB/elements/common_download.jsp?num_id_pk=Nzk0> accessed 13 January 2022.
50. Drugs Consultative Committee (DCC), "*MINUTES OF THE 35TH MEETING OF THE DRUGS CONSULTATIVE COMMITTEE HELD ON 29TH & 30TH APRIL, 2004*" (2004) 470. <https://cdsco.gov.in/opencms/opencms/system/modules/CDSCO.WEB/elements/common_download.jsp?num_id_pk=Nzk3> accessed 13 January 2022.
51. Drugs Consultative Committee (DCC), "*MINUTES OF 38TH MEETING OF DRUGS CONSULTATIVE COMMITTEE HELD ON 4TH JUNE 2007 AT NEW DELHI UNDER THE CHAIRMANSHIP OF DR. M. VENKATESWARLU. DRUGS CONTROLLER GENERAL OF INDIA*" (2007) 5.
52. Drugs Consultative Committee (DCC), "*MINUTES OF THE 43rd MEETING OF THE DRUGS CONSULTATIVE COMMITTEE HELD ON 14th NOVEMBER*" 10.
53. Department-Related Parliamentary Standing Committee on Health and Family Welfare, *The Functioning of The Central Drugs Standard Control Organisation (CDCSO)* (Fifty-Ninth Report) (RS 2012) at para 15.11.
54. Ministry of Health & Family Welfare, *Final Action Taken Report on the observations/recommendations contained in the 59th report of the department related parliamentary standing committee on Health & Family Welfare on the functioning of the Central Drugs Standard Control Organisation (CDSCO)* (2012) 25.
55. Central Drugs Standard Control Organisation, *Guidelines on Recall and Rapid Alert System for Drugs (Including Biologicals & Vaccines)* (2012).
56. Usha Sharma, "CDSCO drafts guidelines on recall and rapid alert system for drugs" *Express Pharma* (Mumbai, 22

November 2012) <https://www.expresspharma.in/cdsco-drafts-guidelines-on-recall-and-rapid-alert-system-for-drugs/> accessed 30 May 2021.

57. Drugs Consultative Committee (DCC), "*REPORT OF THE* 45TH *MEETING OF THE DRUGS CONSULTATIVE COMMITTEE HELD ON* 4th *AND* 5th *FEBRUARY 2013 AT THE HOTEL METROPOLITAN NEW DELHI-110001*" (2013) <https://cdsco.gov.in/opencms/opencms/system/modules/CDSCO.WEB/elements/common_download.jsp?num_id_pk=ODA3> accessed 30 May 2021.
58. Dinesh S. Thakur and Prashant Reddy T., *A report on fixing India's broken drug regulatory framework* (4 June 2016) (on file with authors).
59. Peethaambaran Kunnathoor, "Amend D&C Act to make manufacturers accountable for prompt recalling of NSQ drugs from market: Kerala deputy DC" *Pharmabiz* (Chennai, 12 October 2015) <http://www.pharmabiz.com/PrintArticle.aspx?aid=91059&sid=1> accessed 30 May 2021.
60. Drugs Technical Advisory Board (DTAB), "*MINUTES OF THE* 72ND *MEETING OF THE DRUGS TECHNICAL ADVISORY BOARD HELD ON* 27TH *JUNE, 2016 AT NIRMAN BHAWAN, NEW DELHI-110001*" (2016) <https://cdsco.gov.in/opencms/opencms/system/modules/CDSCO.WEB/elements/common_download.jsp?num_id_pk=Nzcy>
61. Drugs Consultative Committee (DCC), "*REPORT OF* 50TH *MEETING OF DRUGS CONSULTATIVE COMMITTEE HELD ON 04 &* 05TH *NOVEMBER, 2016 AT NEW DELHI*" (2016) 22 <https://cdsco.gov.in/opencms/opencms/system/modules/CDSCO.WEB/elements/common_download.jsp?num_id_pk=ODEy> accessed 13 January 2022.
62. Reply to RTI application dated 16 December 2021, Ministry of Health and Family Welfare (Application No CDSCO/R/T/21/00900 filed on 28 October 2021).
63. Thakur and Reddy (n 58).
64. "Medicine: Dangerous Drug" [1941] *Time* <http://content.time.com/time/subscriber/article/0,33009,765439,00.html> accessed 17 March 2022; Swann (n 43).

65. Shri Dharanidhar Basumatari to the Minister of Health & Family Welfare, Rajya Sabha Deb 2 May 1989, Question No 737.
66. Government of India, Ministry of Health & Family Welfare, GSR 431(E)(*Gazette of India Extraordinary*, Part II – s 3(i), 30 June, 2005)(publishing Drugs & Cosmetics (5th Amendment) Rules, 2005).
67. Chittabratta Mazumdar and Dipankar Mukherjee on the "Revision of Schedule M of Drugs and Cosmetics Act", Rajya Sabha Deb 10 December 2004, Question No 874.
68. Sushmi Dey, "If I follow US Standards, I will have to shut almost all drug facilities: G.N. Singh", *Business Standard*, (30 January, 2004) *available at* https://www.business-standard.com/article/economy-policy/if-i-follow-us-standards-i-will-have-to-shut-almost-all-drug-facilities-g-n-singh-114013000034_1.html.
69. K.L. Sharma, *Healing the Pharmacy of the World: An Inside Story of Medical Products Manufacturing and Regulation in India* (Notion Press 2021) 104.
70. Katherine Eban, *Bottle of Lies: The Inside Story of the Generic Drug Boom* (HarperCollins 2020).
71. PTI, "Dr Reddy's Gets a Breather after USFDA Gives More Time to Respond to Warning Letter-Business News" *Firstpost* (Hyderabad, 26 November 2015) <https://www.firstpost.com/business/dr-reddys-gets-a-breather-after-usfda-gives-more-time-to-respond-to-warning-letter-2522724.html> accessed 17 March 2022.
72. Eban (n 70) 361, 366-67 & 324.
73. Sharma (n 69) 104.
74. Reply to RTI application dated 26 May 2022, Karnataka Drug Control Department (Application No DCD/RTI/114/2021-2022 dated 26 May, 2022).

CHAPTER FIVE

New Drugs and "The Persistent Insolence of the CDSCO..."[1]

One of the landmark events in the history of Indian drug regulation is a report from the Department Related Parliamentary Standing Committee on Health & Family Welfare that was tabled before Parliament on 8 May 2012. This report, which was titled rather drably as the "Fifty-Ninth Report on The Functioning of the Central Drugs Standards Control Organisation (CDSCO)" contained one of the most scathing indictments of India's national drug regulator, the CDSCO, and the DCGI who heads the CDSCO. The report marked the first ever independent scrutiny of the functioning of India's drug regulator and it was clear from a reading of the report that the CDSCO failed on all counts.

While most parliamentary reports are usually written in bland bureaucratese, this particular report was punctuated with words such as "persistent insolence", "deep concern", "disappointment", "skewed priorities and perceptions" and "collusive nexus" to describe the conduct of the CDSCO. The report contained a laundry list of sins committed by the CDSCO, including misplacing crucial files, irregular approvals, evidence of collusion between doctors and pharmaceutical companies and a lack of transparency in the regulator's functioning.

The most startling allegations in the report pertained to the manner in which the DCGI approved "new drugs" despite the lack of any supporting evidence from rigorous clinical trials demonstrating their safety or efficacy. As a result, all types of "new drugs", which never received approval in the better-regulated markets in developed countries were available for sale in India.

In the world of drug regulation, the task of verifying the safety and efficacy of a drug is considered to be one of the most sacrosanct public duties of the drug regulator. Individual doctors or hospitals lack the time and resources to verify the claims made by pharmaceutical companies about the safety and efficacy of their drugs. This is where drug regulators, financed by public money, step in to lay down the rules of the game and ensure that the pharmaceutical companies play by these rules. Historically, the first challenge in this context was to decide the rules of the game to prove safety and efficacy in a scientifically rigorous manner. This has proved to be a tricky issue not just because of resistance from the pharmaceutical industry but also from patient groups who want faster and quicker access to drugs. The second challenge lies in enforcing these rules in a transparent and efficient manner so as to build public confidence in both the drugs approved and the regulator itself. Confidence in the regulator is precious; it is earned by consistently enforcing regulations in a transparent manner and protecting public health over decades. Drugs are often approved based on a limited set of clinical and safety data collected in controlled conditions; it is the trust in the regulator that inspires confidence amongst both the medical community and patients to consume new drugs that are approved based on a limited data set. When a new drug enters the market, it most often encounters real-world conditions that were never evaluated in the clinical trial. Monitoring the usage of the new drug, its adverse events in the population at large, all go to building the credibility of the drug regulator step by step over decades, to a point where those who do this consistently and faithfully are held as a gold standard in the industry.

India has gone from not having any rules for several decades on the approval of new drugs, to creating rules which were never applied transparently by the regulator. In order to understand the scale of the incompetence of the Indian system, it will help if we understand the American system as a useful reference point, especially the manner in which it evolved to become the gold standard of the world.

The gold standard for approving new drugs

The original gold standard for drug approvals is the system put in place in 1962, by the Kefauver-Harris Amendments to the Federal Food, Drugs & Cosmetic

Act in the USA, post the thalidomide tragedy. The Senate Committee headed by Kefauver that had conducted an inquiry into the functioning of the American pharmaceutical industry in the years prior to the enactment of this law, had heard repeated complaints from doctors that "detail-men" from the pharmaceutical industry, who were selling them drugs, often made greatly exaggerated claims of the efficacy of their drugs and that there was no way for doctors themselves to verify these claims. A simple strategy used in the pre-1962 era to validate the efficacy of a new drug was to publish case-studies based on how new drugs were perceived to act on individual patients. The case-study would then be published in medical journals and more often than not be used as a marketing tool by pharmaceutical companies in order to promote the drug. From a scientific viewpoint, such individual case studies were akin to anecdotal evidence and were plagued by problems ranging from "bias" of the investigators to the "placebo effect" to "statistical insignificance" of the test group. The system, however, worked well for pharmaceutical companies as there was little scientific accountability and they could get away with making exaggerated claims about their new drugs.[2]

It was thus not surprising when more than one doctor appearing before the Senate sub-committee recommended that a government body like the USFDA or the National Institute of Health (NIH) be vested with the responsibility to vet the claims of the pharmaceutical industry.[3] Eventually that is exactly what the US

Congress did when it enacted the Kefauver-Harris Act in 1962.

This law set a global benchmark for approving new drugs. For the first time ever, the law required pharmaceutical companies to provide "substantial evidence" that a new drug would have the therapeutic effect advertised on the proposed labelling of the drug.[4] Further, "substantial evidence" was defined in the law as "adequate and well-controlled investigations, including clinical investigations, by experts qualified by scientific training and experience to evaluate the effectiveness of the drug".[5] The power to decide the requirements of an "adequate and well-controlled investigation" was delegated to the USFDA.

The original regulations drafted by the USFDA back in 1965 required all new drugs to go through a three-phase clinical trial process after the investigational drug completed basic in-vitro (in the laboratory) and animal testing. Phase I required testing the new drug on only healthy humans to determine toxicity, metabolism, absorption, elimination, safe dosage range etc. The aim was to determine the dose response in healthy volunteers especially from a safety perspective, which could be used to assess the dosage for testing on actual patients in the next phase. Phase II trials were meant to test efficacy of the new drug on a small number of human patients suffering from the disease that was the target of the new drug. Finally, if the new drug demonstrated promising results in the Phase II trial, the innovator could conduct Phase III trials on a larger number of patients to generate statistically significant safety and efficacy data for the drug. The investigators conducting the study were expected to develop protocols for the Phase III study with the aim of producing "well-controlled clinical data". The regulations left enough flexibility for academia and industry to design their own controls for each trial, subject to the regulator's approval.[6]

Over the years, the research methodology that eventually came to be trusted by both academia and regulators was the double-blind randomized clinical trial (RCT). The British Medical Research Council conducted the first double-blind randomized comparative clinical trial in 1948 to test the effectiveness of the newly discovered antibiotic Streptomycin on tuberculosis.[7] This trial brought together, for the first time, the following three important scientific methodologies in the context of clinical trials.

The first was the idea of "comparator trials". Comparator trials have been used by scientists since the 18th century, when James Lind divided twelve sick sailors on HMS Salisbury, who were diagnosed with scurvy, into two groups and gave citrus fruits like oranges and lemons to one of these two groups. When only the group that received the oranges and lemons (the treatment group) recovered from scurvy, Lind had proof that citrus fruits could prevent scurvy.[8] In picking a therapy to compare the new drug with, it is up to investigators conducting the clinical trial to either pick the existing standard of care or alternatively a "placebo".

The second methodological innovation was the process of "randomization" of patients between the control group and the treatment group. Simply put, the volunteer patients for the clinical trial would be randomly assigned to the control group and the treatment group by persons other than those who were responsible for conducting the clinical trial without consideration of their individual symptoms. The idea of randomization in experiments has existed since the 1920s and was meant to avoid not just subconscious "bias" on part of the treating doctors but also ensure that patients have an equal chance of getting the treatment in question.[9]

The third methodological innovation was the process of "double blinding" wherein neither the doctors conducting the trial nor the patients would be informed about the identity of the patients in the control group and the treatment group. This was meant to guard against both the biases of the investigating doctors and the "placebo effect".

The placebo effect, also known as the "psychic influence" manifests when patients report feeling better after being administered therapy or medicines that in reality have no curative effects. Doctors have for many centuries given their patients "sham" medicines, also known as placebos, just to please rather than benefit the patient.[10] In 1801, John Haygarth demonstrated the importance of placebos while trying to establish whether metallic rods could relieve symptoms through their electro-magnetic influence. The control group in this case were administered regular wooden rods rather than metallic rods and yet reported feeling better post the "treatment" causing Haygarth to remark about "the wonderful and powerful influence of the passions of the mind upon the state and disorder of the body".[11] "Blinding" the patient to whether they were in the control group or the treatment group would reduce the possibility of the placebo effect. Similarly, it was important to "blind" even investigating doctors from the identity of patients in the treatment and control groups, so as to prevent their own biases from interfering with their recording of the study's clinical observations. Hence the phrase "double blind". The patients in both groups would be "unblinded" only after the trial was completed in order to analyze the results of the treatment group against that of the control group, which received either a placebo or the prevailing "standard of care".[12] If patients in the treatment group receiving the new drug demonstrated better treatment outcomes than those in the control group who received the placebo or prevailing standard of care in a statistically significant manner, the researchers in question would have concrete proof that the new drug was in fact more beneficial than existing treatment.

After the first double blind RCT by the British Medical Research Council, RCTs gained increasing legitimacy amongst scientific and government circles such as the influential NIH in the USA. The endorsement of RCTs by the scientific community as a reliable method to produce medical knowledge about the efficacy of new drugs is viewed by many as an attempt by the medical community to hold pharmaceutical companies to account for the highly exaggerated claims made by their salespersons to doctors. The pharmaceutical industry itself was not an enthusiastic supporter of the idea of RCTs because it greatly increased the costs and risks of bringing a new drug to the market.[13]

By the 1980s, RCTs came to be known as the "gold standard" for generating the quality of clinical evidence required for approvals from regulators. The USFDA amended its existing regulations in 1985 to incorporate more elements of RCTs into its existing framework.[14] For example, the amendments in 1985 specifically mentioned the kind of control groups that should be used and that patients should ideally be assigned to groups in a manner that reduced bias etc.

Incorporating rigorous scientific standards into the law was only one component of the new American approach to evaluating the efficacy of new drugs. There are three other important components to this framework.

The first component was the creation of a well-staffed, inter-disciplinary bureaucracy of scientists and administrators, headed by a public health professional, usually a medical doctor. As of 2020, the USFDA employed approximately 7,000 personnel in the Centre for Drug Evaluation and Research (CDER) as well as the Centre for Biologics Evaluation and Research (CBER), whose responsibility it is to vet applications for the marketing of new drugs.[15] Within CDER, there are different divisions which evaluate each new drug application from the perspective of chemistry, pharmacology, microbiology, clinical pharmacology as well as a statistical review.

The second important component was a participatory framework which provided both the medical profession and the general population a chance to participate in the approval of new drugs. The USFDA creates "advisory committees" consisting of independent scientists and doctors as well as consumer and industry representatives to provide the agency with outside opinions on each new drug application. In addition, the members of the general public can provide their inputs at public hearings or through written comments to the agency.[16]

The third important component of this regulatory framework was a legal guarantee of transparency which was previously circumscribed to an extent by trade secret considerations. The scientific evaluations of new drug applications by the CBER and CDER were made publicly available subject to certain redactions to protect proprietary information. Similarly, deliberations of the committees and public hearings were transcribed and made publicly available subject to redactions to protect proprietary information.

The approval process for new drugs at the USFDA was not always so participatory or transparent. A Review Panel on New Drug Regulation which had been setup by the American government, which published its report in 1977, called upon Congress to amend the law to provide for more transparency in disclosure of scientific data during the approval process.[17]

The opaque, non-participatory scenario painted in the 1977 report was partly reformed by the enactment of the Drug Regulation Reform Act, 1978 which made the approval process more participatory by allowing for experts and citizens to be heard during the approval process.[18] Subsequent laws like the Food and Drug Administration Amendments Act, 2007 encouraged even more transparency. Despite these reforms, crucial safety and efficacy data submitted by pharmaceutical companies to the USFDA remains confidential and shielded from disclosure. American academics, doctors and journalists continue to demand more transparency through litigation and other advocacy measures.[19] For these reasons, the USFDA continues to be the "gold standard" around the world. It is the benchmark against which most countries peg their own drug regulatory system.

The struggle to introduce safety and efficacy requirement for "new drugs" in India

While the Thalidomide tragedy catalyzed regulatory reform across developed countries during the 1960s, Indian law saw little reform during the same period.

The only provision that existed in Indian law at the time to regulate the import of "new drugs" was Rule 30A of the Drugs & Cosmetics Rules, 1945. This rule, which was inserted into Indian law in 1952 required the submission of all documentary evidence related to standards of quality, purity and strength of the drug along with "such other information as may be required by the licensing authority including the results of therapeutic trials carried out with it".[20] An identical requirement was extended to even domestically manufactured "new drugs" in 1961, through Rule 69B.[21]

In both instances, the law was silent on whether these "new drugs" necessarily had to be "safe" and "effective" in order to be approved for sale in India. In other words, the law outlined the documentary requirements but not the clinical standards required to approve "new drugs". Hence there was nobody in government actually verifying the therapeutic claims being made by manufacturers of new drugs before they were introduced in the market.

Due to the lax regulatory requirements, all kinds of dangerous drugs not approved elsewhere in developed markets were being sold in India with little evidence of safety or efficacy. By the late 1970s, it became clear that India had a problem due to the sale of dangerous or irrational drugs. The nature of the problem was two-fold.

The *first* was the continued sale of dangerous drugs that had been prohibited in other countries. An illustrative example is Amidopyrine which was first synthesized in the late 1890s by German scientists and sold widely as an anti-fever medicine until countries like Australia and the USA banned it in 1964 and 1977 respectively because it causes agranulocytosis, a life-threatening blood disorder in many patients.[22] The Indian medical community had flagged this drug in medical journals as early as 1955 but the Government of India had not taken any action in this regard.[23]

The *second* problem, which continues till date, is the sale of multiple fixed dose combinations (FDCs) in India. These drugs are usually combinations of two or more drugs into one pill or syrup. The purpose of FDCs is to improve compliance of patients who have to take multiple drugs for a single, or similar ailments. For example, patients diagnosed with HIV or tuberculosis are required to take many different drugs every day. Patients are more likely to take one pill on time, rather than two or three different pills. In these circumstances, FDCs can improve compliance which in turn can significantly improve treatment outcomes.[24] The problem in India is that pharmaceutical companies started marketing all kinds of irrational FDCs (meaning the combination of drugs does not make clinical sense) lacking in any therapeutic rationale or clinical evidence. This was possible because the country lacked regulations that required demonstration of safety and efficacy of new drugs, including FDCs, prior to their marketing. For example, a combination of vitamins with anti-diarrheals or the combination of vitamins with anti-inflammatory agents and tranquilizers is "irrational" and makes little sense, yet these were combinations actually sold in India. Apart from the concern about the lack of any therapeutic rationale, the other problem with combining different drugs into a FDC is that these drugs may interact adversely with each other or neutralize each other, thereby negating any therapeutic effectiveness, or worse, lead to serious adverse events. Since at the time there was no legal mandate to evaluate these combinations under clinically controlled conditions, it was largely up to the creative instincts of the pharmaceutical industry on how these FDCs were marketed and prescribed.

One of the primary reasons for the presence of numerous FDCs in India is that these drugs are a convenient tactic to avoid price regulation under the Drug Price Control Order (DPCO).[25] Since the DPCO historically applied only to single ingredient drugs and not FDCs, it is possible that the Indian pharmaceutical industry turned to creating FDCs in order to evade the price control dragnet. The other possible reason for the tsunami of FDCs in India is that they are used as a marketing tactic similar to the earlier practice of the pharmaceutical industry in the USA.[26] Since there are only a limited range of approved new drugs in each therapeutic class, pharmaceutical companies can compete over price only to a certain extent. The other way to distinguish themselves from competition is through innovation and creating new products. Most Indian pharmaceutical companies lack the R&D skills to create new molecules, it is possible that they attempted to innovate by creating new FDCs of existing drugs to distinguish their products from their competitors and command a higher price.

Both the issues identified above—the continued sale of drugs with dangerous and unknown side-effects as well as the tsunami of FDCs in the Indian market—raised questions about the efficacy of India's drug regulatory framework. The Indian Government was aware of some of these issues as far back as the late 1970s after one of its expert committees, the Hathi Committee (also known as The Committee on Drugs & Pharmaceutical Industry) pointed out in its report, in 1975, that "according to medical opinion, in a large number of cases the therapeutic usefulness of particular drug combinations" was "doubtful".[27] In a statement laying the new drug policy before Parliament in 1978, the Minister from the government commanded the drug regulator to "immediately go into the various drug combinations and take prompt measures to eliminate irrational drug combinations or use of ingredients far in excess of what is required."[28]

In the same year, at the meeting of the Drugs Consultative Committee (DCC), which has amongst its members, representatives from all the state drug controllers, there was acknowledgment in the minutes that the government was coming under criticism for its failure to properly regulate the entry of new drugs into the Indian market.[29]

In an ideal world, the continued sale in India of drugs with dangerous side-effects like Amidopyrine as well as the presence of hundreds of irrational FDCs should have provoked the Government of India to move swiftly to prohibit these drugs. Further, the Government should have revamped the entire procedure to vet the safety and efficacy of new drugs before any manufacturing licences were granted for new drugs in the country. Surprisingly, the government concentrated only on prohibiting harmful drugs from the market, without putting in place a rigorous clinical trial framework to assess the safety and efficacy of new drugs. This included the cancellation of import licences for drugs like Amidopyrine[30] and the issuance of orders banning drugs under Section 26A, a provision that had been inserted into the law in 1982 by Parliament in order to provide the Ministry of Health with the legal power to prohibit the manufacture and sale of existing drugs.[31]

It would take until the announcement of the new Drugs Policy,1986 for the Government of India to agree that the system in place was "far from being adequate" and committing to examining the safety and efficacy data for all new drugs being introduced in India in the future.[32]

Further, taking aim at FDCs, the new Drug Policy,1986 declared that new formulations of already approved drugs "would not be allowed to be manufactured unless their therapeutic efficacy and rationality are adequately tested and proved".[33]

Two years later, in 1988, the Government of India moved to implement the promises announced in the Drugs Policy, 1986, through the route of delegated legislation; i.e., instead of moving legislation in Parliament to amend the Drugs & Cosmetics Act, it used its executive powers to enact the Drugs & Cosmetics (Eighth Amendment) Rules, 1988.[34] These amendments replaced the existing Rule 30A which defined "new drugs" with a new definition that included for the first time in Indian history, a requirement for the new drug to be "effective and safe for the proposed claims".[35]

In order to be approved under the new rules, an application for a new drug would now have to be complemented with a lengthy list of clinical trial data collected through rigorous three-phased clinical trials, much like the requirements under American law that was referenced earlier in this chapter.[36] These amendments also introduced a legal framework for regulating clinical trials in India.[37] Further, the approval of all "new drugs" (which now included FDCs) was centralized with the DCGI for the first four years of the drug's availability in India, after which the drug controllers operating under the state governments could directly issue manufacturing licences for the manufacture of those drugs.[38] This regulatory architecture has remained largely untouched save for a few form-changing amendments in 2005 and 2019. Surprisingly, this new regulatory framework was entirely silent on any kind of transitory framework for drugs already on the market prior to 1988.

Despite the amendments in 1988, creating on paper a regulatory standard for "new drug" approvals that was similar to the system followed in the USA, in practice, the new system proved to be a spectacular failure. This was obvious from the fact that the Ministry of Health continued issuing hundreds of orders under Section 26A for several decades after 1988, banning a number of drugs, especially FDCs. In one instance, in 2007, the Government of India banned 294 FDCs in one go, only for those orders to be stayed by a court of law where the matter simply lingered on for years together.[39] In the following decade, it issued hundreds of orders prohibiting hundreds of FDCs already being sold but did nothing to plug the entry of new irrational FDCs into the market.

Equally worrying was the fact that some Indian doctors continued to complain about the approval of dubious new drugs by the DCGI which had not been approved in developed countries.[40] The lurking suspicion in many quarters was that pharmaceutical companies were exploiting poor regulation in markets like India to sell drugs to unsuspecting patients which they knew would not pass regulatory scrutiny in the developed countries that had robust approval procedures for new drugs. The worst, however, was yet to be exposed.

Parliamentary wrath exposes the new drug approval process

The full extent of the rot in the approval process of "new drugs" within the CDSCO became evident only in the year 2012, when the Parliamentary Standing Committee on Health & Family Welfare, consisting of 31 Members of Parliament drawn from both the Lok Sabha and Rajya Sabha, tabled before Parliament a stunning investigation into the functioning of the CDSCO. This report remains till date one of the most scathing and astonishing official reports on the abject failure of India's drug regulatory structure.[41]

One of the focus areas of the parliamentary committee in its 59th report was the process by which the CDSCO and its head—the DCGI—were approving new drugs. Since parliamentary committees can summon records from the government, the committee was able to scrutinize records that have never been made public by the CDSCO. The exception of course were cases where the files went "missing", which is regrettably a frequent occurrence at the CDSCO's office.[42]

The drug approval files that were accessed by the parliamentary committee revealed a worrying state of affairs. Of the 39 drugs scrutinized by the committee, 13 did not have permission for sale in the better regulated markets of developed countries. Other drugs were approved without any Phase III clinical trial data (where the efficacy of the drug is established) or without any consultation with experts in the field. In many cases, the CDSCO was faulted with an over-reliance on a small number of Delhi-based experts for consultation on "new drug" approvals.[43]

A closer examination of the manner in which these "new drugs" were approved reveals the jarring realities about the manner in which the drug approval process works in India. In particular, we selected and tracked in detail two approvals that had been red-flagged by the parliamentary committee based on its investigation. These following case-studies reveal the extent of the "rot" within the CDSCO:

1. Buclizine

Buclizine was a drug developed by a Belgian company called UCB Pharma and has since been marketed in India by companies such as Mankind Pharma. Originally approved in India as an anti-histamine on 3 August 1982 to treat allergies, Buclizine was later approved in 2006 by the DCGI to be used as an appetite stimulant for children.[44] Apparently, the marketing literature accompanying the drug claimed that evidence from three clinical trials supported the claim that the drug was effective as an appetite stimulant.

These claims have been met with a lot of scepticism by the Indian medical community. Writing in the *Indian Journal of Pharmacology*, an Indian doctor questioned whether the lack of appetite was even a condition that could be "cured". He also questioned the methodology of the three clinical trials cited by the manufacturer, criticizing them for being underpowered and poorly designed.[45] The same doctor also explained how a literature survey of studies regarding Buclizine failed to identify any convincing literature justifying the use of the drug as an appetite stimulant.[46]

During the course of its investigation, the parliamentary committee sent a questionnaire to the Ministry of Health asking it to respond to their questions about these approvals. On receiving the replies from the Ministry, the parliamentary committee accused the Ministry of giving "incorrect and misleading information" about the regulatory status of the drug in other countries. The committee also levelled the serious allegation that the Ministry "went out of the way to volunteer incorrect information".[47] Further, the committee alleged that the company's own "core data sheet" had stated that it lacked clinical studies and scientific data to market the drug as an appetite stimulant.[48] Each of these allegations levelled by the parliamentary committee against the Ministry was stunning. The parliamentary committee concluded its examination of the Buclizine approval with a demand that the DCGI reconsider the continued sale of the drug.[49]

2. Approval of dubious Fixed Dose Combinations (FDCs):

As discussed earlier, the presence of numerous FDCs in India has been a problematic issue in the country since at least the mid-1970s. The parliamentary committee examined this issue at two levels.

First, the committee examined files of two specific FDCs approved by the DCGI. In the case of the first FDC of Aceclofenac and Drotaverine approved by the DCGI, the committee noted that the combination was not approved in any of the well-regulated markets in North America, Europe or Australia.[50] While Aceclofenac is a nonsteroidal, anti-inflammatory drug (NSAID), generally used for the treatment of pain and inflammation, Drotaverine is an "antispasmodic" drug. Neither drug was approved in lucrative and well-regulated markets such as the USA. So why was it approved in India? The committee, during its investigation, discovered that the six "expert opinions" provided by Themis Medicare, to justify its application for the sale of the drug in India were identical to each other despite the fact that the doctors who signed the opinions were in six different parts of the country, from Chandigarh to Hyderabad. The committee alleged that the expert opinions were basically written by the pharmaceutical company that applied for the approval and merely signed by the doctors in question without any study of the clinical evidence.[51]

In the case of a second FDC, consisting of Flupenthixol and Melitracen that was initially marketed by Lundbeck, a Danish company, the parliamentary committee again made a series of worrying allegations. It first stated that, "...the Ministry failed to provide any documents and information on the regulatory process that led to its approval".[52] The committee also alleged that this FDC was not approved for sale in the better-regulated markets in the West, including in Denmark, the home country of the drug's manufacturer and that the drug was being sold primarily in poorly regulated markets.[53] A third allegation by the committee claimed that the product-insert for the drug included indications other than those for which the drug had been officially approved by the DCGI. Apparently, the drug was officially approved for the following indications: (i) Psychogenic depression, (ii) Depressive neuroses, (iii) Masked depression and (iv) Psychosomatic affections, but its package insert promoted the drugs for two unapproved indications: "Menopausal depression" and "Dysphoria and depression in alcoholics and drug addicts".[54] In most developed countries, it is a criminal offence to market a drug for indications that are not approved by the drug regulator.

(The company has refuted most of these allegations in an advertisement published in the newspapers and even sued the doctor who wrote about the drug for criminal defamation before a court in Bangalore.[55] Eventually the Ministry of Health banned the drug on two occasions under Section 26A except on both occasions the Karnataka High Court set aside the ban on procedural grounds.)

After scrutinizing the manner in which the DCGI was approving FDCs, the committee turned its sights to the various state drug controllers who were indiscriminately issuing manufacturing licences for FDCs despite the fact that they lacked the authority to issue these licences unless the FDC was first approved by the DCGI. In rather blunt language, the parliamentary committee accused some state drug regulators of issuing manufacturing licences for FDCs, not approved by the DCGI.

The aftermath of the 59th report of the Parliamentary Standing Committee

The tabling of the 59th report before Parliament, in May 2012, sent shockwaves through the Indian pharmaceutical industry and medical community. Never before had a parliamentary committee in India conducted such an in-depth investigation into the functioning of India's drug regulatory system and revealed so many of its darkest secrets to the world. Apart from receiving extensive coverage in the press, the committee's findings attracted a lot of attention from the international academic community with a number of foreign academics publishing studies on various problems with the drug regulatory framework in India, with a special focus on the flood of irrational FDCs in India and its consequences for global public health, especially on the rise of antibiotic-resistant bacteria.[56] One study published in the *Lancet* in 2014 specifically called upon the Government of India to enact a new drug regulatory law to replace the Drugs & Cosmetics Act, 1940.[57]

The fact that the parliamentary report got extensive coverage in the press meant that the government of the day was under pressure to demonstrate that it was taking some steps to overhaul the drug regulatory mechanism in India, especially the proliferation of FDCs and the process by which new drugs were being approved by the CDSCO. The immediate response was typically bureaucratic. A number of committees were setup to examine different issues, many of which turned in reports of varying quality, most of which were ignored by the Ministry of Health. The other response was draft legislation that pushed for greater centralization of drug regulation but that legislative effort lost steam quickly.[58]

On the issue of FDCs, a few years after the tabling of the parliamentary report, the Ministry of Health issued orders under Section 26A prohibiting the sale and manufacture of 344 FDCs in 2016.[59] These actions prompted massive litigation before the courts leading to some orders being set aside and reissued once against in 2018. Yet, the FDC problem is far from being resolved in India as evidenced by the fact that as late as 2024, the government was still issuing orders under Section 26A prohibiting another 156 FDCs. Academics tracking the sales of FDCs have alleged in published studies that there are several hundred unapproved FDCs being sold in India in different therapeutic categories.

More worrying was the government's response to the allegations of illegal drug approvals. Given the Parliamentary Committee's scathing indictment of the manner in which the CDSCO was approving new drugs, one would have expected a swift inquiry from the government so that it could pin accountability on the officers responsible for taking some of these disastrous decisions.

Since there was little reporting in the press on steps taken by the Ministry of Health to fix responsibility on officials responsible for these drug approvals, we filed a series of RTI applications asking the government for records of the action that it had taken to fix accountability on officers involved in the granting of these irregular approvals. This was an arduous process that involved drafting precise queries to be filed with the Ministry and then sifting through a ton of information that the Ministry of Health provided us in response to our request for information. Thanks to an eagle-eyed research assistant, we discovered that the

Ministry of Health had informed Parliament that the DCGI had setup a four-member expert committee under Dr Tribhuban Mohan Mohapatra to investigate the suspicious drug approvals identified in the parliamentary report. Some more research led us to discover on the internet a poorly scanned order by the DCGI from 2013 constituting an inquiry committee under the chairmanship of Dr Mohapatra with a specific mandate to examine the manner in which the above-mentioned drugs in question were approved.[60]

Equipped with this new information, we filed two more requests for information under the RTI Act with the Ministry of Health and the CDSCO in May 2018, asking both authorities for a final copy of the inquiry committee's report. The replies that we received were stunning! The CDSCO informed us that the committee report was "not readily available"[61] and that it was transferring our application to the Ministry of Health, which in turn informed us it had "checked all its records" and it was able to confirm that the information sought by us was "not available" with it.[62] The report of the Mohapatra committee had apparently disappeared into thin air. The RTI Act provides for a departmental appeal, which also failed to turn up any results, after which we filed an appeal before the Central Information Commission (CIC).

Thanks to the CIC's huge backlog, it took us almost two years to get a hearing. Our appeal finally came up for a hearing on 12 May 2020 during the first lockdown of the COVID pandemic. The hearing was to take place via "Whatsapp" since the pandemic made it difficult to travel to the CIC's office in New Delhi. Approximately 15 hours prior to the hearing scheduled before the CIC, we received an email from the CDSCO late in the night, informing us that they had procured a copy of the report from Dr Mohapatra himself and were providing a copy of the same to us![63] The CDSCO could have done this back in 2018 when we first asked it for the report but chose to keep the matter pending for almost two years before trying to procure the report from Dr Mohapatra. Even this version of the report was not signed by its authors and the annexures to the report, which were copies of the drug approval files (and contained the names of the relevant bureaucrats), were missing.

The CDSCO's conduct was brought to the CIC's attention the next day during the hearing which resulted in the CIC expressing "serious concern" about the record keeping procedures at the CDSCO. The commission also ordered the CDSCO to digitize its records as soon as possible.[64] Even after the CIC ordered the DCGI to provide us with a copy of the annexures to the report, the DCGI failed to do so, necessitating another lawsuit before the Delhi High Court.[65] After almost two years of delays and diversions before the court, the government conceded in court, via an oral submission, that it had lost half the annexures (which were the most incriminating records that could be used in criminal proceedings). It took another two years for the government to make this admission on affidavit.

The reason the CDSCO and the Ministry of Health 'misplaced' the Mohapatra committee report for seven long years was evident from a reading of the report. The report had named and accused three former DCGIs for their dubious role in approving some of the drugs identified by the parliamentary committee. The committee's report painted a picture of utter callousness within the DCGI's office while it reviewed applications for new drugs. Take for example the approval of Buclizine as an appetite stimulant in 2006. It was initially approved only as an anti-histamine, although as noted by the Mohapatra committee, "...the document relating to the first approval is not available".[66] With regard to the additional approval as an appetite stimulant, the Mohapatra committee noted a litany of problems with the drug's approval, including the fact that the published trial reports focused on "body weight gain" and not on appetite stimulation leading to better intake of food, which in turn would result in gain of body weight. Additionally, the committee noted that the standard practice of requiring the status of regulatory approvals in other jurisdictions was also allegedly ignored by the DCGI while processing this application. As per the committee, when warning bells were reportedly rung within the DCGI's office in 2007 by a Joint Drug Controller who informed the DCGI in writing that the drug had faced adverse regulatory action in the USA, the DCGI simply ignored the issue.[67]

The Mohapatra committee concluded that the DCGI did not follow the law and ignored objections raised by other bureaucrats, while approving Buclizine as an appetite stimulant.[68]

If this report had been made public in 2013, as soon as it had been submitted to the DCGI, it would have immediately paved the way for prohibiting the use of Buclizine as an appetite stimulant. Instead, the fate of this drug bounced around different sub-committees setup by the DTAB until one of us, Dinesh Thakur, sued the Ministry of Health and DCGI in 2018 demanding the government take a decision on the continued sale of Buclizine.[69] In less than a week of the Delhi High Court issuing notice to the government, asking it to respond to our petition, the Ministry of Health issued a ban order under Section 26A prohibiting the sale of Buclizine as an appetite stimulant (its approval as an anti-histamine has not been disturbed).[70]

The second drug scrutinized by the Mohapatra committee was the FDC of Aceclofenac and Drotaverine, which were also red-flagged by the parliamentary committee. After investigating the approval, the Mohapatra committee made the stunning allegation that this FDC was approved by the DCGI despite the company failing to provide any clinical trial data to support the efficacy of the drug. Once again, if the Mohapatra committee report had been made public in 2013, the Ministry of Health would have been compelled to prohibit the sale of this particular FDC. Instead, after Dinesh sued the Ministry of Health before the Delhi High Court asking it to take a decision to ban this drug, the government replied stating that the company that sought the approval had on 14 March 2019 "surrendered" the "permission" granted to it to market the drug.[71] However the same FDC continues to be sold by other pharmaceutical companies since the government has not yet prohibited the marketing of this drug in India.

With regard to the approval of the third drug—Letrozole—as a fertility treatment, the Mohapatra committee made the allegation that the DCGI completely ignored the recommendation of a joint drug controller to ask Sun Pharmaceuticals for animal toxicity data before approving its application for human clinical trials. This was important because Novartis, which had invented the drug, had warned against the use of the drug as a fertility treatment.[72] As with the other cases, the Mohapatra committee notes that the DCGI ignored the recommendations of the junior officer without providing any reasons in writing and simply referred the clinical trial protocol to handpicked experts for their opinion. Similarly, with regard to the requirement imposed by the DCGI for providing post-marketing surveillance (PMS) reports on the use of Letrozole on the general population, the Mohapatra committee notes that there was a complete failure within the CDSCO to insist on the submission of PMS data by pharmaceutical companies to the CDSCO.[73]

It is worth noting that the Mohapatra committee concluded its report stating that "...there was no proper system in place to deal with matters pertaining to approval of New Drugs." In particular, the committee pointed out that, "...the exercise of the discretionary power by the DCGI without stating any reason is totally irregular and undesirable." It found the practice of the DCGI simply ignoring written objections by joint drug controllers and other staff, without stating any reasons, to be a "serious misuse/abuse of power on the part of the DCGI." The committee also concluded that "commercial needs of the industry" were given "more focus than the regulatory norms." Even something as basic as record keeping and archiving of files by the CDSCO was found to be wanting by the Mahapatra committee.[74] The irony, of course, was that the Mohapatra Report itself went missing for seven years.

If the recommendations of the Mohapatra committee had been implemented by the Ministry of Health in 2013, the system may have become more transparent and streamlined. However, since the Ministry of Health and the CDSCO "misplaced" this report for more than seven years, there was no opportunity for policymakers to consider its recommendations. As a result, when the Ministry of Health introduced a new set of New Drugs and Clinical Trial Rules in 2019 it did not have an opportunity to learn from the recommendations of the Mohapatra committee's report. The new rules introduced in 2019 thus represent a continuance of the old status-quo.

The only seemingly substantive change brought about after the scathing observations of the 59th report was the creation of "Subject Expert Committees" consisting of external medical experts to provide non-binding recommendations to the DCGI about applications for new drug approvals. This is largely a superficial reform measure since there is no transparency in how these committees operate.

The pandemic stress test

The year after the New Drugs and Clinical Trials Rules, 2019 came into effect, with the aim of streamlining the drug approval process, the COVID-19 pandemic swept the world. The pharmaceutical industry responded to the pandemic by investing in the creation of new vaccines as well as in the creation of new drugs and repurposing existing treatments to treat COVID-19 patients. Across the world, the pandemic was the ultimate stress test for drug regulators because most of them were under immense political pressure to approve new treatments for COVID-19 regardless of whether clinical evidence substantiated their therapeutic efficacy. Even the much-vaunted USFDA granted a very contentious emergency use authorization (EUA) for the use of Hydroxychloroquine (HCQ) to treat COVID-19 on the basis of an open-label non-randomized French study on 36 patients, after American President Donald Trump began advocating for HCQ's benefits. Eventually this EUA was revoked after more rigorous randomized clinical trials demonstrated that HCQ had no therapeutic effect on patients affected by COVID-19.[75]

The DCGI's streak of approvals during this same time period was far more controversial.

The first problem was that the DCGI began granting

drug approvals in various "modes" that did not find any mention in the New Drugs and Clinical Trial Rules, 2019 and way before the completion of Phase III clinical trials. For example, the DCGI announced that it was granting "Restricted Emergency Use Authorization" to three drugs—Favipiravir, Itolizumab and Virafin—despite the fact that the phrase "Restricted Emergency Use Authorization" does not find any mention in the New Drugs and Clinical Trial Rules, 2019.[76]

We filed applications under the RTI Act asking the CDSCO under which provision of the law it was granting "Restricted Emergency Use Authorization". The CDSCO was unable to give a straight answer on how exactly it was circumventing the legal requirement in Indian law that a new drug necessarily complete a three-phased clinical trial to substantiate its safety and efficacy. In its reply, the Ministry of Health pointed us to a chapter rather than a specific rule in the law. Its reply is reproduced below:

> Details of regulatory requirements and guidelines for permission to Import and/ or Manufacture of new drugs for sale are specified in Chapter X and Second Schedule of the New Drugs and Clinical Trials Rules, 2019.[77]

But the fact of the matter is that neither the chapter nor schedule mentioned in the Ministry's reply contain the phrase "restricted emergency use authorisation"! Simply put, there was no legal basis for these approvals without adequate Phase III clinical trial data. It also quickly became obvious that even the pharmaceutical industry had no clue about the happenings in the DCGI office. There was one instance where a pharmaceutical company claimed that its drug received approval under Section 26B (which is a provision that can be invoked by the government during epidemics) but when we asked the CDSCO, it replied to us saying that the drug was not approved under Section 26B.

We then had to speculate that perhaps the DCGI was granting "accelerated approvals", which is a regulatory pathway recognized in the New Drugs and Clinical Trial Rules, 2019 for drugs treating conditions/diseases lacking adequate treatments. Under this pathway, these drugs could be approved after conclusion of Phase II trials, provided that Phase II clinical trials demonstrated "remarkable efficacy".[78] None of the aforementioned drugs met this milestone. This became evident when the government's own National COVID Taskforce consisting of experts from elite Indian medical institutions like AIIMs and ICMR, did not recommend the inclusion of Favipiravir, Itolizumab and Virafin in the national COVID-19 treatment guidelines that were being updated periodically to guide doctors in making treatment decisions for patients infected with COVID-19.[79] The decision of this taskforce not to include these drugs in the treatment protocol when the drug regulator had approved them for COVID-19 treatment was never publicly explained. We suspect the reason for non-inclusion of these drugs was that the clinical trials that formed the basis of the DCGI's approvals had come under heavy criticism for being underpowered or poorly designed.[80]

Notwithstanding the non-inclusion of these drugs in the treatment guidelines laid down by the government's COVID-19 taskforce, the fact that the DCGI had approved them was sufficient for people to hanker after these drugs leading to some of these companies raking in a fortune. For example, the Indian pharmaceutical companies selling Favipiravir, led by Glenmark Pharmaceuticals, earned a stunning ₹762 crores from the sale of Favipiravir making it the top selling drug in India during the pandemic.[81] In many cases, municipal corporations and state governments were placing huge orders for Favipiravir.[82] This transfer of wealth from the middle and working classes to the pharmaceutical industry was facilitated by the DCGI through its opaque regulatory process.

The questionable approvals did not stop with just new drugs. There was plenty of controversy regarding the DCGI's approval of vaccines. For example, when the DCGI approved Covaxin, the vaccine developed by Bharat Biotech with support from ICMR to combat COVID-19, it announced that it was granting the vaccine "restricted emergency use authorization" under "clinical trial mode" despite the company not having completed its Phase III trials.[83] Separate from the scandal of approving a vaccine before the conclusion of Phase III trials was the fact that the phrase "clinical trial mode" did not find any mention in the New Drugs and Clinical Trial Rules, 2019!

The use of such random legal terminology that does not find mention in the official law and the refusal of the DCGI to identify the provision of law under which such approvals were granted represented a new pinnacle of arbitrariness in the functioning of the DCGI.

The second set of problems with the DCGI's approvals during the pandemic was the lack of transparency. The only information available to the public was a tightly condensed summary of the minutes of the "Subject Expert Committee" (SEC). These committees were created after the 59th report of the Parliamentary Standing Committee and were staffed by external experts who were to advise the DCGI on approvals of different drugs. The minutes of each committee meeting, which are published by the DCGI are barely 250-words long and are completely inadequate to understand all the complexities of the approval process. Even something as simple as membership of this committee was not made public despite repeated demands by the public health community.[84] It took a parliamentary question by an MP from the opposition to force the government to reveal the membership of one such committee to the public, during the course of the pandemic.[85] In an ideal world, the DCGI would transcribe verbatim the discussions of the committee and publish the same or alternatively, like some other regulators, live-stream discussions of the SEC to the public on the internet. In addition, the DCGI should have released its own records pertaining to the approval of these medicines so that the medical community could understand the basis of its approval. Unfortunately, the New Drugs and Clinical Trial Rules, 2019 does not require the release of such records, although there is a strong case to argue that Section 4 of the RTI Act, 2005 mandates the proactive disclosure of such records by the DCGI.

The only silver lining of the COVID-19-related controversies over new drug approvals in India is the fact that many of the controversial approvals granted during the pandemic were meticulously documented by Indian science journalists, doctors and public health activists. Never before had the DCGI and the pharmaceutical industry faced such scrutiny in India. It certainly helped that both the journalists and doctors had an easy reference point in the actions of foreign regulators in the USA and Europe while approving new drugs.

The absence of evidence-based medicine in India

In our opinion, the heart of the problem in India with the wide availability and sale of dubious drugs of doubtful safety and efficacy is not just an indifferent regulator but also the lack of widespread understanding within the Indian medical community of the basics of "evidence-based medicine". The foremost principle of evidence-based medicine is to insist on the production of high-quality evidence to substantiate the safety and efficacy of a new drug, rather than depending merely on "intuition or unsystematic clinical experience", as the basis of treatment decisions.[86] In the hierarchy of knowledge recognized by evidence-based medicine, data generated through randomized double blind clinical trials is placed on a higher pedestal; much above anecdotal evidence generated through individual case studies.

Individual doctors have been making an effort to spread the principles of evidence-based medicine in India but an institutional push appears to be lacking. As reported by one Indian practitioner of evidence-based medicine at an elite Indian medical institution, attempts to integrate evidence-based medicine into the curriculum at medical schools has not met with much success.[87]

One possible reason for the lack of awareness of the principles of evidence-based medicine is that most Indian doctors actually have very little exposure to rigorous clinical research. Until 2005, it was rather difficult to conduct clinical trials in India, meaning that doctors and medical students in India never participated in or designed clinical trials. This is because in 1988 when the Drugs & Cosmetics Rules were amended to create a regulatory framework for clinical trials, a rule was inserted requiring clinical trials in India to always be one step behind clinical trials conducted elsewhere in the world. This is to say that a Phase II clinical trial for a new drug could be conducted in India only if Phase III trials had begun elsewhere in the world for the same new drug. From a research perspective, it made no sense to be conducting a Phase II trial in India, if Phase III trials are taking place elsewhere in the world unless it was for a different indication. It is possible that this regulatory structure was created with an intent to dissuade pharmaceutical companies from conducting clinical trials in India because of fears of exploitation of the Indian population by powerful pharmaceutical companies. This position in the law changed in 2005 when the Government of India, upon the recommendations of the Mashelkar Committee amended the law to "harness [the] country's potential to participate in global multi-centric clinical trials."[88]

Once the law was changed in 2005 to make it easier to conduct clinical trials in India, the nascent clinical research establishment here was rocked by a series of scandals over data integrity, informed consent and even some deaths of volunteers.[89] These scandals, which were inevitable due to the lack of any credible regulatory mechanism to ensure the conduct of ethical clinical trials, eventually led to the Supreme Court imposing a temporary ban on clinical trials in India with an exception for only those trials approved by the Secretary of Health.[90] Ultimately, the government did create a new framework under the New Drugs And Clinical Trial Rules, 2019 to regulate clinical trials. Like many other Indian laws, it borrows extensively from the American system of self-regulation without the accompanying stress on transparency or accountability. We do not expect these rules to make any long-term difference.

Perhaps due to these reasons listed above, evidence-based medicine has not spread amongst the medical community in India and Indian doctors continue to prescribe dubiously approved drugs. Any sustained long-term reform will depend on overhauling the curriculum taught at medical schools, to ensure that every graduating doctor has a rigorous understanding of evidence-based medicine.

The future of reform of the new drug approval process—transparency, transparency, transparency

The only short-term solution to combat the arbitrariness with which new drugs are approved in India is to insist on transparency at every level of the drug approval process. Bureaucrats who are aware that their decisions are going to be publicly accessible are more likely to behave themselves and follow the law. Sunlight, after all, is the best disinfectant. Such transparency measures also make it easier for doctors, journalists and academics to track the functioning of the institutions responsible for drug approvals. The situation today is such that the average Indian has to really fight with the bureaucracy in order to get access to even basic information related to drug approvals. Despite multiple requests that we have made to access the approval dossiers of some of the controversial drugs discussed in the chapter, we were never given access.

Contrast the difficulty of accessing such information in India, to the information made public by the American or European drug regulators. The USFDA publishes on its website different reviews of new drug applications, which includes a medical review, chemistry review, pharmacology review, statistical review, microbiology review and a clinical pharmacology biopharmaceutics review. Detailed notes on approvals of the proprietary name, the labelling and all communications between the USFDA and the pharmaceutical company are also made publicly available. Similarly, the European Medical Agency (EMA) makes available a detailed European Public Assessment Report (EPAR) explaining all the scientific reasons underlying its decision to approve a new drug. In contrast, the CDSCO makes available barely 250 words worth of information, summarizing the recommendation of the subject expert committees. There appears to be little to no understanding within the Ministry of Health on the worth of transparency or for that matter, the fact that Section 4 of the Right to Information Act, 2005, actually requires all government offices to proactively publish their records online.

It of course helps the government that not many people in civil society or Parliament are asking it to make transparency the cornerstone of future reform. Hopefully more doctors and ordinary citizens will make similar demands for transparency, creating pressure on the Ministry of Health to publish all records pertaining to drug approvals. Once information is available for public scrutiny, we expect the quality of drug approvals to improve incrementally until it reaches the standards followed in developed countries.

Notes

1. Department Related Parliamentary Standing Committee on Health and Family Welfare, *The Functioning of The Central Drugs Standard Control Organisation (CDCSO)* (Fifty-Ninth Report) (RS 2012) para 7.51.
2. Laura E. Bothwell and others, "Assessing the Gold Standard—Lessons from the History of RCTs" (2016) 374 *New England Journal of Medicine* 2175.
3. United States Senate (Sub-committee on Antitrust and Monopoly), *Study of Administered Prices in the Drug Industry* (Rep No 448, 1961) 156.
4. Jeremy A. Greene and Scott H. Podolsky, "Reform, Regulation, and Pharmaceuticals—The Kefauver–Harris Amendments at 50" (2012) 367 *New England Journal of Medicine* 1481.
5. Public Law 87-871, 1962, s 505(d) (21 U.S.C. 355 (d)).
6. New Drugs, 21 CFR § 130.3 (1965).
7. P. D'Arcy Hart, "A Change in Scientific Approach: From Alternation to Randomised Allocation in Clinical Trials in the 1940s" (1999) 319 *BMJ* 572.
8. Graham Sutton, "Putrid Gums and 'Dead Men's Cloaths': James Lind Aboard the Salisbury" (2003) 96 *Journal of the Royal Society of Medicine* 605.
9. Peter Armitage, "Fisher, Bradford Hill, and Randomization" (2003) 32 *International Journal of Epidemiology* 925.
10. A.J. de Craen and others, "Placebos and Placebo Effects in Medicine: Historical Overview." (1999) 92 *Journal of the Royal Society of Medicine* 511.
11. ibid.
12. Ted J. Kaptchuk, "Intentional Ignorance: A History of Blind Assessment and Placebo Controls in Medicine" (1998) 72 *Bulletin of the History of Medicine* 389.
13. Bothwell (n 2).
14. David S. Jones and Scott H. Podolsky, "The History and Fate of the Gold Standard" (2015) 385 *Lancet* (London, England) 1502; 21 CFR § 314.126.

15. US Food & Drug Administration, "Detail of full-time Equivalents (FY 2020)" (2020).
16. Office of the Commissioner, "Learn About FDA Advisory Committees" [2020] FDA <https://www.fda.gov/patients/about-office-patient-affairs/learn-about-fda-advisory-committees> accessed 14 July 2021.
17. United States (ed), *Review Panel on New Drug Regulation: Final Report* (Dept of Health, Education, and Welfare, Review Panel on New Drug Regulation 1977) 2-3.
18. N. Dorsen and J.M. Miller, "The Drug Regulation Process and the Challenge of Regulatory Reform" (1979) 91 *Annals of Internal Medicine* 908, 911.
19. Christopher Morten and Amy Kapczynski, "The Big Data Regulator, Rebooted: Why and How the FDA Can and Should Disclose Confidential Data on Prescription Drugs and Vaccines" (*Social Science Research Network* 2020) SSRN Scholarly Paper ID 3696503 <https://papers.ssrn.com/abstract=3696503> accessed 14 July 2021; "UPDATE 1-GSK Promises to Publish Detailed Drug Trial Data" *Reuters* (5 February 2013) <https://www.reuters.com/article/gsk-data-idUSL5N0B5CV920130205> accessed 14 July 2021; "Unreported Clinical Trial Results: Lost Opportunities for FDA, NIH" (*STAT*, 13 April 2020) <https://www.statnews.com/2020/04/13/lost-opportunities-clinical-trial-results-unreported-lost-opportunities/> accessed 14 July 2021.
20. Government of India, Ministry of Health, *SRO 694* (*Gazette of India Weekly*, Part II–s 3, 14 April 1952) published on 19 April 1952.
21. Drugs Third (Amendment) Rules, 1961; Government of India, Ministry of Health, *SO 1449* (*Gazette of India Weekly*, Part II–s 3, 13 June 1961) published on 24 June 1961.
22. T.Y. Chan and A.W. Chan, "Aminopyrine-Induced Blood Dyscrasias—Still a Problem in Many Parts of the World" (1996) 5 *Pharmacoepidemiology and Drug Safety* 215.
23. R.M. Kapadia and A.D. Desai, "Amidopyrine (Dipyrone) and Its Toxicity" (1955) 43 *The Indian Journal of Medical Research* 297.

24. "Guidelines for Registration of Fixed-Dose Combination Medicinal Products" (World Health Organization 2005) WHO Technical Report Series 929.
25. "What Are FDC Drugs and Why Has the Govt Decided to Ban Them?" *Business Today* (13 September 2018) <https://www.businesstoday.in/industry/pharma/story/what-are-fdc-drugs-and-why-has-the-govt-decided-to-ban-them-110595-2018-09-13> accessed 18 July 2021.
26. William Rosen, *Miracle Cure: The Creation of Antibiotics and the Birth of Modern Medicine* (Penguin 2017) 272.
27. Government of India, Ministry of Petroleum & Chemicals, *Report of The Committee on Drugs and Pharmaceutical Industry (Hathi Committee Report)* (1975) 174.
28. Government of India, *Drug Policy, 1978* (1978) para 101.
29. Drugs Consultative Committee (DCC), "*Minutes of the 20TH Meeting of The Drugs Consultative Committee Held at New Delhi on the 4th & 5th July, 1978*" (1978) 37, para 3 <https://cdsco.gov.in/opencms/opencms/system/modules/CDSCO.WEB/elements/common_download.jsp?num_id_pk=ODUz> accessed 17 July 2021.
30. Question raised by Shri Suresh Kalmadi and Shri Arvind Kulkarni, Lok Sabha Deb 30 April 1982, Question No 478, 122.
31. Government of India, Ministry of Health & Family Welfare, *GSR 578(E)* (Gazette of India Extraordinary, Part II–s 3(i), 23 July 1983).
32. Government of India, *Drug Policy, 1986: Measures for Rationalisation, Quality Control and Growth of Drugs & Pharmaceutical Industry In India* (1986).
33. ibid.
34. Government of India, Ministry of Health & Family Welfare, *GSR 944(E)* (*Gazette of India Extraordinary*, Part II–s 3(i), 21 September 1988) 10.
35. Rule 122E (c) contained the new definition of "new drugs".
36. This criterion was laid down in the new Rule 122A, Rule 122B, Rule 122C & Rule 122D.

37. This framework was laid down in the new Schedule Y to the Drugs & Cosmetics Rules 1945.
38. All applications for new drugs had to be approved by the licensing authority appointed by the Government of India under Rule 21 of the Drugs & Cosmetics Rules, 1945.
39. Noemie Bisserbe and Khomba Singh, "DCGI Likely to Invoke Special Provisions to Ban 294 Drugs" *The Economic Times* (New Delhi, 21 November 2007) <https://economictimes.indiatimes.com/industry/healthcare/biotech/pharmaceuticals/dcgi-likely-to-invoke-special-provisions-to-ban-294-drugs/articleshow/2557395.cms?from=mdr> accessed 18 July 2021.
40. These allegations were documented in detail in the 59th report of the Department Related Parliamentary Standing Committee on Health and Family Welfare: *The Functioning of The Central Drugs Standard Control Organisation (CDCSO)* (n 1).
41. ibid.
42. ibid para 7.12.
43. ibid para 7.14.
44. New Drugs Approved by CDSCO, *Buclizine HCl tablet (25mg) & Syrup 6mg/5ml* (Sr No 3277, 28 June 2006) <https://cdscoonline.gov.in/CDSCO/Drugs> accessed 3 August 2021.
45. Thirunavukkarasu Arun Babu, "Buclizine Is Back Again! This Time as a Pediatric Appetite Stimulant" (2011) 43 *Indian Journal of Pharmacology* 219.
46. ibid.
47. *The Functioning of The Central Drugs Standard Control Organisation (CDCSO)* (n 1) para 7.39.
48. ibid.
49. ibid para 7.41.
50. ibid para 7.32.
51. ibid para 7.34.
52. ibid para 7.44.
53. ibid para 7.45-7.46.
54. ibid para 7.44.

55. *M/S Lundbeck India Private Limited vs Dr Chandra M. Gulhati* Criminal Petition No 4683/2011 before the Karnataka HC (26 July 2012) <https://indiankanoon.org/doc/183428285/> last accessed 2 May 2022.
56. Patricia McGettigan et. al., "Use of Fixed Dose Combination (FDC) Drugs in India: Central Regulatory Approval and Sales of FDCs Containing Non-Steroidal Anti-Inflammatory Drugs (NSAIDs), Metformin, or Psychotropic Drugs" (2015) 12 *PLOS Medicine* e1001826; Patricia McGettigan and others, "Threats to Global Antimicrobial Resistance Control: Centrally Approved and Unapproved Antibiotic Formulations Sold in India" (2019) 85 *British Journal of Clinical Pharmacology* 59.
57. *See* Peter Roderick and others, "India Should Introduce a New Drugs Act" (2014) 383 *The Lancet* 203.
58. The Drugs and Cosmetics (Amendment) Bill 2013 (Bill No LVIII of 2013).
59. Press Trust of India, "Health Ministry Bans 344 Fixed Dose Combination Drugs", *Business Standard India* (New Delhi, 14 March 2016) <https://www.business-standard.com/article/pti-stories/health-ministry-bans-344-fixed-dose-combination-drugs-116031400523_1.html> accessed 4 August 2021.
60. DCGI Dr G.N. Singh ordering the "Constitution of a Committee to review the procedure and practices followed by CDSCO for granting marketing approval and clinical trials on certain drugs" (Order no DCG(I) Misc/2013-18, 26 March 2013) (On file with authors).
61. Reply to RTI application, Office of the DCGI (Application No CDSCO/R/20/2018/50052, 30 May 2018) (On file with Authors).
62. Reply to transferred RTI application, Drug Regulation Branch, Ministry of Health (Application No CDSCO/R/20/2018/50052, 21 June 2018) (On file with Authors).
63. Email from the RTI Cell of the CDSCO to one of the authors (11 May 2020 at 9:28 PM) (On file with Authors).

64. *Prashant Reddy vs Ministry of Health & Family Welfare* Second Appeal No CIC/MH&FW/A/2018/159460-BJ (26 May 2020) <https://indiankanoon.org/doc/115080764/> accessed 5 August 2021.
65. *Prashant Reddy T. vs Drug Controller General of India* W.P. No. 7213 of 2020 before the High Court of Delhi.
66. T.M. Mahapatra et. al, *Report of the Committee Constituted to Review the Procedures and Practices followed by CDSCO for granting approval and clinical trials on certain drugs (Mahapatra Committee Report)* (2013) para 5.2 (On file with authors).
67. ibid.
68. ibid.
69. *Dinesh Thakur vs Union of India* W.P.(C) 11107/2018.
70. Government of India, Ministry of Health & Family Welfare, *SO 6161(E)* (*Gazette of India Extraordinary*, Part II–s 3(ii), 13 December 2018).
71. Counter-Affidavit dated 24 April 2019 filed by the Ministry of Health and DCGI in LPA No 687 of 2018 filed before the High Court of Delhi at New Delhi (On file with authors).
72. *Mohapatra Committee Report* (n 66) para 5.3.
73. ibid.
74. *Mohapatra Committee Report* (n 66) para 6-7.
75. The United States Food and Drug Administration (FDA), "Coronavirus (COVID-19) Update: FDA Revokes Emergency Use Authorization for Chloroquine and Hydroxychloroquine" (15 June 2020)<https://www.fda.gov/news-events/press-announcements/coronavirus-covid-19-update-fda-revokes-emergency-use-authorization-chloroquine-and> accessed 5 August 2021.
76. Drug Controller General of India (DCGI), "Notice: Approval of Favipiravir Tablets to Glenmark Pharmaceuticals and Remdesivir Injection to Cipla Ltd, Hetero Drugs and Mylan Labs" (2 July 2020) <https://cdsco.gov.in/opencms/resources/UploadCDSCOWeb/2018/UploadPublic_NoticesFiles/faviNOTICE.pdf> accessed 5 August 2021; Press

Information Bureau, Government of India, "DCGI Gives Nod for Restricted Emergency Use to Itolizumab for Moderate to Severe COVID-19 Patients" (11 July 2020) <https://pib.gov.in/pib.gov.in/Pressreleaseshare.aspx?PRID=1637926> accessed 5 August 2021; Staff Writer, "Covid Treatment: Zydus Gets Emergency Use Approval for Virafin" *Mint* (23 April 2021) <https://www.livemint.com/companies/news/covid-treatment-zydus-gets-emergency-use-approval-for-use-of-virafin-11619169889774.html> accessed 5 August 2021.

77. Reply to RTI application, Central Drugs Standard Control Organisation (Application No CDSCO/R/E/20/00315).
78. The New Drugs & Clinical Trial Rules 2019, Second Schedule.
79. AIIMS/ICMR-COVID-19 National Task Force/Joint Monitoring Group, Ministry of Health & Family Welfare, Government of India, "CLINICAL GUIDANCE FOR MANAGEMENT OF ADULT COVID-19 PATIENTS" (17 May 2021) <https://www.icmr.gov.in/pdf/covid/techdoc/COVID_Management_Algorithm_17052021.pdf> accessed 5 August 2021.
80. Gayathri Vaidyanathan, "Scientists Criticize Use of Unproven COVID Drugs in India" (2020) 587 Nature 187; Priyanka Pulla, "Is Favipiravir Good for COVID-19? Clinical Trial Says No, Press Release Says Yes", *The Wire Science*, (25 November 2020) <https://science.thewire.in/the-sciences/favipiravir-glenmark-open-label-trial-primary-endpoints-efficacy-cure-times-misleading-press-release/> accessed 5 August 2021; Priyanka Pulla, "The Worrying Ways in Which Biocon's Itolizumab Trial Was Deeply Flawed", *The Wire Science*, (24 August 2020) <https://science.thewire.in/the-sciences/biocon-itolizumab-phase-ii-clinical-trial-cdsco-simon-two-stage-inconsistencies/> accessed 5 August 2021; Ronak Borana, "DCGI Approves Virafin for Moderate COVID. Where's the Evidence It Works?", *The Wire Science* (24 April 2021). <https://science.thewire.in/the-sciences/zydus-virafin-pegylated-interferon-alpha-2b-india-dcgi-approve-covid-trial-methods-flaw/> accessed 5 August 2021.

81. Rupali Mukherjee, "Anti-Covid drug now top-selling pharma brand" *Times of India* (11 May 2021) <https://timesofindia.indiatimes.com/business/india-business/anti-covid-drug-now-top-selling-pharma-brand/articleshow/82540028.cms> accessed 1 October 2021.
82. Prabin Kalita, "Assam 'First State' to Procure Itolizumab for Covid Patients" *The Times of India* (17 July 2020) <https://timesofindia.indiatimes.com/city/guwahati/assam-first-state-to-procure-itolizumab-for-covid-patients/articleshow/77016405.cms> accessed 1 May 2022; "Coronavirus in Mumbai: BMC to Buy 27 Lakh Favipiravir Tablets for Rs 80 per Tablet from Glenmark" *Business Today* (2 July 2020) <https://www.businesstoday.in/latest/economy-politics/story/coronavirus-in-mumbai-bmc-to-buy-27-lakh-favipiravir-tablets-for-rs-80-per-tablet-from-glenmark-262915-2020-07-02> accessed 1 May 2022.
83. Press Information Bureau, Government of India, "Press Statement by the Drugs Controller General of India (DCGI) on Restricted Emergency approval of COVID-19 virus vaccine" (3 January 2021) <https://www.icmr.gov.in/pdf/press_realease_files/HFW_DCGI_energency_use_authorisation_03012021_2.pdf> accessed 5 August 2021.
84. Shreya Dasgupta, "India Needs More Transparency in Its COVID-19 Vaccine Trials, Critics Say" (*Science* | *AAAS*, 25 November 2020) <https://www.sciencemag.org/news/2020/11/india-needs-more-transparency-its-covid-19-vaccine-trials-critics-say> accessed 5 August 2021.
85. R. Prasad, "Government Releases Names of Vaccine Expert Panel" *The Hindu* (Chennai, 5 April 2021) <https://www.thehindu.com/news/national/coronavirus-government-releases-names-of-vaccine-expert-panel/article34246372.ece> accessed 5 August 2021.
86. Gordon Guyatt and others, "Evidence-Based Medicine: A New Approach to Teaching the Practice of Medicine" (1992) 268 *JAMA* 2420.
87. Kameshwar Prasad, "Evidence-Based Medicine in India" (2012) 66 *Journal of Clinical Epidemiology* 6, 8.

88. Government of India, Ministry of Health and Family Welfare, *Report of The Expert Committee on a Comprehensive Examination of Drug Regulatory Issues, including the problem of Spurious Drugs (Mashelkar Committee Report)* (No Z.28015/112/2002-D/DMS&PFA, 2003) 30.
89. T.N.N., "Clinical Trials: DCGI Faults 9 More CROs" *The Times of India* (Hyderabad, 20 July 2011) <https://timesofindia.indiatimes.com/city/hyderabad/clinical-trials-dcgi-faults-9-more-cros/articleshow/9290503.cms> accessed 5 August 2021.
90. Sanjeet Bagcchi, "Indian Supreme Court Halts Approval of New Clinical Trials until Regulatory Framework Is Set Up" (2013) 347 *BMJ* f5996.

CHAPTER SIX

Can "Made in India" Generic Medicine Be Trusted?

On 2 August 2023, the National Medical Commission (NMC), sparked a massive controversy amongst the medical community when it announced a new rule that would mandatorily require all doctors to prescribe drugs solely by their generic names, instead of the prevailing practice of prescribing drugs by their "brand names".[1] To illustrate with an example, instead of writing Crocin® (which is a brand name owned by one specific company) every time they want to prescribe Acetaminophen (the chemical name of Paracetamol), Indian doctors would now be required by law, to write only Paracetamol on the prescription.

The aim of such a rule, as articulated by Prime Minister Narendra Modi at a public speech in 2017, was to break the alleged nexus between pharmaceutical companies and doctors, wherein doctors are bribed by pharmaceutical companies to prescribe their brand of medicine.[2] By forcing doctors to write only generic names in the prescription, the hope of the government was that the pharmacist would then dispense the lowest-priced brand to the patient, resulting in savings for the patient. The government was obviously presuming that the pharmacist would behave honestly and not have his own arrangements with pharmaceutical companies.

The backlash to this new rule from the doctors was almost instant and the NMC had to announce a rollback of the rule in less than a month.[3] While the cynics accused doctors of opposing the rule because it would supposedly break their alleged corrupt nexus with pharmaceutical companies, most doctors cited their concerns with the quality of medicine sold in India as the reason for their opposition to the rule. Simply put, most doctors did not trust that all brands of drugs available in the Indian market, containing the same active ingredient, would have the same therapeutic effect on their patients. This lack of trust in the quality of drugs in India was, in effect, an indictment of India's drug regulatory framework.

Over the decades, several Indian doctors have complained in journals and other writings, about a lack of faith in India's drug regulatory framework.[4] Based on their own experience with treatment outcomes for patients under their care, Indian doctors are aware that many formulations of Indian generic medicines do not have the expected therapeutic effect on their patients. These doctors have figured out, through "trial and error" based on patient feedback, the specific brands of generic medicine that have the expected therapeutic effect and prescribe only those to their patients. This anecdotal evidence from individual doctors is also reflected in market pricing of generic drugs in India, where different brands of the same generic drug command different prices, with the price differentials in some cases being anywhere between 100% to 200%. For example, a study in 2005, noted that the brand of Ciprofloxacin owned by one company was being sold at a price that was 194% higher than the cheapest substitute in the market. Similarly, the most expensive brand of Nimesulide was 150% higher than the cheapest brand on the market.[5] These price differences between different brands of generics continue to persist in the Indian market even today.

From a theoretical viewpoint, a significant difference in price between different brands of generic drugs makes little sense because these different brands are supposed to contain the same active ingredient and are therefore the same product with the same therapeutic properties. Generic drugs are not like different brands of toothpaste or soap where companies justify price differences based on claims that their product is superior to other brands. Generic drugs with the same ingredients, once approved by the regulators are supposed to be exact copies of each other and therefore should have an identical therapeutic effect on patients. Rationally acting patients and doctors should therefore buy or prescribe the more affordable generic drug forcing the more expensive generic drugs to reduce their price in order to continue competing in the market. But this did not happen in the Indian market for many reasons. One such reason offered by economists is that consumers of drugs as well as doctors do not perceive all generic formulations to be of the same quality and hence interchangeable with each other or with the innovator brand.[6] Hence, pharmaceutical companies that were presumed to be more "trustworthy" could charge a premium for the trust reposed by patients in their products. These "perceptions" of Indian doctors have been moulded by their clinical experience wherein they have observed different brands of generic medicines have varying therapeutic effects on their patients. The reason they have seen such varying patterns lies in the lax regulatory requirements in India for the approval of generics drugs.

As we will demonstrate through the course of this chapter, the Government of India slumbered while the rest of the world, especially the Americans, worked hard at creating a rigorous scientific and legal framework that would instill confidence in both doctors and patients that all generics approved by the American drug regulator were interchangeable with each other. Understanding these challenges and the gradual evolution of the regulatory framework for generics is important in order to understand the resistance of Indian doctors to mandatory generic substitution of drugs in India. An excellent starting point to this discussion is the evolution and pioneering role of American regulatory law on the approval of generic drugs.

The birth and science behind the rise of generic medicines in the USA

The first half of the 20th century gave rise to a number of pharmaceutical giants like Pfizer, Merck, Eli Lilly, GlaxoSmithKline, Parker Davis, Schering, etc. This tremendous growth of the pharmaceutical industry was fueled by greater public and private investment into scientific research that led to marvelous new medical discoveries especially in the field of antibiotics. This period also saw many countries amend their patent laws to protect these pharmaceutical inventions. Since patent terms were mostly limited to 14 years in that era, many of the patents for the breakthrough discoveries in the 1940s and 1950s were set to expire in the 1950s and 1960s, thereby opening the door for other companies to manufacture generic copies of the same drug.

The entry of multiple generic drugs after the expiry of a patent monopoly had the potential to drive down prices by increasing competition. The possibility of hefty price erosion in the pharmaceutical sector was largely welcomed in the 1950s by American lawmakers who were shocked by the profit margins of the pharmaceutical industry, especially in contrast with other industries selling essential commodities to the general population.[7]

The innovator pharmaceutical industry in the USA, whose patents had guaranteed them a monopoly so far, was not as enthusiastic about welcoming competition. As documented in detail by Jeremy A. Greene in his extensively researched book on the history of the generic drug industry, *Generic: The Unbranding of Modern Medicine*, the innovator drug industry adopted several "dirty tricks" to slow down the entry and acceptance of generic drugs in the USA, including choosing complicated generic names and painting all generic drugs as being manufactured in dirty and unsafe facilities.

"Dirty tricks" aside, there was also serious scientific uncertainty regarding the manner in which regulators would approve generic versions of innovator drugs once the patents expired. Starting in 1962, after the enactment of the Kefauver-Harris amendments, innovator companies in the USA had to demonstrate safety and efficacy of new drugs ("innovator drug") through a system of rigorous clinical trials on patients. These trials were both expensive and risky. The question now was whether generic drugs would have to go through similar trials to establish its safety and efficacy?

Although all generic versions of the innovator drug would have the same "active ingredient" as the innovator drug, it was possible that different manufacturers would use different binders, stabilizers, disintegrating agents, tasting agents and would be compressed by different tablet punching machines.[8] For extended-release formulations, which release the drug over a longer period of time in the gut of the human body, the use of different excipients by the innovator and generic manufacturers could significantly influence the timing and the rate at which the drug is released. Each of these factors had the potential to influence the manner in which the generic drug dissolved in the blood stream of patients. Any variations in the way the drug was formulated or in the use of different excipients or compression/milling using a tablet punching machine could affect the rate at which the drug dissolves and is absorbed by the bloodstream of a patient. Depending on the drug in question, this difference in absorption rates can have a material effect on treatment outcomes in patients. If a drug fails to dissolve at the same rate as the innovator, it may lead to a differing amount of the drug reaching the site of action in the human body, thereby impeding the expected therapeutic effect of the medication. A lower amount of drug dissolving in the bloodstream may not be adequate to generate a proper dose response, which is instrumental to the therapeutic outcome. Alternately, if too much of the drug dissolved into the bloodstream too quickly, it could be potentially toxic for the patient.

One possible regulatory solution to guarantee the efficacy of generic drugs was to put these generic formulations through the same set of clinical trials that the innovator drug was subjected to by law, in order to generate the required efficacy data. This solution was, however, both unethical and expensive. The use of placebos during such clinical trials entails depriving one set of patients the best available treatment that has already been scientifically validated by the innovator's clinical trials and is therefore unethical. From a cost perspective, the repetition of clinical trials would be quite expensive, thereby increasing the costs of generic medicine to patients. As a result, repetition of clinical trials for generic formulations did not make any sense if the objective was to introduce competition and drive down prices of generic medicine.

Instead, focus shifted towards the working hypothesis that chemical equivalence between the innovator drug and generic drugs could be established in the laboratory through standard pharmacopeial methods laid down in pharmacopeias (these are official compilations prescribing testing methods to establish the quality of a drug). The tests generally prescribed at the time by a pharmacopeia to test a drug included assay, identification, weight variation, content uniformity, purity and disintegration. These tests could be carried out in the laboratory at a relatively low cost, especially when compared to the prospect of repeating clinical trials for generic formulations.[9]

This hypothesis came into question in the 1960s when scientists began testing the extent to which generic medicines manufactured by different companies were dissolving and being absorbed by patients. These tests were conducted by examining blood or urine samples from volunteers who consumed the generic medicines in question. By testing the amount of the drug available in these blood or urine samples, scientists could calculate the extent to which these drugs were being absorbed into the blood stream and otherwise metabolized in the body. This is called the bioavailability of the drug in the human body. These experiments demonstrated that despite the pharmacopeial equivalence of these drugs when tested in the lab, there was a significant variability in the rate at which these drugs were being absorbed into the bloodstream of human volunteers. These experiments led to an entirely new area of research called biopharmaceutics, which can be further divided into pharmacodynamics studies (PD) and pharmacokinetics studies (PK).[10]

Canadian researchers J.A. Campbell and D.G. Chapman who worked at the Canadian Food and Drug Laboratories in Ottawa in the 1960s were pioneers in this area of research. In one of their first experiments, when Chapman compared eight different versions of shellac-coated Amphetamine, all manufactured by different companies, it was discovered that the amount of drug excreted in the urine of volunteers varied widely. From the urine tests, it was determined that one tablet delivered only 5 mg, while another delivered the full 15 mg at once.[11] This was likely because the shellac coatings used for extended-release formulations were disintegrating at different times that were not uniform. From a clinical viewpoint, this could be deeply problematic as it would adversely affect treatment outcomes.

In a different set of experiments, a pharmacologist, John H. Wagner tested time-release capsules and enteric-coated tablets, containing a radiopaque contrast agent on dogs trained to lay still on X-ray tables. The aim was to assess the speed at which the drug was being released in the digestive tract of the dogs. This experiment demonstrated that the supposedly identical pills were being released at varying time periods. This meant that although the drugs demonstrated chemical equivalence in the laboratory when tested through standard pharmacopeial techniques, the bioavailability of the drug in the blood stream or urine of dogs was not equivalent to the innovator drug.[12]

These studies raised questions about whether "in-vitro" testing i.e., testing in the laboratory, using standard pharmacopeial methods could actually replace "in-vivo" testing i.e., on human volunteers in order to establish the bioequivalence of the generic with the innovator drug.

This issue of bioequivalence between the innovator drug and generic drugs became an actual regulatory concern in 1967 when the patents for Parke Davis's Chloromycetin expired. Many generic versions of the drug entered the market but due to a series of events involving poorly dissolving generic Chloromycetin, the USFDA decided to test various generic versions of Chloromycetin on human volunteers to examine the bioavailability of the generic versions. Those tests revealed that generic versions of the drugs were being absorbed into the blood at widely varying rates. As a result, the USFDA suspended permission for all generic versions of Chloromycetin until it could work out a revised protocol to grant approval for generic medicines.[13] Similar problems were discovered with different brands of Tetracycline and Oxytetracycline, which failed to demonstrate bioequivalence despite showing equivalence in the laboratory when subjected to standard pharmacopeial tests.[14] There was now enough evidence that equivalence as established through existing pharmacopeial tests in the laboratory did not always guarantee bioequivalence in the human body and hence therapeutic equivalence could not be guaranteed with only in-vitro testing.

One proposed solution to this problem was to require manufacturers of generic pharmaceutical drugs to test their drugs on human volunteers (not patients but volunteers) in order to generate bio-availability data i.e., the rate of absorption of the drug into the bloodstream of human volunteers. This is measured by testing the blood and urine of the volunteers at different time-intervals to compute the dissolution profile of the generic formulation in the human body over a time period. As long as the dissolution curve plotted on a graph is the same or substantially similar to that of the innovator drug, the generic formulation can be presumed to be bioequivalent to the innovator drug. The scope for acceptable differences in dissolution profiles reduces in the case of "narrow therapeutic index" (NTI) drugs where even a small change in dosage may have a significantly large therapeutic effect on the patient. But for broad therapeutic index drugs, for example, standard antibiotics, once bioequivalence is established between the innovator and its generic formulation, doctors and pharmacists can safely substitute the innovator drug with the generic formulation as it is presumed that both versions would guarantee the same therapeutic effect. Although mandating bioequivalence testing through in-vivo methods i.e., on human volunteers was more expensive than using in-vitro methods in the lab i.e., pharmacopeial testing, bioequivalence studies cost only a fraction of full-fledged clinical trials involving patients.

Given the burning importance of creating a simple regulatory pathway for generics and the financial implications of such a policy for medical costs, a number of expert committees were setup in the USA to study the issue of bioequivalence from a regulatory perspective.[15]

After much debate and deliberation, in 1977, the USFDA published regulations to make in-vivo bioequivalence testing on human volunteers the default rule for approving all generic drugs, save for some exceptions.[16] For example, ointments, injections, etc. were excluded from the requirement of bioequivalence testing. The onus was now on the pharmaceutical company manufacturing generics drugs to request for an exemption or waiver from the requirement of conducting in-vivo bioequivalence testing. For those drugs, where in-vivo bioequivalence studies were required to be conducted, the generic drug formulation was to be evaluated on a small number of healthy volunteers and as long as the dissolution profile of the generic formulation was in the range of 75% to 125% of the innovator's dissolution profile, it would be deemed bioequivalent to the innovator drug. The USFDA also published a list of drugs for which in-vitro data would suffice.[17] These bioequivalence standards that evolved within the USFDA gradually proliferated around the world into other jurisdictions.[18] To guarantee better dissemination of information about approved generics, the USFDA also began the process of publishing the "Orange Book", which listed all the bioequivalent generics for every "new drug" that had been approved by the USFDA.

This new regulatory structure put in place by the USFDA, guaranteeing the therapeutic equivalence of generics with the innovator drug, cleared the deck for many American states to pass new laws allowing, or mandating pharmacists to substitute innovator drugs with generic formulations, thereby lowering healthcare costs across the USA.[19]

This regulatory concept of "bioequivalence" also became one of the central tenets of the Drug Price Competition and Patent Term Restoration Act, 1984 better known as the Hatch-Waxman Act. A study on the effect of the Hatch-Waxman Act on drug prices revealed that the prices of generics reduced by 51% to 80% over a period of five years after the entry of generics was permitted.[20] The American experience highlights the importance of having credible regulatory pathways for generic drugs to enter the market and more importantly, win the confidence of the medical community, pharmacists and patients.

The lethargic Indian approach to mandatory in-vivo bioequivalence studies

Indian regulatory authorities were made aware of many of the above problems regarding varying bioavailability of generic drugs as early as in 1972 when the DCC, which has as its members representatives of all the state drug controllers and the DCGI, circulated amongst its members a paper published by the World Health Organization (WHO). This WHO paper warned that several generic drugs of some formulations were not having the expected therapeutic effect due to differing rates of bioavailability. The WHO paper struck a warning note in the very first paragraph, which is reproduced below:

> During the last few years reports have appeared in the literature concerning drugs which either have not given the expected clinical results or which have caused unexpected toxic reactions. This has been more noticeable in patients who have been stabilized on drug for a period of time and, after taking—a new batch or brand, have experienced a change in the clinical effectiveness of their medication. A suspected cause of malabsorption or enhanced absorption is the variation of release characteristics of the final product.

The paper also warned how changing brands during the course of treatment could affect treatment outcomes. In pertinent part it stated:

> The decision as to which drugs (and dosage forms) require dissolution tests depends upon a number of factors. It has been shown that changes in formulation may produce clinical hazards, e.g. increased toxicity of phenytoin with change of excipient; ineffective control of blood sugar with some brands of tolbutamide. The number of drugs and formulations where a

> dissolution test should be included is probably not great. Where a patient is being treated for a chronic illness or requiring continuous replacement therapy, a change in formulation between batches or brands may result in lack of clinical efficacy or in an increase in toxicity....[21]

The WHO paper ended with a recommendation for greater international coordination to study the correlation between dissolution tests and "physiological availability" of drugs. In simple English, the WHO paper pointed out that many brands of drugs were not dissolving in the human body as expected, thereby leading to differing treatment outcomes. Given these serious revelations, one would have expected the DCC and the Ministry of Health to sincerely consider reforming existing regulations in India. Yet, no action was taken.

In 1975, the Hathi Committee Report on Drugs & Pharmaceutical Industry, which was commissioned by the Government of India to study the pharmaceutical industry made a fleeting reference to the WHO paper while flagging the issue of bioavailability of different brands of drugs. The committee made the following pertinent observation on the importance of bioequivalence studies, without exactly laying down any specific standards to be followed in the future:

> It is often argued that bioavailability is an important factor in the efficiency of a drug. The W.H.O. Technical Series Report on bioavailability has highlighted different facets of this problem, particularly, the fact

> that as yet there are no established and accepted methods for evaluation of bioavailability of different brands of drugs. A drug manufactured by a firm, may differ from batch to batch in its bioavailability. Bioavailability is particularly important in the case of oral preparations and that too with respect to only a very few drugs. It cannot be denied, that in case of drugs like digoxin, phenytoin etc. bioavailability is important, but this has nothing to do with brand or generic names. The Drug Control authorities will have to exercise effective control over the standards of such drugs which will need bioavailability studies as per recommendations of the W.H.O., whether these drugs are introduced under generic or brand names."[22]

Despite this warning, the Ministry of Health took no remedial action. More astonishing however is that in 1981, the Ministry of Health selectively enforced a recommendation made by the Hathi Committee to abolish the use of brand names for select generic drugs, without paying any heed to the recommendations pertaining to the issue of varying bioavailability amongst generic drugs. Issued on 17 January 1981, this notification of the Ministry of Health amended the law to prohibit the pharmaceutical industry from using their brand names on the packaging of the following drugs: Analgin, Aspirin, Chlorpromazine and its salts, Ferrous Sulphate, Piperazine and its salts. The same set of amendments also declared that all future drugs licensed for manufacture or import in India could no longer feature the trade name on the labelling of the drug.[23] This was an astonishingly radical policy since it meant that pharmaceutical companies would have to sell their drugs without any brand names on the packaging. It was hoped that with brand names abolished and no way for patients to distinguish between drugs manufactured by different pharmaceutical companies they would buy the most affordable. The Hathi Committee had recommended this move as part of its recommendation to lower drug costs but it was also careful to explain how other quality control measures, including the issue of bioavailability, had to be addressed before taking the aforementioned steps.[24] The government selectively chose to enforce only the recommendation to abolish brand names without taking action on any of the committee's other recommendations to address issues related to bioavailability of generic drugs.

This decision to do away with brand names for most drugs was challenged by pharmaceutical companies like Pfizer, Hoescht, Cyanamid India Ltd. and Cosme Farma Laboratories before the Delhi High Court on a number of grounds. The High Court ultimately struck down the policy in August 1982 as unconstitutional after the government was unable to present a coherent defense of its policy.[25] One of the factors that contributed to the court's decision was the argument by the industry that not all generic drugs were equivalent because of concerns regarding bioavailability and that it was important for industry to be able to distinguish their drugs from those of competitors. In pertinent part, the court's reasoning is reproduced as follows:

> Similarly, we cannot accept the contention that there would be no difference in formulations made by different formulators out of the same bulk drug. High-powered advertisement techniques apart, it is common knowledge and is well supported by medical opinion that two different patients may react differently on taking the same drug. Obviously, this is because of the difference in what the petitioners call the bio-availability, i.e. therapeutic impact. Respondent No. 4's contention in support of what has been said by first three respondents that there is no particular difference in therapeutic impact of various formulations manufactured from the same bulk drug cannot be accepted. We are inclined to agree with what the petitioners say because that is not only based on reason but also on experience.[26]

Even after this loss before the courts, the government did not take steps to tackle the issue of bioequivalence despite the issue coming up in Parliament during Question Hour. For example, in the Rajya Sabha, an MP by the name Raique Alam asked the Government of India, during "Question Hour" on 5 November 1986, whether it proposed to make bioequivalence testing compulsory. The Minister responded by stating that, "There is no immediate proposal to make bio-equivalence test compulsory."[27]

The requirement of bioequivalence studies as precondition for manufacturing approval of generics finally made its debut in Indian law only in 2001[28] but in a very convoluted and limited manner. The new rule introduced in 2001 required evidence of bioequivalence for only generic drugs approved by the DCGI for an initial four-year period while the drug maintained a "new drug" status under Indian law. After the expiry of the arbitrary four-year period, applications to manufacture generic copies of the erstwhile "new drug" were required to be filed with state drug controllers rather than the DCGI and would no longer require bioequivalence data.

To illustrate this requirement with the help of an example, if a new drug, "Formula X", got approved in 2001 by the DCGI, all companies seeking permission to manufacture generic versions of "Formula X" till 2005 would first have to seek approval from the DCGI by submitting the necessary data, including bioequivalence data and then seek a manufacturing licence from the state drug controller. Therefore, if a different pharmaceutical company wanted to manufacture generic versions of "Formula X" after 2005, it could directly seek a manufacturing licence from the state drug controller, without conducting/providing any proof of bioequivalence testing to the DCGI or state drug controllers.

There is no scientific rationale for this bizarre distinction where manufacturers of generic drugs entering the market after the expiry of the "four years" period did not have to establish the bioequivalence of their formulations with the innovator drug. The only possible explanation for this bizarre distinction in regulatory standards is that the powerful domestic pharmaceutical industry leaned on the government in order to avoid conducting the more expensive in-vivo bioequivalence testing on human volunteers and also reduce the probability of their applications for manufacturing licences being rejected due to their inability to formulate bioequivalent formulations.

In 2013, after the scathing 59th report of the Parliamentary Standing Committee on Health, the government setup an expert committee under Professor Ranjit Roy Choudhury to "formulate policy and guidelines for approval of new drugs, clinical trials and banning of drugs." While remaining silent on the absurdity of the "four year" cut-off for bioequivalence testing, the Ranjit Roy Choudhury Committee did make a recommendation that all generic drugs (regardless of whether they were in the "new drug" status) being manufactured in India be subject to mandatory bioequivalence testing on human volunteers.[29] These recommendations began a process of deliberations within the government on the issue of making bioequivalence testing mandatory for all generics.

When the above recommendations were deliberated upon in 2014 by the DCC, which has representatives of all state drug controllers and the DCGI, the recommendation made by the Ranjit Roy Choudhury Committee was opposed at the meeting on the astonishing ground that the "infrastructure" for conducting such bioequivalence testing was not "uniformly available" in India.[30]

This argument was quite simply a lie, since by 2014 many foreign pharmaceutical companies were outsourcing their bioequivalence studies to Indian clinical research organizations. As usual, the DCC never provided any empirical evidence to back its claim regarding the "shortage of infrastructure".

The fact that the DCC so blatantly placed the interests of the pharmaceutical companies over and above the public health requirements of the people of India is worrying and perhaps reflective of the cozy relationships between the pharmaceutical industry and drug regulators in India.

The issue was revived in 2016, coincidentally after we submitted a report to the Ministry of Health pointing out the absurdity of requiring bioequivalence testing for only generics in the "new drug" phase and not for those entering the market after the "four year" period.[31] A few weeks after the submission of our report, the issue was taken up by the DTAB at its 72nd meeting held in June 2016. Unlike the DCC, the DTAB, which is staffed primarily by experts from different government institutions, recommended to the government that bioequivalence testing be made mandatory for all Indian generic medicine subject to the Biopharmaceutical Classification System (BCS).[32]

The BCS, which was developed by scientists working for the USFDA's Division of Biopharmaceutics, is basically a framework that helps determine which generic drugs are required to go through in-vivo bioequivalence testing on humans as opposed to in-vitro testing in the laboratories (which is cheaper), based on the solubility and permeability of drugs.[33]

The BCS classified all formulations into four categories as explained below:

Class	*Solubility*	*Permeability*
Class I	High	High
Class II	Low	High
Class III	High	Low
Class IV	Low	Low

The classification of drugs on the basis of solubility and permeability was due to the fact that these two factors contribute the most to the bioavailability of a formulation in the human body. "Availability" of the drug, i.e., its concentration in the blood stream post ingestion is largely determined by how effectively the formulation dissolves in the stomach-acid (for oral formulations) and its ability to permeate through the intestinal tissue. The higher the solubility and permeability, the easier it is for the drug to enter the bloodstream. Drugs with high solubility are typically easier to test through in-vitro methods and hence it has been argued that these drugs be given a waiver from being evaluated through in-vivo bioequivalence testing.

The BCS system was then used by the USFDA to evolve guidelines on bio-waivers; i.e., if a formulation fell within Class I or Class III, where it demonstrated high solubility, the manufacturer could apply for a biowaiver from in-vivo bioequivalence studies and instead produce only in-vitro data i.e., data collected through laboratory tests.[34] This would reduce the costs of bringing a generic to the market since "in-vivo" bioequivalence studies on humans are more expensive than "in-vitro" testing conducted in laboratories.

As per one published study, which attempted to classify the top 200 selling drugs in the USA, EU and Japan, according to the BCS methodology, it was found that more than 55% fell within Class I and Class III, meaning that they would likely qualify for biowaiver.[35] An earlier study by the same authors, found a similar percentage of drugs on the WHO's Essential Drug List qualifying for possible bio-waivers.[36]

Although these drugs qualify for biowaivers, it does not mean that pharmaceutical companies automatically get a biowaiver in either the USA or Europe. The regulators in these countries allow for biowaivers on a case-by-case basis and will continues to do so until the process of classifying all formulations into the four categories of the BCS is completed. As a result, the biowaiver pathway is not invoked very frequently by the generic pharmaceutical industry in most countries.[37]

These nuances regarding the adoption of the BCS system were missed entirely by the DTAB. Instead, the DTAB recommended mandatory bioequivalence studies only for drugs in Categories II and IV thereby implying blanket biowaivers for all drugs in Categories I and III. By 3 April 2017 the Ministry of Health notified the Drugs & Cosmetics (Ninth Amendment) Rules, 2017 making bioequivalence testing compulsory on the lines suggested by the DTAB.

The incorporation of the BCS into Indian law and the blanket exemption for drugs in Categories I and

III was problematic for many reasons. To begin with, the amendments do not provide a legal definition of the phrases "highly soluble" or "highly permeable" or define the parameters for each of the "categories" in the BCS system. Neither does Indian law classify all known drugs in these four categories of the BCS. Given this ambiguity, it is still not clear how the 28 state drug controllers and eight drug controllers in the union territories who issue manufacturing licences for generic drugs, are going to interpret the meaning of "high solubility" and "high permeability" in a uniform and consistent manner across the country. To make matters worse, the DTAB and Ministry of Health missed the fact that regulators like the USFDA, which developed the BCS, prohibit biowaivers for drugs with a NTI. These are drugs where even a small dosage variation can have significant variations in therapeutic outcomes. Given this variability, these drug formulations are always subject to in-vivo bioequivalence studies in the USA. The Indian regulations are entirely silent on whether drugs with a NTI can get approved through the route of biowaivers.

Equally concerning, is the silence of the government on DTAB's recommendation that all existing generic drugs (approved prior to the bioequivalence regulations coming into effect in 2017) be required to go through bioequivalence testing within three years.[38] This was an essential recommendation by the DTAB to guarantee that all Indian generics approved prior to 2017 were in fact bioequivalent to the innovator drugs. Unfortunately, this recommendation has not been enforced by the Ministry of Health.

We have no idea why the Ministry chose to ignore this recommendation but it is very likely that the generic pharmaceutical industry lobbied the Ministry to ignore it. It is no secret that the Indian generic pharmaceutical industry is not in favour of mandatory in-vivo bioequivalence testing. In fact, the generic drug industry has reportedly lobbied the Ministry of Health to do away with this requirement for drugs that are being exported to other countries.[39] It would be unethical for India to exempt exports from such a key parameter used to assess drug quality.

Many of the issues described above, including the poor drafting of the 2017 amendments that brought in the BCS and biowaiver system, were clearly identified in a petition that one of us, Dinesh Thakur, sent to the Ministry of Health in June 2020.[40] As usual, the Ministry did not even bother acknowledging receipt of the petition, much less implement the recommendations contained in it.

We will never know the true human cost of not having put in place a well-designed bioequivalence framework since 1968 when there was clear evidence that in-vitro testing techniques were inferior to in-vivo testing for a number of generic medicines. Suffice it to say that the lack of mandatory bioequivalence testing has resulted in the approvals of hundreds if not thousands of brands of generics manufactured in India and it is very likely that many of these brands have adversely affected the lives of patients, whether Indian or foreign, who consumed these Indian medicines.

The large-scale data fabrication of bioequivalence data by Indian CRO for export markets

Although Indian law did not require bioequivalence testing till a few years ago, most of the developed countries in the West, which are the main export markets for the biggest Indian pharmaceutical companies, have always required bioequivalence testing for any generic drug being sold in their markets. It is a general practice for most Indian pharmaceutical companies exporting drugs to the West to outsource bioequivalence studies to external clinical research organizations (CROs) in order to generate data required to acquire approvals from American and European regulators to sell their generic medicine in those markets.

In order to conduct these bioequivalence tests, CROs recruit healthy volunteers on whom the generic drug is administered so as to generate data on its dissolution profile in human bodies and measure whether it is equivalent to the innovator drug.

However, if the generic formulation of the innovator drug fails to demonstrate bioequivalence with the innovator drug during the course of a bioequivalence study, the pharmaceutical company would necessarily have to go back to the drawing board and improve its formulation for a second round of tests. In a hyper-competitive market, these delays could cause millions of dollars in losses. This is especially true for countries like the USA, which has a unique regulatory mechanism under the Hatch Waxman Act, where launching the first generic formulation can result in a windfall gain.

Given these financial implications, there is a huge incentive for generic pharmaceutical companies to collude with CROs to fabricate bioequivalence data. The simpler scam is to pass off the innovator's drug as the generic drug i.e., instead of providing its own generic formulation to the CRO, the manufacturer of the generic drug seeking approval will misrepresent the innovator drug as its own generic drug to the CRO. This will virtually ensure a finding of bioequivalence in favour of the generic drug without having to necessarily collude with the management of the CRO. For example, in 1989, Bolar Pharmaceuticals, one of the pioneers in the American generic pharmaceutical industry, was caught red-handed passing off to a CRO an innovator drug as its own generic formulation for the purposes of a bioequivalence study.[41] Less than two decades later, a pioneer of the Indian generics pharmaceutical industry, Ranbaxy Laboratories, was suspected of indulging in similar fraud.[42]

The genesis of the Ranbaxy scandal was at a Hyderabad-based CRO, called Vimta Labs, which had been contracted by Ranbaxy to generate the required bioequivalence data for a number of its generic AIDS drugs. An inspection was conducted by the WHO on behalf of the South African government, which was buying anti-retrovirals drugs from Indian generic manufacturers. A French Inspector by the name of

Olivier LeBlaye, who led one of the inspections on Vimta Labs in 2003 on behalf of the WHO, questioned the integrity of the bioequivalence and other data generated by the CRO for Ranbaxy's drugs.[43] That one inspection opened the can of worms for Ranbaxy, culminating in its guilty plea in 2013.

In the years that followed the guilty plea by Ranbaxy, drug regulators around the world began focusing their attention not just on manufacturing facilities owned by Indian pharmaceutical companies but also Indian CROs. The object of such inspections was to examine whether the CROs were adhering to Good Clinical Practices (GCP) while conducting bioequivalence testing on behalf of generic pharmaceutical companies and not fabricating quality data. GCPs are designed to create a system of documentation that can be inspected in order to assess the data-integrity of the bioequivalence study. This includes the use of software and equipment that creates an audit trail making it difficult for the staff at CROs to engage in retrospective manipulation of data.

Typically, CROs may fabricate data for one of two reasons. The first is if the generic drug fails the bioequivalence study; in which case the client-generic company may pressure the CRO to manipulate records to demonstrate bioequivalence so as to not delay launch plans for the generic drug. The second reason for manipulation may just be poorly trained staff who cut corners without any pressure from the client-generic pharmaceutical company. Since proof of outright fraud is usually difficult to collect, unless a whistleblower can provide such information, in most of these cases evidence of a pattern of poor documentation practices at a CRO can lead to a presumption of poor data integrity practices at the CRO. Foreign regulators can be unforgiving of data integrity issues.

During the course of the last eight years, at least seven Indian CROs have been accused of significant failures to adhere to GCPs by American and European regulators. The seven CROs in question were Alkem Laboratories Ltd.[44], Semler Research Centre Pvt. Ltd.[45], Quest Life Sciences Pvt. Ltd.[46], GVK BioSciences Pvt. Ltd.[47], Micro Therapeutic Research Pvt. Ltd.[48], Panexcell Clinical Lab Pvt. Ltd.[49] and Synchron Research Services Pvt. Ltd.[50].

It is interesting to note that in each of these cases, different foreign regulators had investigated the Indian CROs. While Semler and Synchron was investigated by the USFDA, Quest Life Sciences was investigated first by British, Spanish and German regulators[51] followed by representatives of WHO. GVK Biosciences was investigated by the French regulator and the Micro Therapeutic Research was jointly investigated by Austrian and Dutch regulators. Panexcell was investigated by Austrian, German and American regulators, at different times and accused of irregularities by all three regulators.

A recurring allegation during the inspections of Quest Life Sciences, GVK Biosciences and others was the suspected fabrication of electro cardiogram (ECG) data. It is generally standard practice to record ECG data as part of a bioequivalence study in order to monitor the health of the volunteers. Monitoring the health of volunteers is particularly important in the Indian context because it has been well documented that many volunteers sign up for multiple bioequivalence studies and clinical trials at the same time because of the financial incentives offered by CROs.[52] This is dangerous for the volunteers. There is at least one reported instance of a volunteer dying during a bioequivalence study, allegedly, at GVK Biosciences.[53] Rather than actually monitoring the health of these volunteers, staff at Indian CROs tend to fabricate ECG data by recording the names of different volunteers against the ECG of a single patient. Such fabrication likely takes place in order to save time and effort but at the cost of safety of the volunteers. Fabricated ECGs reflect very poorly on CROs because it demonstrates a cavalier approach toward both the safety of volunteers, raising suspicions in the minds of regulators about the rigour with which the rest of the data has been recorded.

A second problem with the Indian CROs has been the failure of staff to maintain records in a timely and accurate manner. This is a problem across the CRO sector in India. An illustrative example of poor documentation practices from the "Notice of Concern" issued by the WHO after inspecting Quest Life Sciences is as follows:

> As inspectors entered the bioanalytical laboratory, laboratory staff members were seen in the process

> of completing records, some of them back-dated. An apparent attempt was made to hide documents from inspectors.[54]

Similarly, the EMA while announcing action against Micro Therapeutics Research Labs alleged that inspections by Austrian and Dutch regulators "identified several concerns at the company's sites regarding misrepresentation of study data and deficiencies in documentation and data handling."[55] As per the EMA, the problems with handling data included "...the practice to generate source data retrospectively, documentation of incorrect information, overwriting and changing raw data without ensuring the readability of the initial entry and the practice to apply implausible changes without giving a sound justification."[56]

This issue of poor documentation, fabrication of data and back-dating of records is an endemic problem across CROs and manufacturing facilities reflecting a culture of poor training and compliance across the board.

A third problem identified with Indian CROs has been the fabrication of the final results of the bioequivalence studies i.e., the drug likely failed the bioequivalence testing but the results were manipulated in order to enable the client pharmaceutical corporations to obtain regulatory approval. Finding evidence of such fabrication is very difficult unless there is a whistleblower. In the case of the USFDA's inspection of Semler Research Centre, the American inspectors claimed to have found a spreadsheet on one of the computers documenting in detail data manipulation in some of the older bioequivalence studies. Semler Research Centre, of course, denied the allegation levelled against it, claiming that a former rogue employee who had left to work for a competitor had covertly placed the spread sheet on its computers.[57]

A similar allegation was made by a whistleblower against GVK Biosciences accusing his supervisors of replacing the dissolution profiles of 14 volunteers participating in a bioequivalence study for a generic drug in order to make it look like the generic formulation was indeed bioequivalent to the innovator drug. The trial was being conducted for a major Indian pharmaceutical company that was looking to launch its generic version of a drug in the USA. The French regulator found the accusations made by the whistleblower to be credible.[58] Although the USFDA, which was the recipient of the fabricated data, did not take any public action against the Indian company in question, it is worthwhile to note that the pharmaceutical company in question withdrew its marketing application for the generic drug flagged by the whistleblower, which was pending before the American regulator.

Similarly, both Panexcell and Synchron were accused by the USFDA of submitting "falsified study data" thereby raising doubts about the bioavailability data generated at the firms.[59]

The nature of these regulatory actions is such that the regulator conducts the inquiry and provides an opportunity to the company to respond before deciding to take action. There is no trial or jury in such cases and the punishments can vary depending on the issues discovered during inspections. These alleged infractions by Indian CROs were punished by foreign regulators in different ways. In many of these cases, regulators announced the cancellation of all drug approvals granted on the basis of studies at the CRO found to be in violation of GCPs. This hurts the pharmaceutical companies that have engaged these CROs to generate regulatory data for their drugs and also damages the reputation of the CRO affecting its business.

After the French investigation into GVK Biosciences, the EMA on 15 July 2015 cancelled the approval of 700 drugs whose manufacturers had relied on GVK Biosciences for generating data that was submitted to various European regulators.[60] Two years later, the EMA suspended 300 drugs approvals because these approvals were based on unreliable data from Micro Therapeutics.[61] Similarly in 2016, the USFDA cancelled approvals secured on the basis of studies at Semler.[62] In July 2020, the EMA recommended the cancellation of all marketing authorizations of all generic medicine that were approved on the basis of bioequivalence studies at Panexcell.[63] The USFDA, in September 2021, announced the cancellation of all drug authorizations based on data generated at Synchron Research Services and Panexcell Clinical Lab because of data integrity issues.[64]

These cancellations affected not just Indian pharmaceutical companies but also a significant number of American and European pharmaceutical companies outsourcing their bioequivalence studies to Indian CROs because of the lower costs of such studies in India. Apart from scorching the reputation of these CROs in the eyes of their clientele, cancellation of drug approvals by foreign regulators also triggers contractual litigation between the CROs and their customers who can now legitimately sue for damages suffered due to the regulatory action.

In some cases, CROs like Semler Research Centre tried suing the USFDA before a federal court in the USA demanding damages for the loss of business it suffered as a result of the USFDA's public announcement. The case was eventually dismissed in 2019.[65]

The most controversial fallout of an Indian CRO scandal was in the GVK Bio case. After the European regulator ended up cancelling approval of approximately 700 generic drugs of various Indian and foreign pharmaceutical companies because of suspect data from GVK Biosciences, the matter quickly escalated with the Indian Government getting involved and threatening to sue the EU before the World Trade Organization (WTO). The basis of such action before the WTO was never clear, especially since regulatory issues are not covered by the WTO Agreement. The Indian government also called off ongoing free trade talks with the EU in retaliation to the action taken against GVK Biosciences. Some senior officials from the Indian Government including the then-incumbent DCGI, G.N. Singh, made some truly bizarre statements on the controversy. He stated in pertinent part, "One must understand that there is a bigger game being played out here. I have repeatedly stated that multinational pharmaceutical companies constantly use incidents like this to bring disrepute to Indian generic drug makers."[66] There was no evidence to indicate that multinational pharmaceutical companies were behind the EMA's moves. The Europeans did not blink in this stand-off. The Indian government never did sue the EU before the WTO and eventually restarted trade talks.

Many years later, in 2021, after much wrangling, obfuscation and an appeal under the RTI Act, the CDSCO finally gave us a copy of the report of the investigating committee setup by the DCGI to investigate GVK Bio after the EU accused the company of manipulating data. The report was barely two pages long and appears to have found some merit in the allegations made by ANSM (the French Regulator) about fabrication of ECG reports but then, rather bizarrely, concludes that such fabrication would not affect the safety of the subjects. This was a bizarre conclusion because if the ECG reports were being fabricated, it meant that the health of patients was not being monitored as per the approved study protocols. If the health of the volunteers was not being monitored and the approved study protocols were not being followed, how could anybody assume the integrity of the rest of the study data?

We also filed requests under the RTI Act with the CDSCO asking whether it investigated these

CRO scandals in India. At the first level, the Public Information Officer often refused to give us any information by invoking exceptions in the RTI Act, such as ongoing investigations. The only information we received at this level was that Quest Life Sciences was investigated by the CDSCO and its licence to conduct bioequivalence studies was suspended for a grand total of 15 days![67] When we filed an appeal before a senior officer at the CDSCO, we were given a list of remedial action taken by Quest Life Sciences but were not told of any action taken by the CDSCO against Quest Life Sciences. We followed up with another request for information under the RTI Act, more than four years later in 2021, asking the DCGI's office whether it had completed its investigation into Quest Life Sciences and if so, to provide us with a copy of the report. We received a one-line reply stating that the information sought could not be provided because of the exemptions in Section 8(1)(e) and (h) of the RTI Act i.e., it would impede an ongoing investigation as well as be in violation of the fiduciary duty owed by the DCGI to Quest Life Sciences.[68] Apart from the surprising fact that the investigation continued for more than four years without an outcome, there is also the fact that the DCGI as a regulator does not owe any fiduciary duty to these companies.

Even with regard to a publicly announced probe into nine CROs by the CDSCO in the year 2011, after reports of various malpractices and at least one death during clinical trials, the CDSCO refused to provide us with any information on the outcome of the probe merely stating that a show-cause notice had been served on two of the CROs and that information about an ongoing investigation could not be shared under the RTI Act.[69] This, despite the fact that our request for information had been filed in 2017, several years after the scandal was reported in the press in 2011.[70] The fact that the investigation was not completed six years later is telling of the regulator's lackadaisical attitude towards this crisis at Indian CROs; but the story does not end over there. We filed another request for information under the RTI Act in October 2021, asking for a copy of the final investigation report into the nine CROs. This time, the CDSCO claimed that it did not have any information about the investigation, despite claiming in its previous reply that the investigation was underway. An appeal to the departmental appellate authority resulted in a similar answer.[71]

Some of the other replies received were even more bizarre. For example, when we asked the CDSCO for a copy of its inspection report into Semler Research, we were told that while the CDSCO had been informed of the USFDA investigation and that it had proposed its own investigation, "...no information with respect to further action is available. Hence no investigation report is available."[72] We were not provided with a reason as to why the proposed investigation never took place.

In the end, the only two reports given to us by the CDSCO under the RTI Act pertained to the investigations conducted into Micro Therapeutics Research Labs and another CRO for which we did not even request any information.[73] Stunningly, the CDSCO redacted the names of the officers who carried out the investigations! From the final reports, it was clear that the CDSCO officials did not really follow up on accusations by foreign regulators against Micro Therapeutics Research Labs. The CDSCO's investigation report did not strike us as rigorous or aimed at unearthing data integrity issues.

As should be obvious by now, the CDSCO has traditionally done a poor job in regulating CROs. With the enactment of the New Drugs and Clinical Trial Rules, 2019 the Ministry of Health has on paper introduced a marginally better legal framework for CROs conducting BA/BE studies. However as of 2024, the European and American drug regulators continued to flag serious data integrity problems, including data fabrication, at Indian CROs. We are yet to hear of any serious remedial or punitive action by the Indian regulators, in terms of more rigorous inspections or licensing of CROs in India or punishments for those CROs found to be fabricating data.

The stability question: How 'stable' are Indian generic medicines?

Separate from bioequivalence, the other critical problem with Indian generics is the issue of stability testing, which is the most basic of quality regulations in most countries. That has unfortunately not been the case with

Indian law or its pharmaceutical industry. Anecdotally, it should be mentioned that one of the main charges against Ranbaxy Laboratories by the USA government and its agencies, leading to the historic guilty plea by the company in 2013, was the failure of Ranbaxy to comply with mandatory regulatory requirements in America for "stability testing" of each batch of drugs being shipped to the American market.[74]

There is a reason that the American legal system takes the failure to comply with regulations on stability testing so seriously. A poorly synthesized and formulated drug that is not stable will degrade as it travels through the supply chain. An unstable drug can break down for a number of reasons that include changes in temperature, humidity and exposure to sunlight. The degradation can also happen due to the type of ingredients used in the drug. This includes the Active Pharmaceutical Ingredient (API), the binder used to increase adhesion of the formulation, additives such as flavouring agents, etc. If any of these ingredients degrade, it can either cause impurities in the drug or reduce the therapeutic efficacy of the drug. For example, "wax" which is used as a binder may degrade into oil at high temperatures and this oil can become rancid over time reacting with the API to generate chemical substances that may have unintended consequences for patients.

In most instances, patients themselves will not know that a drug has become unstable unless the degradation manifests itself in the form of visual dis-colouration or emanates some kind of odour or it simply crumbles upon being removed from packaging. It is therefore imperative that pharmaceutical companies be required to submit stability data to the regulator as part of their application to manufacture the drug to establish that they have mastered the ability to formulate the drug.

Further, pharmaceutical companies must conduct stability testing before they release a batch of their product to the market and continue such testing throughout the lifecycle of the batch until the expiry date. Before batch release, this stability testing is conducted in special chambers by exposing formulations to elements like heat, light and humidity, in an effort to replicate the conditions that shipped consignments may face while travelling through the supply chain. After the batch is subjected to these conditions in these special chambers, the samples are subjected to regular pharmacopeial testing in the laboratory to check for impurities, the rate of dissolution, an assay test, etc.

After batch release, retained samples of each batch are tested through the life-cycle until expiry. If a batch that has been released fails any of this pharmacopeial testing, the manufacturer should publicly announce the recall of the batch from the market. If a batch fails stability testing before it is released in the market, the manufacturer should be required to destroy the batch. In both instances, the manufacturer faces a loss of revenue and at times, a loss of face because of which there is very little incentive for manufacturers to carry out stability testing or announce recalls unless mandated by the law.

In a country like India, with its heat, humidity and stressed supply chains, it is absolutely vital to mandatorily conduct stability testing before and after batch release to ensure that every formulation shipping out to the market is stable and remains that way for the duration of its expected journey, till it reaches the patient.

Shockingly however India for the longest time, simply did not mandate stability testing for all generic drugs being sold in the country, as a precondition to being issued a manufacturing licence. As explained earlier, India essentially has two different regulatory regimes—one for "new drugs", which last for "four years" and another for drugs that have been in the Indian market for more than "four years". For the first four years, the DCGI must approve a "new drug" before the state drug controller issues a manufacturing licence. Thereafter, from the fifth year onward, manufacturers are only required to approach the state drug controllers for manufacturing licenses. Rather absurdly, the regulatory data requirements until recently have been different for both these categories. Thus, while all drugs, even generics, in the "new drugs" phase have been required to submit stability data to the DCGI since 2001[75] as a condition for regulatory approval, there was no requirement for manufacturers seeking approval from state drug controllers from the fifth year to submit the same kind of stability data to state drug controllers as precursor to being granted a manufacturing licence.

From a regulatory standpoint, it is absurd to subject the same type of drugs to different regulatory requirements. The policy silence on stability testing was particularly worrying because of the safety and efficacy implications for patients.

In 2013 at a meeting of the DCC, the lack of stability testing for all generics entering the market after the four years mark was identified as a "serious lacuna" by the committee and it was resolved to make stability testing mandatory for all generics being approved for sale in India.[76]

A few weeks later, this proposal to make stability testing mandatory for all generics, including those securing approval from state drug controllers, was approved even by the DTAB.[77] Despite this bureaucratic consensus in 2013 on making stability testing mandatory for all generic drugs, it would take until 2015 for the Ministry of Health to publish draft stability testing rules in the *Gazette of India* for public comment.[78] Astonishingly, even these draft rules were never converted into law for years! As explained in the minutes of later meetings of the DTAB, the pharmaceutical lobby had complained that such a requirement would affect the small and medium enterprises manufacturing drugs, and increase the cost of drugs.[79]

This successful opposition from the pharmaceutical industry is revealing of both the influence wielded by it on drug regulation in India as well as its complete indifference towards patient safety. In any event, it is likely that this opposition from the industry appears to have been enough to paralyze the decision-making machinery at the Ministry of Health. Industry profits had triumphed over concerns for public health; and not for the first time.

In 2016, we red-flagged this lack of mandatory stability testing in a report that we sent to the Ministry of Health containing recommendations for reform of the drug regulatory framework in India.[80] In the same year, the issue of compulsory stability testing was taken up once again by both DTAB and DCC. The DTAB reiterated its earlier recommendation to make stability testing compulsory.[81] The DCC which specifically stated that "representations" had been received regarding the lack of compulsory stability studies for all generic drugs in India, accepted the importance of stability testing but did not specifically reiterate its support for the pending amendment to make "stability testing" compulsory for all generics.[82]

On 2 May 2017, the Ministry of Health once again published another set of draft rules on stability testing, inviting public comments.[83] These rules were, however, very vague. Unlike the draft rules from 2015, which simply extended the existing (albeit inadequate) stability testing requirements for "new drugs" to even those generic drugs approved by state drug controllers, the new draft rules proposed making stability testing mandatory but without prescribing any standards or parameters that were to be met during the course of such testing! For example, it is necessary to state the conditions for which the drug's stability has to be tested. A country like India is classified as a Zone IV country, which means that drugs have to be stable for atmospheric conditions of 30 degree Celsius. Similarly, it is necessary for the law to provide some guidance on the batch strength from which the samples for testing are to be drawn. Most importantly, the draft rule was silent on drug approvals already granted over the last several decades. Drafting a new law is pointless without such details and it appears that the Ministry of Health was unaware of these nuances of policy making.

Nevertheless, a year after the draft rules were published, the Ministry of Health officially notified the Drugs & Cosmetics (Third Amendment) Rules, 2018 on 10 April 2018, making stability testing compulsory for all generic medicine manufactured in India, without mentioning the parameters that were to be met by those seeking manufacturing licences.[84]

Even these diluted requirements are being resisted by the industry. Reporting from 2019 indicates that lobbies representing the small and medium units within the Indian pharmaceutical industry were publicly lobbying for a rollback of the requirement for mandatory submission of stability data for drug approval.[85]As per another media report, a local pharmaceutical lobbying group in the state of Bihar was on a mission to have the state drug controller for Bihar removed because he sought to enforce the new requirement of stability testing.[86]

Given the opacity of the approval process, it is

impossible for outsiders like us to verify the extent to which stability testing is being enforced by state drug controllers.

One of us, Dinesh Thakur, brought the deficiencies in the new regime for mandatory stability testing to the notice of the Ministry of Health, in two petitions in 2019 and 2020, seeking urgent reform of both the new stability testing rules and also the existing, inadequate stability testing requirements in the law. In those same petitions, we had requested the government to consider setting up an expert committee to study the issues raised by us so that a scientifically sound policy could be put in place to guide state drug controllers.[87] The Ministry has not even acknowledged our petitions; much less provide substantive replies.

Even presuming the Ministry of Health does take corrective action on the policy front, we are doubtful of the extent to which Indian pharmaceutical companies will actually conduct mandatory stability testing after being issued manufacturing licences and whether the Indian regulators, especially state drug controllers, have the capacity to conduct rigorous inspections like American and European regulators to ensure data is not being fabricated by pharmaceutical companies. Our concern is based on a number of allegations made by foreign regulators accusing Indian pharmaceutical companies of regularly fabricating stability data for drugs being exported to their jurisdictions. The Indian pharmaceutical industry has a high incentive to fabricate stability test reports because a batch that fails stability testing will have to be destroyed. This means lost revenues and depending on the size of the batch such financial loss can be massive, especially if it triggers other contractual violations. Creating deterrents against breaking the law, be it through threat of prosecution or cancellation of licences, requires building capacity of Indian regulators to detect data fabrication, and more importantly, political will to enforce the law without worrying about the implications of such enforcement measures on the growth of the Indian pharmaceutical industry. As of today, India is nowhere close to building such regulatory capacity, primarily due to a lack of political will.

The future of generics in India—An interim labelling requirement for bioequivalent and stability-tested drugs

Despite the rollback of the NMC rule on mandatory generic names in prescriptions, similar instructions issued by the Ministry of Health to the doctors in government hospitals run by the Government of India remain undisturbed. The question remains as to whether the Indian state and its regulators can guarantee to the medical profession and patient community that generic drugs manufactured in India are therapeutically equivalent and interchangeable with the innovator drug. We think not.

This is not because we doubt the science of similarity between generics and innovator drugs. We absolutely believe that it is possible for most generics to be interchangeable with their innovator counterpart. Our concern rather is with the shoddily drafted regulations, poorly equipped regulators and the overwhelming political might of the pharmaceutical industry, that has already delayed implementation of these essential regulations for way too long.

We need to ask ourselves as to why bioequivalence testing was made mandatory in India for all generic drugs only in the year 2017 when the USA had made it compulsory as early as in 1977? We need to ask similar questions on why stability testing was made mandatory for all generics in India only in the year 2018 when the rest of the world had mandated such testing since the birth of the modern pharmaceutical industry? Why was such a crucial quality-control measure delayed for so long, especially in a country like India, with its climate and challenging supply chain?

One possible answer to the above questions is the fact that the Ministry of Health simply lacks the expertise to make the necessary regulations. This would not be surprising since it is well documented that the Indian Government lacks "state capacity" in several areas of governance. In fact, even in cases where it commissions external "experts" to study the issue and provide advise; as we have seen in many instances, the chosen experts deliver reports lacking in the rigour required of policy documents and legal regulations.

The other possible answer to these questions is the simple fact that the Government of India favours the growth of the Indian pharmaceutical industry over the health of its citizens and foreign trade partners because it has been "captured" by the powerful pharmaceutical industry lobby in the country. Breaking the hold of industry over the government will require political intervention and that is quite difficult despite health being a politically sensitive subject. Changing the status quo will take consistent and renewed public pressure from doctors and ordinary citizens invested in building a regulatory framework that privileges public health over the profits of the pharmaceutical industry.

In the meantime, there is the very real problem faced by doctors and patients in identifying the formulations of generic drugs that have been properly tested on quality parameters. It is doubtful if the new bioequivalence and stability regulations introduced over the last few years apply retrospectively, meaning that formulations approved prior to these regulations coming into effect have not been tested for bioequivalence and stability. If 95% of the generic drugs in the Indian market were approved prior to these regulations coming into effect in 2017 and 2018, then it would mean that 95% of the generic drugs in the Indian market have likely not gone through bioequivalence or stability testing. The government currently is showing no indication of enforcing these regulations retrospectively, possibly because of industry pressure. So how then are doctors and patients to identify those generic drugs that have successfully cleared bioequivalence and stability testing?

To help doctors and patients on this count, we propose that the government should introduce a mandatory labelling requirement for all drugs sold in India indicating whether the drug in question has successfully undergone bioequivalence and stability testing. Such a labelling requirement combined with a mandatory requirement to publicly disclose bioequivalence and stability data will give doctors the necessary information to ascertain the trustworthy formulations for themselves. Hopefully, such a labelling requirement will create pressure on the industry to voluntarily adhere to the bioequivalence and stability testing requirements even if the government does not enforce the regulations retrospectively.

We also need to keep an eagle eye on the possibility of government relaxing the bioequivalence requirement for those drugs manufactured in India for the purpose of export. As per news reports, the Ministry of Health was at one point seriously considering the possibility of waiving the requirement of bioequivalence testing for drugs meant to be exported to countries that do not have such a requirement in their domestic law.[88] This recommendation was supposedly made by the Ministry of Commerce and industry lobbies. The mere fact that such a waiver was even proposed to the Ministry of Health is an indicator of the moral bankruptcy of the pharmaceutical industry. Such a waiver is both immoral and unethical because it would mean allowing Indian industry to export generic drugs that could not be sold in India because bioequivalence testing is now mandatory for the domestic market.

Notes

1. Vicky Pathare, "IMA labels NMC directive to prescribe only generic drugs as 'unjust'" *Hindustan Times* (Pune, 14 August 2023) <https://www.hindustantimes.com/cities/pune-news/indian-medical-association-raises-concerns-over-national-medical-council-s-decision-on-generic-medicines-101692035977952.html> accessed 3 October 2024.
2. Joe C. Mathew, "PM Modi Wants to End the Unholy Doctor-Drug Industry Nexus, but There Are Many Challenges" *Business Today* (New Delhi, 20 April 2017) <https://www.businesstoday.in/latest/economy-politics/story/modis-generic-drug-pitch-is-noble-but-at-what-cost-80042-2017-04-20> accessed 16 August 2021.
3. Saubhadra Chatterji, "Modi Says Govt Will Bring Law to Push Doctors to Prescribe Generic Medicines" *Hindustan Times* (New Delhi, 17 April 2017) <https://www.hindustantimes.com/india-news/pm-modi-says-govt-will-bring-law-to-push-doctors-to-prescribe-generic-medicines/story-g6kv0LZefi8KG2EcuyiPOP.html> accessed 16 August 2021.
4. Rhishikesh Thakre and Pralhad Patil, "Generic Drugs: A Call for Balanced Approach" (2017) 54 *Indian Pediatrics* 692; Anup Soans, "Quality, Not Price, Is the Key Issue When Prescribing Generic Drugs in India" *The Wire* (1 May 2017) <https://thewire.in/health/drugs-generics-branded-health> accessed 16 August 2021; Yash Paul, "Why Should I Not Prescribe Branded Drugs?" (2012) 9 *Indian Journal of Medical Ethics* 138; Elizabeth Gourd, "India's Generics-Only Drug Policy Could Put Health at Risk" (2017) 18 *The Lancet Oncology* e373.
5. Sudip Chaudhuri, *The WTO and India's Pharmaceuticals Industry: Patent Protection, TRIPS, and Developing Countries* (Oxford University Press 2005) 246.
6. ibid 247. Other reasons include information asymmetry wherein consumers may not have enough information about different brands.

7. United States Senate (Sub-committee on Antitrust and Monopoly), *Study of Administered Prices in the Drug Industry* (Rep No 448, 1961).
8. ibid 93-94.
9. ibid 96.
10. Jerome Philip Skelly, "A History of Biopharmaceutics in the Food and Drug Administration 1968–1993" (2009) 12 *The AAPS Journa*l 44.
11. Jeremy A. Greene, *Generic: The Unbranding of Modern Medicine* (John Hopkins University Press 2014) 99-100.
12. ibid 100.
13. ibid 111.
14. Skelly (n 10) 46.
15. Skelly (n 10).
16. "Bioavailability and Bioequivalence Requirements" 21 CFR 117 (1977).
17. Bernard E Cabana, "Bioavailability/ Bioequivalence" (1977) 32 *Food, Drug, Cosmetic Law Journal* 512, 519.
18. Roger L. Nation and Lloyd N. Sansom, "Bioequivalence Requirements for Generic Products" (1994) 62 *Pharmacology & Therapeutics* 41.
19. Greene (n 11) 137-154.
20. "Price Declines after Branded Medicines Lose Exclusivity in the U.S." (IMS Institute for Healthcare Informatics 2016).
21. Dr. G.B. Engel, The Introduction of a Dissolution Test in Pharmacopoeial Specifications, World Health Organisation WHO/PHARM/70.459 as reproduced in Annexure II of the Drugs Consultative Committee (DCC), *"REPORT OF THE 15th MEETING OF THE DRUGS CONSULTATIVE COMMITTEE HELD ON 9th AND 10th March, 1972 AT NEW DELHI"* (1972) 308-312.
22. Government of India, Ministry of Petroleum & Chemicals, *Report of The Committee on Drugs and Pharmaceutical Industry (Hathi Committee Report)* (1975) 254.
23. Government of India, Ministry of Health and Family Welfare, *GSR 27(E)* (Gazette of India Extraordinary, Part

II–s 3(i), 17 January 1981)–Drugs & Cosmetics (Amendment) Rules 1981.

24. Hathi Committee (n 22).
25. *Hoechst Pharmaceuticals vs C.V.S. Mani* ILR 1983 Delhi 548 (Delhi HC, 13 August 1982).
26. ibid. para 29.
27. Shri Raique Alam to the Minister of Health and Family Welfare, Rajya Sabha Deb 5 November 1986, Question No 248, 124.
28. Government of India, Ministry of Health and Family Welfare, *GSR 900(E)* (*Gazette of India Extraordinary*, Part II–s 3(i), 12 December 2001) (inserting Form 44 and Appendix 1A into the Drugs & Cosmetics Rules 1945).
29. Government of India, Ministry of Health and Family Welfare, *Report of the Prof. Ranjit Roy Chaudhury Expert Committee to Formulate Policy and Guidelines for Approval of New Drugs, Clinical Trials and Banning of Drugs* (2013) 5.
30. Drugs Consultative Committee (DCC), "*REPORT OF THE 47th MEETING OF THE DRUGS CONSULTATIVE COMMITTEE HELD ON 30TH AND 31ST JULY, 2014 AT NEW DELHI*" (2014) 9-10. <https://cdsco.gov.in/opencms/opencms/system/modules/CDSCO.WEB/elements/common_download.jsp?num_id_pk=ODA5> accessed 17 August 2021.
31. Dinesh S. Thakur and Prashant Reddy T., *A report on fixing India's broken drug regulatory framework* (4 June 2016) (on file with authors).
32. Drugs Technical Advisory Board (DTAB), "*MINUTES OF THE 72ND MEETING OF DRUGS TECHNICAL ADVISORY BOARD HELD ON 27TH JUNE, 2016 AT NIRMAN BHAWAN, NEW DELHI*" (2016) 8-9 <https://cdsco.gov.in/opencms/opencms/system/modules/CDSCO.WEB/elements/common_download.jsp?num_id_pk=Nzcy> accessed 17 August 2021.
33. Vinod P. Shah and Gordon L. Amidon, "G.L. Amidon,

H. Lennernas, V.P. Shah, and J.R. Crison. A Theoretical Basis for a Biopharmaceutic Drug Classification: The Correlation of In Vitro Drug Product Dissolution and In Vivo Bioavailability, Pharm Res 12, 413–420, 1995—Backstory of BCS" (2014) 16 *The AAPS Journal* 894.

34. Office of Pharmaceutical Quality and the Office of Translational Sciences, Center for Drug Evaluation and Research (CDER), "Waiver of In Vivo Bioavailability and Bioequivalence Studies for Immediate-Release Solid Oral Dosage Forms Based on a Biopharmaceutics Classification System Guidance for Industry" (Food and Drug Administration (USFDA) 2017).
35. Toshihide Takagi and others, "A Provisional Biopharmaceutical Classification of the Top 200 Oral Drug Products in the United States, Great Britain, Spain, and Japan" (2006) 3 *Molecular Pharmaceutics* 631.
36. Nehal A. Kasim and others, "Molecular Properties of WHO Essential Drugs and Provisional Biopharmaceutical Classification" (2004) 1 *Molecular Pharmaceutics* 85.
37. Lorena Barbosa Arrunátegui and others, "Biopharmaceutics Classification System: Importance and Inclusion in Biowaiver Guidance" (2015) 51 *Brazilian Journal of Pharmaceutical Sciences* 143 ("Although there was an increase in the number of applications of biowaiver based on BCS, this progress has been tempered by the lack of international harmonization and the reluctance of companies to adhere to the methodology due to fears raised by a possible delay in the registers."); Ines Lenić and others, "Overview of the European Medicines Agency's Experience With Biowaivers in Centralized Applications" (2019) 12 *Clinical and Translational Science* 490; Barbara M. Davit and others, "BCS Biowaivers: Similarities and Differences Among EMA, FDA, and WHO Requirements" (2016) 18 *The AAPS Journal* 612.
38. Drugs Technical Advisory Board (DTAB) (n 32) 9, para 4.7.
39. Shardul Nautiyal, "Health Ministry Soon to Exempt BA/

BE Studies for Drugs Manufactured Solely for Export Purpose" *Pharmabiz* (Mumbai, 10 December 2020) <http://www.pharmabiz.com/NewsDetails.aspx?aid=134044&sid=1> accessed 30 September 2021.

40. Dinesh Thakur to the Union Minister for Health, "Petition to Setup Expert Committee to Amend the Bioequivalence Framework Put in Place by the Drugs & Cosmetics (Ninth Amendment) Rules, 2017" (7 June 2020) (on file with author).
41. Greene (n 11) 4.
42. Katherine Eban, *Bottle of Lies: The Inside Story of the Generic Drug Boom* (HarperCollins 2020) 127.
43. ibid 63.
44. E.J. Lane, "India's Alkem to Respond to European Data Fraud Probe" *FiercePharma* (17 April 2016) <https://www.fiercepharma.com/pharma-asia/india-s-alkem-to-respond-to-european-data-fraud-probe> accessed 18 August 2021.
45. Zachary Brennan, "A Rogue CRO Employee, a Suspect Spreadsheet, and Now a $50m Lawsuit Against FDA" (*Regulatory Affairs Professionals Society (RAPS)*, 29 January 2018) <https://www.raps.org/news-and-articles/news-articles/2018/1/a-rogue-cro-employee,-a-suspect-spreadsheet,-and-n> accessed 18 August 2021.
46. Bureau, "WHO Questions Integrity of Clinical Trials Data of Quest Life Sciences" *Business Line* (Chennai, 24 January 2018) <https://www.thehindubusinessline.com/companies/who-questions-integrity-of-clinical-trials-data-of-quest-life-sciences/article7395881.ece> accessed 18 August 2021.
47. PTI, "GVK Bio Manipulated Clinical Trials of Generic Drugs: Reports" *The Economic Times* (Berlin, 5 December 2014) <https://economictimes.indiatimes.com/industry/healthcare/biotech/pharmaceuticals/gvk-bio-manipulated-clinical-trials-of-generic-drugs-reports/articleshow/45385764.cms?from=mdr> accessed 18 August 2021.
48. PTI, "EMA Recommends Suspending 300 Drugs Tested by Indian CRO Firm" *Business Line* (New Delhi, 15 January 2018) <https://www.thehindubusinessline.com/companies/

ema-recommends-suspending-300-drugs-tested-by-indian-cro-firm/article9601315.ece> accessed 18 August 2021.

49. "EMA Recommends Suspension of Panexcell-Tested Meds" *thepharmaletter* (28 July 2020) <https://www.thepharmaletter.com/article/ema-recommends-suspension-of-panexcell-tested-meds> accessed 30 September 2021.
50. Press Release, "Questions and Answers Regarding Data Integrity Violations at Panexcell Clinical Lab and Synchron Research Services", *United States Food & Drug Administration* (16 September 2021) <https://www.fda.gov/drugs/drug-safety-and-availability/questions-and-answers-regarding-data-integrity-violations-panexcell-clinical-lab-and-synchron> accessed 23 September 2021.
51. Zeba Siddiqui, "Serial Testers and Cursory Checks: India's Flawed Generic Drug Trials Business" *Reuters* (Hyderabad, 28 December 2016) <https://www.reuters.com/article/us-india-drug-testing-insight-idUSKBN14G1U6> accessed 18 August 2021.
52. Priyanka Pulla, "Lured by Blood Money: Serial Volunteers Set a Disturbing Trend" *The Hindu* (30 December 2017) <https://www.thehindu.com/opinion/op-ed/lured-by-blood-money-clinical-trials/article22328296.ece> accessed 18 August 2021.
53. "Man Undergoing Drug Test Dies in Andhra" *The New Indian Express* (Hyderabad, 7 December 2008) <https://www.newindianexpress.com/states/andhra-pradesh/2008/dec/07/man-undergoing-drug-test-dies-in-andhra-8853.html> accessed 18 August 2021.
54. Letter from Dr Mark McDonald, Coordinator, Prequalification Team, World Health Organisation to Dr Sivakumar, Quest Life Sciences Pvt Ltd (No P5-447-3/DM/MM/SC, 30 June 2015).
55. EMA Press Office, "EMA Recommends Suspension of Medicines Due to Unreliable Studies from Micro Therapeutic Research Labs" *European Medicines Agency* (24 March 2017) <https://www.ema.europa.eu/en/news/ema-recommends-

suspension-medicines-due-unreliable-studies-micro-therapeutic-research-labs> accessed 18 August 2021.

56. Committee for Medicinal Products for Human Use (CHMP), "CHMP Assessment Report" (European Medicines Agency (EMA) 2017) EMA/420215/2017.
57. Brennan (n 45).
58. ANSM, *Final Inspection Report of GVK Biosciences* (Inspection Reference No: GCP-121501-FR, 11 July 2013).
59. Letter from Sean Kassim, Director, Office of Study Integrity and Surveillance, USFDA to Mr. Umesh Mishra, CEO of Panexcell Cinical Lab Pvt. Ltd. at p.3 undated <https://www.fda.gov/media/151569/download> accessed 24 September, 2021; Letter from Sean Kassim, Director, Office of Study Integrity and Surveillance, USFDA to Dr. Shivprakash Rathnam, Managing Director, Synchron Research Services Pvt. Ltd. at p.3. undated <https://www.fda.gov/media/151570/download> accessed 24 September 2021.
60. Asit Ranjan Mishra & Udgirkar Trushna, "EU Defends Ban on 700 GVK Biosciences Drugs" *Mint* (8 August 2015) <https://www.livemint.com/Politics/BB5yiv1k6Upq6vB2z385JI/EU-defends-ban-on-700-GVK-Biosciences-drugs.html> accessed 18 August 2021.
61. EMA Press Office (n 55).
62. The United States Food and Drug Administration (USFDA), "Notification to Pharmaceutical Companies: Clinical and Bioanalytical Studies Conducted by Semler Research Are Unacceptable" (20 April 2016) <https://www.fda.gov/drugs/drug-safety-and-availability/notification-pharmaceutical-companies-clinical-and-bioanalytical-studies-conducted-semler-research> accessed 18 August 2021.
63. EMA Press Office, "Panexcell Clinical Laboratories: suspension of medicines over flawed studies" *European Medicines Agency* (24 July 2020) < https://www.ema.europa.eu/en/news/panexcell-clinical-laboratories-suspension-medicines-over-flawed-studies> accessed 30 September 2021.
64. The United States Food and Drug Administration (USFDA),

"Notification to Pharmaceutical Companies: Clinical and Bioanalytical Studies Conducted by Panexcell Clinical Lab or Synchron Research Services are Are Unacceptable" (16 September 2021) <https://www.fda.gov/drugs/drug-safety-and-availability/notification-pharmaceutical-companies-clinical-and-bioanalytical-studies-conducted-panexcell> accessed 30 September 2021.

65. *Semler Research Center Pvt Ltd v United States Food and Drug Administration and Ors* [2018] United States District Court for the Central District of California 2:18-CV-00534.
66. Vidya Krishnan, "A Love Story That Cost GVK Its International Reputation" *The Hindu* (New Delhi, 8 October 2015) <https://www.thehindu.com/news/national/A-love-story-that-cost-GVK-its-international-reputation/article60296519.ece> accessed 21 April 2022.
67. Reply to RTI application dated 12 December 2017, CDSCO (Application No DTGHS/R/2017/80446, 8 November 2017) (On file with authors).
68. Reply to RTI application dated 21 September 2021, CDSCO (Application No CDSCO/R/E/21/00393, 17 August 2021) (On file with authors).
69. Reply to RTI application dated 13 December 2017, CDSCO (Application No DTGHS/R/2017/80448, 8 November 2017) (On file with authors); TNN, "Clinical Trials: DCGI Faults 9 More CROs" *The Times of India* (Hyderabad, 20 July 2011) <https://timesofindia.indiatimes.com/city/hyderabad/clinical-trials-dcgi-faults-9-more-cros/articleshow/9290503.cms> accessed 21 April 2022.
70. ibid.
71. Reply to RTI application dated 19 December 2021, CDSCO (Application No CDSCO/A/E/21/00118, 12 October 2021).
72. Reply to RTI application dated 7 December 2021, CDSCO (Application No CDSCO/A/E/21/00116, 12 October 2021).
73. ibid.
74. *United States of America vs Ranbaxy USA, Inc* [2013] United States District Court for the District of Maryland

1:13-cr-00238-JFM, 10; *The United States of America ex rel Dinesh S Thakur vs Ranbaxy USA, Inc* [2012] United States District Court for the District of Maryland 1:07-cv-00962-JFM, 19.

75. Government of India, Ministry of Health and Family Welfare, *GSR 900(E)* (*Gazette of India Extraordinary*, Part II–s 3(i), 12 December 2001) (inserting Form 44 and Appendix 1A into the Drugs & Cosmetics Rules 1945).
76. Drugs Consultative Committee (DCC), "*REPORT OF THE 46TH MEETING OF THE DRUGS CONSULTATIVE COMMITTEE HELD ON 12TH AND 13TH NOVEMBER, 2013 AT THE HOTEL METROPOLITAN NEW DELHI-110001*" (2013) 28 <https://cdsco.gov.in/opencms/opencms/system/modules/CDSCO.WEB/elements/common_download.jsp?num_id_pk=ODA4> accessed 21 August 2021.
77. Drugs Technical Advisory Board (DTAB), "*MINUTES OF THE 65TH MEETING OF DRUGS TECHNICAL ADVISORY BOARD HELD ON 25TH NOVEMBER, 2013 IN THE CHAMBER OF DGHS, NIRMAN BHAWAN, NEW DELHI–110002*" (2013) <https://cdsco.gov.in/opencms/opencms/system/modules/CDSCO.WEB/elements/common_download.jsp?num_id_pk=NzY1> accessed 21 August 2021.
78. Government of India, Ministry of Health and Family Welfare, *GSR 68(E)* (*Gazette of India Extraordinary*, Part II–s 3(i), 3 February 2015).
79. Drugs Technical Advisory Board (DTAB), "*MINUTES OF THE 72ND MEETING OF DRUGS TECHNICAL ADVISORY BOARD HELD ON 27TH JUNE, 2016 AT NIRMAN BHAWAN, NEW DELHI*" (2016) 5 <https://cdsco.gov.in/opencms/opencms/system/modules/CDSCO.WEB/elements/common_download.jsp?num_id_pk=Nzcy> accessed 21 August 2021.
80. Thakur and Reddy (n 31).
81. Drugs Technical Advisory Board (DTAB), *MINUTES OF THE 72ND MEETING* (n 32) 5, 25.
82. Drugs Consultative Committee (DCC), "*REPORT OF 50TH MEETING OF DRUGS CONSULTATIVE*

COMMITTEE HELD ON 04 & 05TH NOVEMBER, 2016 AT NEW DELHI" (2016) 25-27 <https://cdsco.gov.in/opencms/opencms/system/modules/CDSCO.WEB/elements/common_download.jsp?num_id_pk=ODEy> accessed 21 August 2021.

83. Government of India, Ministry of Health and Family Welfare, *GSR 429(E)* (*Gazette of India Extraordinary*, Part II–s 3(i), 2 May 2017).
84. Government of India, Ministry of Health and Family Welfare, *GSR 360(E)* (*Gazette of India Extraordinary*, Part II–s 3(i), 10 April 2018).
85. Laxmi Yadav, "Pharma SMEs Seek Rollback of Mandatory Submission of Stability Test for Drug Approval" *Pharmabiz* (Mumbai, 11 February 2019) <http://pharmabiz.com/ArticleDetails.aspx?aid=114054&sid=1> accessed 21 August 2021.
86. Peethaambaran Kunnathoor, "Drug Manufacturers in Bihar to Approach DCGI to Complain against State DC for Anti-Industry Policies" *Pharmabiz* (Chennai, 17 April 2019) <http://www.pharmabiz.com/NewsDetails.aspx?aid=115253&sid=1> accessed 21 August 2021.
87. Dinesh Thakur to the Union Minister for Health, "Petition to setup Expert Committee to amend the framework put in place by the Drugs & Cosmetics (Third Amendment) Rules, 2018 for stability testing of drugs" (7 June 2020); Dinesh Thakur to the Union Health Secretary Preeti Sudan, "Petition regarding stability testing" (25 April 2019).
88. Shardul Nautiyal, "Health Ministry soon to exempt BA/BE studies for drugs manufactured solely for export purposes", *PharmBiz* (Mumbai, 10 December 2020) <http://www.pharmabiz.com/NewsDetails.aspx?aid=134044&sid=1> accessed 27 April 2022.

CHAPTER SEVEN

Regulating the Nightmare that Is Traditional Medicine

At the height of the first wave of the COVID-19 pandemic in India in 2020, the Indian media aired a most extraordinary press conference by the yoga-guru-turned-entrepreneur, Baba Ramdev, in his avatar as the founder of Patanjali Ayurved, a company that shot into fame for its herbal, ayurvedic and *swadeshi* products ranging from toothpaste to ayurvedic "cures". At the press conference, Ramdev proclaimed to the world the discovery of an Ayurvedic remedy, Coronil, that had apparently proved its "effectiveness" in treating COVID-19 during "clinical trials". In the ensuing publicity campaign, Patanjali claimed to the press that Coronil had proven 100% effective during clinical trials conducted at its facilities.[1]

At any other time, for any other disease, Ramdev could have made a similar claim and escaped with minimal scrutiny. However, to make such a claim at the height of a pandemic that was claiming thousands of lives daily, especially when the world's best scientific minds were struggling to find a cure for COVID-19, was pushing the boundaries of credulity of even the otherwise gullible Indian population. Initially, the Government of India and various state governments, which were already dealing with the fallout from the pandemic and its mounting death toll, made feeble attempts to restrain Ramdev from making such outlandish claims, only to settle for him marketing his "cure" as an "immunity booster".[2] In the later days of the pandemic, the Minister of Health and Family Welfare Harsh Vardhan appeared alongside Baba Ramdev as the latter released the results of the alleged "clinical trial" for Coronil.[3] The Indian Medical Association representing doctors trained in modern medicine lashed out at the Minister for making such an endorsement of an "unscientific product".[4] Nevertheless, sales of Coronil were reportedly well in the range of ₹250 crores by early November 2020, just as the first wave of the pandemic began to ebb.[5]

Eventually, in 2021, The Resident Doctors Association of AIIMS located in Rishikesh, filed a lawsuit against Baba Ramdev and his associates before the Delhi High Court alleging that the marketing for Coronil posed a "public nuisance" and sought an injunction against him. The court found merit in the argument that the advertisements for Coronil did amount to "public nuisance" and issued a temporary injunction against Baba Ramdev and Patanjali, ordering them to restrain advertising for Coronil.[6] Of course, by the time this injunction was issued, four years later in 2024, the damage was already done and Patanjali had laughed all the way to the bank at the expense of gullible Indian citizens.

But Baba Ramdev and Patanjali were not the only ones making such outlandish claims. There was also the Ministry of Ayush that claimed during the pandemic that Ayush-64, a drug developed by one of its laboratories—the Central Council for Research in Ayurveda and Siddha (CCRAS)—had demonstrated through "multi-centric studies at reputed medical institutions ...[an ability] to help reduce symptoms, disease progression to severe form and duration to become COVID Negative in the management of asymptomatic, mild & moderate cases of Covid 19". However, a few months later, when a group of doctors at AIIMS-Jodhpur carried out an "open label" trial on small group of patients, they concluded that "AYUSH 64 has no significant beneficial effect as compared to control group" while also acknowledging that a larger study was required.[7] When the findings of this study were reported in the press, the Ministry of Ayush lashed out with a childish press release, titled: "Ayush Ministry Strongly Condemns the Tirade Against AYUSH-64 by a Section of Media" with arguments such as the following: "The motivated news articles are a classic case of misinterpreting the facts and seeing the glass half empty."[8] The quieter indictment of Ayush-64 came from the general public who simply ignored the Ministry and its absurd claims.

The fact that the wily entrepreneur and the Ministry

of Ayush were on the same page when it came to making outlandish claims during a public health emergency like COVID-19 should give us a cause for worry. Even more worrisome is the fact that the Ministry of Ayush, whose job it is to promote research and growth of the Ayush industry, is also responsible for regulating the safety of its products and protecting consumers from any harm caused by them. Understanding how India landed at this juncture is important in understanding the nature of the beast that needs to be reined in by the law. Here, we trace the history of how India has struggled since its independence to regulate the Ayush industry.

The post-independence question on Ayush

This discussion must necessarily begin with a mention of the recommendations of a high-profile committee in 1946, called the Health Survey and Development Committee, better known as the Bhore Committee after its Chairperson, Joseph Bhore. This committee, while recognizing that traditional medicine like Ayush was popular with not just the illiterate masses but also large sections of the intelligentsia, clearly batted in favour of modern medicine which was more scientific in its opinion, covering areas of medicine not known to traditional systems of medicine.[9] This of course was a scientific fact. Unlike modern medicine, which by 1946 had made rapid advances in understanding human anatomy and physiology, traditional medicinal systems like Ayurveda and Unani still followed theories that were very similar to the discredited humoural theory developed in ancient Greece. Ayurveda had no understanding of the "cell theory" or "germ theory". Instead, Ayurveda still believed in balancing the *doshas,* much like the "humoural theory" believed in balancing "humours" to cure diseases. Hence the stress on enemas, blood-letting, sweating and purging in humoural theory of medicine.

While these may seem obvious facts that should have tilted the debate in favour of modern medicine, the issue of traditional medicine, especially Ayurveda was politically sensitive in a country like India, which was emerging from the shadows of colonialism after 200 years. Perhaps aware of the danger of being accused of batting in favour of "western medicine", the Bhore Committee also hastened to clarify that the scientific system of medicine that it was recommending should not be viewed as either "eastern" or "western" but rather as a "corpus of scientific knowledge and practice belonging to the whole world."[10] Pointing to how in Japan and China, a timeframe had been announced after which the traditional system of medicine would no longer be recognized, the Bhore committee recommended that the state governments should take a call on the extent to which traditional systems of medicine should feature in their public health systems.[11] In doing so, it steered clear of making its own recommendations on a politically sensitive issue.

The Bhore committee's implicit rejection of indigenous systems of medicine did not go unnoticed by the practitioners of traditional medicine in India.

After a public outcry over this issue, the Government of India set up yet another committee to study indigenous systems of medicine and the manner in which Ayurveda and Unani could be bolstered and perhaps combined with modern medicine.[12] Named the Committee on Indigenous Systems of Medicine, it was headed by Col. Sir R.N. Chopra of the Indian Medical Service. Chopra was a Cambridge-educated pharmacologist who also headed the Drugs Inquiry Committee, 1931 that preceded the Drugs Act, 1940. The other members of the committee were three *vaids* practicing Ayurveda, three *hakims* practicing Unani and two other practitioners of modern medicine. The final report of the committee was unabashed in its praise of Ayurveda, which it described as a "Hindu medicine" dating back to the Vedic age of Indian history. Sample the following extract from the "introduction" of the report:

> About the beginning of the Christian era Ayurveda, (or Hindu Medicine), had reached its apogee and had spread far and wide influencing deeply the systems of medicine in Egypt, Greece, Rome and Arabia. The influence of the Hindu Medicine was not confined to ancient and medieval periods alone. Through its influence on Greek medicine and through the influence of the Greek on Arabian medicine and of the Arabian on the medicine in Europe, the Ayurvedic system can well claim to be the chief, though remote source, from which the mighty river of Western medicine has had its beginnings.[13]

Separate from these declarations of Ayurveda as "Hindu medicine" and the "chief" source of medical knowledge for the rest of the world, the report also declared Ayurveda to be the only "native to soil"[14] medicinal system in India and attributed the decline of Ayurveda to the invasions by the Mughals who brought in their own medicinal system called Unani, which then declined because of British colonialism and its import of western medicine. The following extract from the report makes clear this narrative:

> Ayurveda which is based on the Vedas, was developed systematically more than three thousand years ago, and made great progress both on the preventive and curative side of medicine. When India was subjected to foreign domination Ayurvedic medicine received a setback. The Unani Tibb is not strictly speaking indigenous to India. It came with the Mohammedan rule and gained popularity generally in those areas where Muslims were in the majority and was developed by State support under the Muslim rule. When the British came to India the Western medicine was introduced and came to be adopted as the State system of relief. As a consequence, Ayurveda and Unani Tibb both declined.[15]

Many of the above facts are disputed by modern historians who argue that the Brahmins of Vedic society actively discriminated against traditional healers because the latter were considered to be "impure" given the nature of their profession, especially the requirement to handle bodily fluids like blood or pus. Modern historians claim that these denigrated healers came to join Buddhism, opening the window for institutionalization of medicine in Buddhist monasteries. It is this consolidated body of medical knowledge that came to be reflected in ancient texts like *Charakasamhita* and *Sushrutasamhita*. This school of thought also points out that the knowledge of medicine found in the *vedas* is primarily "magico-religious" (involving prayers and lucky charms) unlike the medicine found in *Charakasamhita* and *Sushrutasamhita*, which is mostly "empirical-rational" and only marginally magico-religious.[16]

It is important to pay attention to the manner in which the Committee on Indigenous Medicine framed the entire issue, especially its unabashed attempt to link specific religions to identified medicinal systems and demarcate the "indigenous" medicinal systems from the "foreign" medicinal systems. Classification of "Ayurveda" as the Hindu medicine and hence its characterization as truly "indigenous" medicine was a crude attempt by the Committee to appeal to the baser political instincts of Hindus by making them view the issue through the communal lens of "Hindu-Muslim" politics that had set the country on fire in the 1940s leading to its partition. Rather than cultivate the idea that the evolution or decline of medicinal systems could be linked to any number of cultural and scientific factors, the report preferred to fall back on the politics of religion; and if anything, was a dog-whistle to the politics of Hindu nationalism that insisted on viewing India as a Hindu country.

In the years that followed the report of the Committee on Indigenous Medicine in 1948, five other committees setup to study the issue of traditional medicine produced five more reports on a variety of topics like research, training and practice of indigenous medicine.

The first was the *Report of the Committee on Research in Ayurveda* setup by the Government of Bombay, Health and Local Government Department (1950). The second was the *Report of the Committee Appointed by the Government of India to Advise them on the Steps to be Taken to Establish a Research Centre in the Indigenous Systems of Medicine and other Cognate Matters* (1951). The third was the *Interim Report of the Committee Appointed by the Government of India to Study and Report on the Question of Establishing Uniform Standards in Respect of Education and Regulation of Practice of Vaidyas, Hakims and Homeopaths* (1956). The fourth was the *Report of the Committee on Ayurveda Research Evaluation* (1958). The fifth was the *Report of the Shuddha Ayurvedic Education Committee* (1963).

Each of these committees were setup with the intent of advocating for traditional medicine, especially Ayurveda, and not to objectively evaluate the effectiveness of Ayurveda in treating patients. From a reading of these reports, it is clear that some of these committees were convinced of the superiority of Ayurveda's *Tridosha* theory over modern medicine as pioneered in the West. Rational scientific evidence had no place in any of these reports. Yet, the political pressure from this lobby of practitioners of traditional medicine appears to have been so great that the Indian state began to take seriously, demands put forth by the practitioners of traditional Indian medicine. Far from announcing a moratorium on traditional medicine, the Indian state embraced traditional medicine. For example, in 1970, a law called the Indian Medicine Central Council Act was enacted by Parliament to officially recognize the right of the Ayurvedic and Unani practitioners to practice Indian medicine by creating a regulatory framework identical to the one for doctors practicing modern medicine. This included a system for setting educational standards for Ayush practitioners and recognition of educational institutions to teach traditional "medicine". India also began dedicating increasingly large amounts of public funds for a mushrooming number of research laboratories dedicated to conducting "research" on traditional medicine. For example, from merely one research body in 1962, India today has four research establishments: the Central Council for Research in Ayurvedic Sciences (CCRAS), the Central Council for Research in Siddha (CCRS), The Central Council for Research in Unani Medicine (CCRUM), the Central Council for Research in Homeopathy (CCRH) and the Central Council for Yoga & Naturopathy (CCRYN). The budget for the entire research establishment has increased steadily from ₹1,088 crores in 2011–12 to ₹2,970 crores in 2021–22. Cumulatively, in the decade between 2011 and 2022 a whopping amount of ₹17,424.51 crores of taxpayer money was spent on these "research" establishments. A correspondingly large bureaucracy was created within the Government of India to administer these new laws and public research establishments dedicated to the growth of Ayush industries. Originally, this bureaucracy operated within the Ministry of Health. In 1995, Prime Minister P.V. Narasimha Rao announced the creation of a separate department within the Ministry of Health, called the Department of Ayush, to oversee this area of traditional Indian medicine.[17] This meant that the Department would be headed by a bureaucrat of the rank of Secretary, thereby increasing its profile within the government. In 2014, Prime Minister Narendra Modi went one step further and upgraded this department to a full-fledged Ministry headed by a Cabinet Minister, giving the Ayush industry and its associated bureaucracy even more heft within the government.[18]

The idea of creating a new Ministry dedicated to Ayush was to encourage the growth of the Ayush industry, except that the same Ministry was also vested with the responsibility of regulating the Ayush industry from a patient-safety perspective. An added dimension was the fact that the research establishment, referenced earlier, also fell within the purview of the same Ministry. In an ideal world, the job of promoting the growth of an industry and regulating it from a safety perspective would not lie with the same industry because of the obvious "conflict of interest". This "conflict of interest" existed even when the Ayush industry was within the purview of Ministry of Health but likely worsened by several degrees with the creation of the Ministry of Ayush. This "conflict of interest" has manifested itself most starkly in the failure of the Indian state to create an effective regulatory framework for Ayush products, as explained in the next few pages.

The regulation of Ayush products post-independence

Since the birth of the modern pharmaceutical industry, governments around the world have exercised five policy levers to ensure quality of medicine. These policy levers are advertising, standardization, safety, efficacy and good manufacturing practices. In India, this playbook has never applied to the Ayush industry. At most, some aspects of advertising of Ayush products have been regulated, albeit ineffectively. The remaining levers have never been applied to the Ayush industry despite its products being marketed like drugs with manufacturers making outlandish claims of curing diseases, Coronil and Ayush-64 being an example each from the private sector and the public sector.

The Ayush industry has traditionally escaped any serious regulation by making a false claim that its products have been used for centuries and therefore have been proven to be safe and efficacious. This is simply not true. Most Ayush products sold in India today are "patent and proprietary" drugs which find no mention in the traditional texts from which the Ayush industry claims its legitimacy. Between 1963 (when Ayush was first included within the ambit of the Drugs & Cosmetics Act) and 1982, the Ayush industry was allowed to manufacture and market only those concoctions listed in 54 Ayurvedic texts, 28 Siddha texts and 12 Unani texts that were listed in the proposed "First Schedule" to the Drugs & Cosmetics Act. These texts include the ancient *Charaka Samhita* which is presumed to have been first written between 100 BCE and 200 CE and subsequently revised by different practitioners. While this was a flimsy mode of regulation since it ignored issues such as safety and efficacy of these products, it did narrow the type of products marketed by the Ayush industry.

In 1982, for reasons still not clear to us, Parliament removed these restrictions on the Ayush industry by allowing it to create and sell "patent and proprietary" products not listed anywhere in traditional texts. Logically, these new products should have been subject to the same regulatory pathways as modern medicine that is, proof of safety and efficacy generated through well-designed clinical trials. But that never happened.

On the twin counts of safety and efficacy, the regulatory apparatus imposes no requirements upon the Ayush industry despite significant cost to public health. Three of these levers: efficacy, safety and advertising, require a more detailed explanation so as to demonstrate just how ineffective the government has been in regulating the Ayush industry.

The question of efficacy of Ayush products

Let us first tackle the question of *efficacy* of Ayush products making therapeutic claims. Simply put, the question is whether the government knows whether these products work as claimed by the manufacturer. For the longest time, there was simply no requirement in the law to establish the efficacy of either traditional or "patent and proprietary" Ayush products. Then in 2010, a new Rule 158B was inserted into the Drugs & Cosmetics Rules by the Ministry of Health. This new rule required all manufacturers making new treatment claims for old formulations or manufacturing new "patent or proprietary" medicine to submit proof of "effectiveness" as a precondition for securing a manufacturing licence. This could have been a potentially game-changing regulatory move, except for the fact that the law did not really require the standard double-blind randomized clinical trials that brought so much rigour to modern medicine since the late 1940s. Instead, Rule 158B required "Pilot study as per relevant protocol for Ayurveda, Sidha and Unani drugs". A footnote to this provision adds, "The standard protocol will also include concept of Anupan, Prakriti & Tridosh, etc. published by Central Research Councils Ayurveda, Siddha, Unani and other Government/Research Bodies." Even by the poor standards of drafting of legal and regulatory law within the Indian Government, the aforementioned wording of Rule 158B is abysmally lacking in clarity. If the idea was to generate scientific data, the government should have simply prescribed the same standards prescribed for modern medicine; i.e., a double-blind randomized clinical trial preceded by animal studies for toxicology and to generate some proof of concept. Instead, these rules made bizarre references to vague concepts like "Prakriti" and "Tridosh", which are yet to be established as having any scientific validity.

Perhaps due to the poorly drafted Rule 158B and its lack of guidance on the meaning of "pilot study", the Department of Ayush in the year 2013 released "Good Clinical Practice Guidelines" for "Clinical Trials in Ayurveda, Siddha and Unani Medicine".[19] In essence, these guidelines laid down a framework to guarantee scientifically rigorous ethical clinical trials. While these guidelines were a step in the right direction, the government also made it clear that these guidelines were completely "voluntary".[20]

The absence of clear-cut, binding legal requirements under Rule 158B on the requirement of "pilot studies" led to much confusion with some manufacturers of "patent & proprietary" Ayurvedic, Siddha and Unani formulations going the route of conducting poorly designed, half-baked clinical trials. From anecdotal evidence, we know that most of these trials were tremendously underpowered; i.e., these trials were carried out on very small, statistically insignificant patient populations. Further, these trials also generally lack a comparator product and tend to be open label instead of being double blinded. This increases the possibility of bias.

Then in 2018, the Ministry of Ayush threw up a new surprise when it issued a circular informing state drug regulators that Rule 158B did not require the conduct of any clinical trials, since the phrase "clinical trial" is not mentioned in the legal provision! According to the Ministry's circular, "...experience or evidence of effectiveness of the ASU [Ayurveda, Siddha, Unani] drug based on textual rationale, published literature and pilot study [was] required in support of the claim of indication or use for issue of licence in accordance with the provisions of Rule 158(b)."[21] This circular went against everything contained in the aforementioned guidelines of the Department of Ayush from 2013 which literally had the phrase "clinical trials" in its title while explaining the expectations from Rule 158. The conversion of the Department of Ayush into the Ministry of Ayush appears to have led to greater capture of the policy-making process resulting in such absurd directives.

As a result, despite the Ayush industry now marketing a whole slew of "patent and proprietary" products making all kinds of outrageous claims, the industry is not required by the law to generate and substantiate any rigorous scientific data backing their claims of efficacy as treatments. This has serious consequences for public health as the Ayush establishment, in both the private and public sector, has started making increasingly audacious claims about their new products. A case in point is Ayush-82, which was developed by the CCRAS. This product was supposed to be a treatment of diabetes and in 2014 it was licensed to 10 private companies, through a government-owned technology licensing company for a cumulative sum of ₹1.47 crores.[22] One of the recipients of these licenses for Ayush-82 was Kudos Laboratories India Ltd., a company in the business of selling Ayurvedic products. Kudos sold this product under the brand name "IME-9" which stood for "Insulin Management Expert". The original packaging of the drug stated that it was an "Ayurvedic 'cure' for Diabetes" and that it was a "human clinical trial research product", which contained "Clinically Researched Formulation Technology". The packaging also claimed it was tested on 800 patients. Also featured prominently on the external packaging of the product were the names of the entities associated with developing and marketing it: The Central Council for Research in Ayurvedic Sciences, Ministry of Ayush, National Research Development Corporation, the Department of Science & Technology, the Ministry of Science and Technology and the Government of India. The product was priced at ₹300 for 60 tablets and each tablet contained aqueous extracts of "Amra, Karela, Gudmar, Jamun and Shudh shilajit" along with preservatives such as sodium methylparaben, sodium propyl paraben and approved excipients. The product's packaging conveyed the image that it had the official blessings of the Government of India.

Kudos also kicked off a very vocal marketing campaign describing IME-9 as "India's first wonder drug to treat diabetes globally" and that "IME-9

Tablets bring sugar under complete control".[23] Other companies launched Ayush-82 under their own brand names. The launch of Ayush-82 in these various avatars immediately drew attention because of the grand claims being made in the marketing campaigns for the drug. Once journalists and scientists began digging into how the drug was approved, they discovered that there were no published peer reviewed double-blind randomized clinical trial studies documenting the therapeutic efficacy of the drug, as is usually the case for new drugs seeking approval.[24] Even worse were the complaints being posted online by patients who had consumed the drug. They complained of sugar levels having shot up, constipation, blood in the stools, etc. with some patients even being rushed to the hospital in an emergency situation.[25]

Ultimately, the advertising blitz launched by Kudos for IME-9 was brought to a halt by the Advertising Standards Council of India (ASCI), an industry watchdog. In correspondence between ASCI and Kudos that we accessed under the RTI Act, it was clear that a number of complaints had been received by ASCI from the general public about the advertisements featuring IME-9. Kudos finally informed the ASCI that it would modify its advertisements to drop claims that the IME-9 would bring "sugar under complete control" and that it was the "first wonder drug to treat diabetes globally".[26] It also changed its packaging to remove any reference to diabetes or insulin management.

By the time these changes were implemented,

Drug Inspectors from the Maharashtra FDA had already initiated a criminal prosecution against Kudos Laboratories under the Drug and Magic Remedies (Objectionable Advertisement) Act, 1954 which prohibits any advertisements that claim to cure or prevent certain medical conditions, including diabetes. On 27 August 2018 the proprietor of Kudos Laboratories pled guilty before the Chief Judicial Magistrate of Ahmednagar on charges of violating the Drug and Magic Remedies (Objectionable Advertisement) Act and was slapped with a paltry fine of ₹15,000 even though the legislation provides for imprisonment for violation of the law. The judge reasoned that since the proprietor had pled guilty and the advertisement in question had been rectified, a simple fine was sufficient.[27] And so ended a saga that began at the publicly funded CCRAS.

At around the same time that the controversy around Ayush-82 erupted, there were several other products launched by the Aysuh industry in collaboration with the government research establishment. This included BGR-34, which was developed jointly by the National Botanical Research Institute (NBRI) and Central Institute of Medicinal & Aromatic Plants (CIMAP), both of which function under the ambit of the CSIR. This product, launched in 2016, contained six Ayurvedic ingredients, namely Daruharida, Vijaysar, Giloy, Majeeth, Methika and Gudmar. A box containing 100 tablets was priced at ₹505. According to the claims made by CSIR in the press, the drug released 34 active phytoconstituents to help manage sugar levels for patients afflicted with diabetes.[28] As per information provided to us under the RTI Act by CIMAP, both labs generated efficacy and safety data on small animals. In industry parlance, such a study would be classified as a pre-clinical study. Thereafter, both labs licensed the technology to a private company called AIMIL Pharmaceuticals (India) Ltd., which made claims to have conducted a very small clinical trial on 56 patients (typically new diabetes medication would be tested on hundreds if not thousands of patients).[29] The results of the study were then published in a journal, which was later discovered by journalists to be a "predatory journal".[30] These are low quality, pay-to-publish journals that are generally avoided by the scientific community.

As with IME-9, when BGR-34 reached the market, its packaging prominently featured the names of CSIR labs along with claims that the product had been scientifically validated through clinical trials. Similar to IME-9, the launch of the product was coupled with a very vocal publicity campaign. In 2016, the product even received a mention from Prime Minister Modi at an event held by CSIR.[31]

As with Ayush-82, the launch of BGR-34 met with a fair deal of public criticism in the media. The fact that the drug was targeted at diabetic patients rang alarm bells because of the potential health implications for patients consuming diabetes medication that was not properly tested. Even commentators otherwise sympathetic to Ayurveda, expressed their alarm over the boisterous claims that these Ayurvedic products would cure diabetes.[32]

These concerns were not unfounded. In the months following the launch of BGR-34, scientists and journalists tracking the usage of the drug reported that the most common complaint from patients was that the drug was, quite simply, ineffective in controlling the levels of blood sugar, which in the case of diabetes is a serious problem.[33] Patients also complained that the drug caused gastric problems and severe allergies.[34] Despite these complaints, as of October 2024, BGR-34 continues to be available for sale with online marketing platforms, which report brisk sales of the drug.

The privately owned Ayush industry is never far behind the public sector laboratories when it comes to spinning tales and making money. In the years following the launch of Ayush-82 and BGR-34, private players like Baba Ramdev's Patanjali launched Ayurvedic products to treat diabetes, hypertension and many other diseases, leading to another round of controversy in the media and courts. Since India lacks a robust pharmacovigilance programme, which collects data on adverse events suffered by patients consuming these Ayush products, little to no data on the possible adverse effects experienced by patients consuming these products is available.

Despite the repeated controversies over Ayush-82, BGR-34, Coronil and Ayush 64, the government has done precious little to reform the law related to "patent and proprietary" Ayush products. Given that public-sector laboratories function under the Ministry of Ayush whose remit is to speak for the industry, it is doubtful whether the Ministry has any incentive to fix the problem. This is evident from the circular issued in 2018, referenced earlier, withdrawing the earlier notification that Rule 158B required the manufacturers of Ayush products to substantiate claims about their products through well-designed clinical trials.

The safety question of Ayush products

In addition to efficacy, the other major concern with any product being marketed for consumption by humans is safety. Even if a product does not cure a disease as advertised, it can still cause harm to patients if it contains dangerous ingredients. The traditional argument of the Ayush industry has been that its products are made from natural substances and are not chemically synthesized, thereby guaranteeing safety. This argument is simply not true. Many natural herbs and plants can be toxic for humans. A case in point is Giloy *(Tinospora cordifolia)*, which is found in many Ayurvedic products. Scientists have blamed Giloy for causing liver damage in patients.[35]

Apart from the natural toxicity of some herbs used in Ayush products, the other big problem with these concoctions is the presence of "heavy metals". The rampant presence of "heavy metals" in Ayurvedic products was first reported in the USA after a scientific study published in the *Journal of the American Medical Association (JAMA)* in the year 2004 reported that

20% of primarily "Made in India" Ayurvedic Herbal Medicinal Products (HMPs) sampled by the authors had the presence of potentially harmful levels of lead, mercury and/or arsenic.[36] The study went on to warn that the level of these "heavy metals" could be potentially harmful to humans. A second study published in *JAMA* in 2009 with a sample size of 193 Ayurvedic "medicines" manufactured both in India and the USA (77 from India, 115 from the USA and one from Canada), reported finding unsafe levels of heavy metals such as lead, arsenic and mercury in 20.7% of the samples.[37]

There are two reasons for the presence of heavy metals in Ayurvedic products. The first is that a branch of Ayurveda called *rasa shastra* prescribes the use of heavy metals in conjunction with herbs to treat diseases.[38] Other traditional medicinal systems have also prescribed a similar use of heavy metals for medicinal purposes. The second reason for the presence of heavy metals is likely contamination in the sourcing of ingredients and the manufacturing process.

Over the last two decades, doctors across the world, from British Columbia[39] to Europe[40] to the USA have documented cases of primarily Indian-origin patients falling sick due to heavy metal poisoning after consuming Ayurvedic products.

After the publication of the first study in *JAMA* in the year 2004, the Department of Ayush under the Ministry of Health and Family Welfare issued an order dated 14 October 2005 under Section 33 EEB of the Drugs

& Cosmetics Act, 1940 fixing the permissible limits of heavy metals that can be present in each container of Ayurvedic products at the levels recommended by the WHO in its publication "Quality Control Methods for Medicinal Plants & Materials".[41] We however doubt whether these safety standards are being enforced in India since subsequent studies by scientists in foreign jurisdictions continue to report distressing levels of heavy metal contamination in Ayurvedic products. In one study published in 2017, the authors, who were scientists, reached out to a community of Indians in the USA known to consume Ayurvedic products and herbal supplements that were sourced from a particular clinic in India. The scientists offered to test both the products and the blood samples of volunteers against standards for "heavy metal" consumption as set down by the Environmental Protection Agency (EPA) in the USA. In approximately 50% of the 252 samples tested, the levels of lead, mercury, arsenic, silver and cadmium exceeded the recommended daily exposure limits in the USA. Some of these samples exceeded the exposure limits for heavy metals by a factor of several thousands.[42] These researchers also tested the blood of 115 persons from this community and discovered that 46 of these 115 persons had elevated levels of lead in their blood i.e. greater than ≥10.0 µg/dl. Four individuals were found to have elevated levels of mercury i.e. greater ≥10.0ng/ml.[43] These are startling numbers and India should be deeply concerned about the extent to which the Ayush industry, especially the Ayurvedic industry, is causing wilful heavy-metal poisoning of Indian patients.

Apart from these foreign studies, Indian doctors continue to report with regular frequency in scientific publications, social media as well as the Indian press, cases of metal poisoning in patients with a history of consuming Ayurvedic products.[44] A particularly vocal doctor on social media is Dr Cyriac Abby Philips, a hepatologist based out of Kerala. Tweeting under the moniker @theliverdr, Philips regularly posts anecdotes about the quality of Ayurvedic products consumed by his patients who mostly suffer from liver damage.[45] He has proven to be particularly effective in riling the Ayurvedic industry, with many of them complaining to the government that they are being defamed by Dr Philips' legitimate criticism.[46] His research includes published case studies on patients suffering alcoholic hepatitis after consuming Ayurvedic products. One such case study is of a young patient of just 14 years of age, who was diagnosed with alcoholic hepatitis of the liver, which was most likely caused by an Ayurvedic product that she was consuming and which tested positive for the presence of both alcohol and arsenic.[47] The patient recovered once she discontinued using the product.

Despite the mounting evidence that many Ayush products are dangerous to patients, we have not seen any serious action on part of the Ministry of Ayush in resolving safety related concerns regarding the use of Ayush products.

The advertising of Ayush products and the scandal around Rule 170

While there is almost no regulation regarding the efficacy and safety of Ayush products that make therapeutic claims, there is a law called the Drugs & Magic Remedies (Objectionable Advertisements) Act, 1954 (DMRA) drafted originally for the pharmaceutical industry, which does make it a criminal offence for the Ayush industry to advertise certain therapeutic claims for their products. In essence, this law prohibits the advertisement for 54 diseases or disorders and prescribes a criminal punishment of up to six months imprisonment and a fine for violation.

The problem with the DMRA is that it seems to lack any deterrent effect on either the Ayush industry or the press, many of whom are only too happy to publish advertisements on behalf of the Ayush industry. This lack of any deterrent effect was the most visible when in February 2022, all of India's leading English-language newspapers published on their front pages, advertisements for Ayurvedic products manufactured by Patanjali claiming to cure diseases like diabetes, liver disorders and heart diseases—all three of which are amongst the 54 conditions prohibited by the DMRA. The advertising campaign was so brazen that the matter did eventually land up before the courts but as of October 2024, Patanjali has not faced any serious punishment for the advertisements.

That the DMRA is not particularly effective was known even prior to the episode involving Patanjali.

As far back as 2012, the Parliamentary Standing Committee had flagged misleading advertisements by the Ayush industry as a public health hazard and urged the government to review the working of the DMRA—the only legislation to regulate drug advertisements.[48] The committee noted in pertinent part, the following:

> 13.6 The Committee was given to understand that a considerable number of AYUSH practitioners are making tall claims of very effective cure and treatment of various ailments, viral/bacterial/fungal infections, AIDS, cancer, Hepatitis etc. The Committee recommends that instead of ignoring such claims, the Department should make all out efforts to verify these claims and find out whether there is any substance therein. In case any of these claims are found to be true, the Department should initiate further research thereon and assist such claimants in developing their line of treatment in public interest.[49]

Despite the suggestion of the Parliamentary Standing Committee, the government did little to rectify the situation. The issue was raised by the Parliamentary Standing Committee in three subsequent reports; on one occasion the committee berated the Ministry of Ayush for its "laidback" approach to the issue.[50] Before the publication of that report, the Ministry of Ayush had published a draft amendment aimed at changing the Drugs & Cosmetics Rules, 1945 to regulate advertisements made by the Ayurvedic industry but did not translate it into binding law. When we asked the Ministry of Ayush, via a request for information under the RTI Act in the year 2017 for the reason for the delay in notifying the draft amendment into the law that it had published in the *Gazette of India* for feedback, we received the following reply:

> Draft Rule 170 could not be finalized so far owing to a large number of diverse comments from the stakeholders and the proposed amendment in the Drugs & Cosmetics Rules, 1945 has not been notified.[51]

Stripped of its bureaucratese, the above reply hints at the fact that an immense pushback from the very powerful Ayurvedic industry blocked the government's attempt to enact new rules to hold it accountable. Nevertheless, given the relentless pressure from the Parliamentary Standing Committee, the Ministry pushed through with the amendment on 21 December 2018, and finally amended the Drugs & Cosmetics Rules, 1945 to impose new restrictions on the advertisements for Ayush products.[52] This included a requirement to submit the advertisements to the Ministry of Ayush for prior approval and a outright ban on advertisements that featured certain material.[53] For example, if the marketing material included misleading or exaggerated claims about the therapeutic effectiveness of the Ayurvedic product in question or if it featured references or photographs of any government labs or public officials, the advertisement would be rejected.

In less than a month after the rules were notified into law, the constitutionality of the amendments was challenged before the Delhi High Court by multiple litigants with commercial interests in the Ayush industry.[54] The list of litigants challenging the constitutionality of the rules were not *vaids* and *hakims* who had descended from the Himalayas to protect their craft, but rather were huge pharmaceutical and FMCG companies like Reckitt Benckiser, Perfetti Van Melle India and Mankind Pharma as well as industry groups such as the Ayurvedic Drug Manufacturers Association (ADMA). These litigants argued, amongst other grounds, that the new rules restricting advertisements were an unconstitutional restriction on their fundamental right to speech.[55] Two other petitions were filed before other High Courts and one of them reportedly stayed the operation of the rule until the constitutional challenge was heard and decided by the High Courts.

Rather astonishingly, and in a display of the political might of the Ayush industry, Rule 170 was simply deleted by the Ministry of Ayush in July 2024 via a notification in the *Gazette of India* without ever being enforced for a single day. Most audaciously, this deletion took place during the pendency of high-stakes litigation before the Supreme Court of India where the court was closely scrutinizing the regulatory action taken by the government in response to the brazenly illegal advertisements published by Patanjali in February 2022. The non-enforcement of Rule 170 had come up during the proceedings before the Supreme Court and perhaps anticipating a directive to enforce Rule 170, the Ministry moved to delete the rule from the law.

An astonished Supreme Court "stayed" the deletion of Rule 170 but this is an extraordinary order that is not tenable in the long run.[56] Regardless of the final outcome in this case, the fact that Rule 170 was brought into the rulebook and subsequently deleted without ever being enforced is illustrative of the Ministry of Ayush's cavalier attitude towards curbing dangerous advertising by the Ayush industry and protecting public health.

The deception by the Ayush industry on its use of modern medicine

A fourth problem with the Ayush industry, especially the Ayurvedic industry is that many manufacturers regularly mix modern medicine with its products in a manner that is both illegal and deceptive, thereby misleading patients who specifically buy Ayurvedic products on the belief that these are consuming "natural" medicine. Apart from being deceptive, such adulteration is also dangerous because some consumers may have allergies to certain modern medicines.

The most rampant kind of adulteration appears to be the surreptitious mixing of steroids such as Betamethasone, Dexamethasone and Prednisolone with Ayurvedic products. Steroids have the effect of suppressing the immune system, which results in reducing inflammation and pain, without actually "curing" the underlying disease. Occasionally, some of these cases are successfully prosecuted. We were able to trace one successful prosecution in Punjab where an Ayurvedic product that tested positive for prednisolone, a steroid, ended with the conviction of the manufacturer who was sentenced to imprisonment for three years.[57] In our experience such prosecutions are rare.

The second common type of adulteration of Ayurvedic products is the surreptitious mixing of Sildenafil, better known as Viagra; the brand name for Pfizer's blockbuster treatment for male erectile dysfunction. These Ayurvedic products are then advertised as treating all kinds of sexual disorders. In one particular case that we tracked, there were two Ayurvedic remedies called "3X Men Capsules Morning & Evening" and "3X Men Syrup 3 Times Passion for Intimate Moments" manufactured by the same firm in Rajasthan. Samples of both the capsules and syrup had been drawn from a chemist's shop in Mumbai by a Drug Inspector of the Maharashtra FDA and sent for testing to a government analyst in a drug control laboratory of the state government. The labelling of both the tablet and the syrup, indicated that the drugs contained a number of ingredients common to Ayurvedic products, such as *Makardhwaja*, *Mucuna Pruriens, Sida Cordifolia*, *Swarnmakshik Bhasma*, *Amla*, *Ashwagandha*, *Kesar*, *Kaunch Beej*, etc. However, when the samples were tested, the government analyst discovered that the capsules contained between 18.65mg and 21.27mg of Sildenafil Citrate per capsule, while the syrup contained 15.44 mg of Sildenafil Citrate per 15 ml of the sample syrup! The firm that manufactured these samples denied the charges. The ensuing investigation that took the Drug Inspector till Rajasthan revealed that the manufacturer actually held licences from the Rajasthan Drug Control Organization to manufacture the capsules, although the "ingredients" approved in the licence were not clear. The Maharashtra FDA launched a criminal prosecution against the company before a criminal court in Mumbai.[58] This prosecution, filed on 7 June 2016, was still pending judgement as of October 2024.

The third common type of adulteration in the Ayurvedic market is where powerful painkillers are mixed with Ayurvedic products. We tracked at least one case, where Drugs Inspectors from the Maharashtra FDA in Ahmednagar drew a sample of a drug called "ARTIN Pluse Ayurvedic Capsules" from a medical and general store. As per the labelling on this Ayurvedic product, it was priced at ₹150 and contained standard ingredients found in Ayurvedic products such as *Guggul, Bhasm* and *Pannage Ras* and that it was "most effective in chronic joint pains". On testing by the government analyst, at the drug testing laboratory run by the state government, it was alleged that the sample contained 62.32 milligrams of Nimesulide, a powerful chemical painkiller that can only be bought with a prescription.

Nimesulide has been a controversial drug because of its alleged toxic side-effects on the liver and is prohibited in certain countries.[59] In India, the drug is prohibited for children but can be prescribed for adults.[60] To conceal such a powerful painkiller, without disclosing it on the labelling is a serious issue. During the investigation by the Drug Inspector who drew the sample, it was discovered that the manufacturer listed on the packaging, as well as one of the distributors in the supply chain were fake entities and simply did not exist! The Drug Inspector eventually filed a criminal case against the shopkeeper and one of the distributors in the supply chain with the offence of selling spurious Ayurvedic products, the punishment for which is a jail term of six months and a maximum fine of ₹10,000.[61]

A fourth type of adulteration of Ayurvedic products that we were able to track were Ayurvedic skin creams claiming to be natural but were in reality adulterated with chemical agents. One particular sample drawn by the Drug Inspectors of the Maharashtra FDA was a skin cream that on its label indicated only natural ingredients such as Aloe Vera, etc. for the purpose of treating hyperpigmentation and scars. When the sample was tested by the government analyst, it was discovered to contain Hydroquinone, a chemical depigmentation agent![62]

As things stand today, we know that Ayurvedic products have a dangerous adulteration problem and that Indian patients are being duped and harmed by such adulteration. The issue, however, is that we do not know the extent of the seriousness of this problem on the ground. We dug out the above information after conducting painful and excruciating searches of government databases and filing requests for information under the RTI Act, 2005. The government can easily publish consolidated figures based on the random sampling conducted by its drug inspectors to indicate the extent of this problem but it has not lifted a finger in this regard. The fight against unscrupulous firms indulging in adulteration of Ayurvedic products is left largely to individual drug inspectors and their sense of duty towards protecting public health.

The future of regulating the traditional medicinal industry

Reining in the Ayush industry, especially Ayurveda, is politically challenging because it represents a potent mix of heady Hindu nationalism that revels in ancient India's glory and global capitalism, as is obvious from the fact that multinational companies like Reckitt Benckiser, Perfetti Van Melle and Mankind Pharma, were involved in the constitutional challenge against Rule 170. Any attempt to question the safety and efficacy of these Ayurvedic cures is painted as questioning the glory of ancient Indian civilization. In addition, there are politically powerful companies like Baba Ramdev's Patanjali, which have made huge investments in this area and which have immense influence over governmental policy.

The larger challenge is that public sentiment in India is very sympathetic to the Ayush industry. It is not uncommon to hear highly educated Indians from the Indian middle class voicing their support for Ayurvedic products. This support emerges partly from a distrust of modern medicine, partly in the belief that Ayurveda is "natural" and therefore less toxic and partly due to the marketing of Ayurveda as an example of the genius of ancient Indian civilization. Altering these beliefs in a country where "scientific temper" is fast disappearing is no easy task. Significant reforms will require a political class with the courage of conviction to follow the science on Ayurveda and Unani to its logical conclusion, except both of the largest political parties are steadfast in their support for Ayush, especially Ayurveda. Some of them, especially those on the Parliamentary Standing Committee for Health have repeatedly pressured the Ministry of Ayush on the issue of advertisements by the Ayush industry. However, as the saga with Rule 170 has demonstrated there are limits to the pressure brought upon the Ministry by individual members. Similarly, there are professional organizations of doctors like the Indian Medical Association, which has rarely backed away from a fight with the Ayush industry. Then there are doctors like Dr Abby Cyriac Philips and Dr K.V. Babu, both residents of Kerala, who have proven to be effective in pointing out the excesses of the Ayush industry on social media. Together, these voices of opposition will hopefully be able to check the worst excesses of the Ayush industry but far-reaching reform of the regulatory policies aimed at the Ayush industry is unlikely to take place any time in the near future.

Notes

1. Ravi Prakash Kumar, "Coronavirus Treatment: Ramdev's Patanjali Launches Coronil Kit for ₹545" *Mint* (23 June 2020) <https://www.livemint.com/news/india/coronavirus-vaccine-coronil-patanjali-baba-ramdev-press-conference-live-updates-11592893304534.html> accessed 10 September 2021.
2. Shiv Kumar, "Maharashtra Bans Baba Ramdev's Coronil" *The Tribune* (Mumbai, 25 June 2020) <https://www.tribuneindia.com/news/nation/maharashtra-bans-baba-ramdevs-coronil-104365> accessed 10 September 2021; BQ Desk, "Ayush Ministry Stops Patanjali From Selling, Advertising Purported Covid Medicine" (*Bloomberg Quint*, 23 June 2020) <https://www.bloombergquint.com/business/ayush-ministry-stops-patanjali-from-advertising-purported-covid-medicine> accessed 10 September 2021.
3. "Ramdev Launches Covid-19 Medicine Coronil, Harsh Vardhan Attends Event" *Hindustan Times* (19 February 2021) <https://www.hindustantimes.com/videos/news/watch-ramdev-launches-covid-19-medicine-coronil-harsh-vardhan-attends-event-101613737807861.html> accessed 10 September 2021.
4. "IMA 'Shocked' over Patanjali's Claim on Coronil; Demands Explanation from Harsh Vardhan" *The Hindu* (New Delhi, 22 February 2021) <https://www.thehindu.com/news/national/ima-shocked-over-patanjalis-claim-on-coronil-demands-explanation-from-harsh-vardhan/article33902720.ece> accessed 10 September 2021.
5. Sanjay Sharma, "Patanjali Sold 25 Lakh Coronil Kits Worth Rs 250 Crore in 4 Months" *India Today* (New Delhi, 2 November 2020) <https://www.indiatoday.in/india/story/patanjali-sold-25-lakh-coronil-kits-worth-rs-250-crore-in-4-months-1737229-2020-11-02> accessed 10 September 2021.
6. *Resident Doctors Association of the All India Institute of Medical Sciences (Rishikesh) vs. Ram Kishan Yadav Alias Baba Ramdev* CS (OS) No. 320 of 2021 before the High Court of Delhi at New Delhi (decided on 29th July, 2024).

7. Pankaj Bhardwaj and others, "Efficacy and Safety of Ayurveda Intervention (AYUSH 64) as Add-on Therapy for Patients with COVID-19 Infections—An Open Labelled, Parallel Group, Randomized Controlled Clinical Trial" [2021] medRxiv 2021.08.10.21261836; The Wire Staff, "COVID-19: Small, Preliminary Study Doesn't Find Proof of AYUSH 64's Efficacy" *The Wire Science* (19 August 2021) <https://science.thewire.in/health/covid-19-small-preliminary-study-doesnt-find-proof-of-ayush-64s-efficacy/> accessed 1 October 2021.
8. Press Information Bureau, Government of India, "Ayush Ministry Strongly Condemns the Tirade Against AYUSH-64 by a Section of Media: 'It is Misinterpreting the Facts, Lacking the Understanding of the Matter'" (26 August 2021) <https://pib.gov.in/PressReleaseIframePage.aspx?PRID=1749138> accessed 1 October 2021.
9. Government of India, *Report of the Health Survey & Development Committee* (Bhore Committee Report) (Vol II; 1946) p. 455.
10. ibid. 456.
11. Ibid. 456.
12. Government of India, Ministry of Health, *Report of the Committee on Indigenous Systems of Medicine* (Chopra Committee Report) (Vol I, 1948) 6-7.
13. ibid. 2.
14. ibid. 1.
15. ibid. 8.
16. Kiran Kumbhar, "The Forgotten Buddhist Origins of India's Ayurvedic Medicine" (*Medium*, 18 March 2021) <https://kikumbhar.medium.com/zysk-chattopadhyaya-history-ayurveda-india-medicine-buddhist-hindu-e85712cc9b52> accessed 10 September 2021; Kenneth G. Zysk, *Asceticism and Healing in Ancient India: Medicine in the Buddhist Monastery* (Motilal Banarsidass Publisher 1998); Steven Engler, "'Science' vs. 'Religion' in Classical Ayurveda" (2003) 50 *Numen* 416.
17. Shailaja Chandra, "Status of Indian Medicine and Folk

Healing: With a Focus on Integration of AYUSH Medical Systems in Healthcare Delivery" (2012) 33 *Ayu* 461 (Shailaja Chandra Report), ch 1: 'Historical Perspective', 13.

18. Aditya Kalra, "India Gets Minister for Yoga and Traditional Medicine" *Reuters* (New Delhi, 11 November 2014) <https://www.reuters.com/article/india-health-yoga-ministry-idINKCN0IV13J20141111> accessed 22 September 2021.
19. Government of India, Ministry of Health and Family Welfare, Department of AYUSH, *Good Clinical Practice Guidelines for Clinical Trials in Ayurveda, Siddha and Unani Medicine (GCP-ASU)* (March 2013).
20. ibid. 5.
21. Government of India, Ministry of Ayurveda, Yoga & Naturopathy, Unani, Siddha and Homeopathy (AYUSH), *Government Notification* (No K.11020/03/2017-DCC (AYUSH), 4 July 2018).
22. Government of India, Ministry of AYUSH, *Committee to Review the Functioning of Central Council for Research in Ayurvedic Sciences (CCRAS) and Peripheral Institutes under it: Report and Recommendations* (2017) 43.
23. As noted in the notice issued by Vice-Chairperson Abanti Sankaranarayan, Advertising Standards Council of India to Kudos Laboratories India Ltd. dated 14 October 2016 (accessed via the RTI Act).
24. PTI, "Quality Concern in Herbal Medicine Remains a Challenge: AYUSH Minister" *The Economic Times* (New Delhi, 8 November 2016) <https://economictimes.indiatimes.com/industry/healthcare/biotech/healthcare/quality-concern-in-herbal-medicine-remains-a-challenge-ayush-minister/articleshow/55310370.cms?from=mdr> accessed 23 September 2021; Dr Sumaiya Shaikh, "Are AYUSH Supported BGR-34 and IME-9 Drugs Safe and Effective for Diabetes?" *Alt News* (13 August 2017) <https://www.altnews.in/bgr-34-ime-9-drugs-safe-effective-diabetes/> accessed 23 September 2021; Anoop Misra, Seema Gulati and Atul Luthra,

"Alternative Medicines for Diabetes in India: Maximum Hype, Minimum Science" (2016) 4 *The Lancet Diabetes & Endocrinology* 302.

25. Pratik Sinha, Sumaiya Shaikh & Arjun Sidharth, *India Misinformed—The True Story*, (Harper Collins India 2019) at 232.
26. Reply to RTI application dated 14 November 2017, Ministry of AYUSH (Application No AYUSH/R/2017/50378, 3 October 2017).
27. *State of Maharashtra vs Karan Goomar* R.C.C.No. 2646/2017 before the Court of Civil Judge, Aurangabad (27 August 2018).
28. PTI, "Herbal Drug BGR-34 Helps Cutting down Heart Attack Risk: Study" *ET Healthworld* (New Delhi, 19 May 2018) <https://health.economictimes.indiatimes.com/news/pharma/herbal-drug-bgr-34-helps-cutting-down-heart-attack-risk-study/64236137> accessed 23 September 2021.
29. Reply to RTI application dated 31 October 2017, CIMAP (Application No CIMAP/R/2017/50008, 3 October 2017); Reply to RTI application dated 9 January 2018, CSIR (Application No CSIRH/R/2017/00191, 3 October 2017).
30. Priyanka Pulla, "Big Claims, Little Evidence" *The Hindu* (25 February 2018) <https://www.thehindu.com/sci-tech/health/big-claims-little-evidence/article22847068.ece> accessed 23 September 2021.
31. K.S. Jayaraman, "Did CSIR's Anti-Diabetic Drug Deserve Modi's Praise?" *The Wire* (4 October 2016) <https://thewire.in/health/bgr-34-csir-modi> accessed 23 September 2021.
32. Shailaja Chandra, "Bitter Medicine" *The Indian Express* (1 November 2016) <https://indianexpress.com/article/opinion/columns/ayush-ministry-ayurveda-medicines-education-3731440/> accessed 23 September 2021.
33. Pulla (n 30).
34. Sinha and others (n 25).
35. Anand Kulkarni and others, "*Tinospora Cordifolia* (Giloy)–Induced Liver Injury During the COVID-19

Pandemic—Multicenter Nationwide Study From India", (2022) 6(6) *Hepatology Communications* 1289-1300 <https://www.ncbi.nlm.nih.gov/pmc/articles/PMC9134809/#> accessed on 3 October 2024.

36. Robert B. Saper and others, "Heavy Metal Content of Ayurvedic Herbal Medicine Products" (2004) 292 *JAMA* 2868 (Of the 27 companies whose products were sampled, 26 were Indian and 1 was Pakistani).
37. Robert B. Saper and others, "Lead, Mercury, and Arsenic in US- and Indian-Manufactured Ayurvedic 'cures's Sold via the Internet'" (2008) 300 *JAMA* 915.
38. S.S. Savrikar and B. Ravishankar, "Introduction to 'Rasashaastra' the Iatrochemistry of Ayurveda" (2011) 8 *African Journal of Traditional, Complementary, and Alternative Medicines* 66.
39. Rob Gair, "Heavy Metal Poisoning from Ayurvedic 'cures's'" (2008) 50 *BC Medical Journal* 105.
40. A. Raviraja and others, "Three Cases of Lead Toxicity Associated with Consumption of Ayurvedic 'cures's'" (2010) 25 *Indian Journal of Clinical Biochemistry* 326.
41. Government of India, Ministry of Health & Family Welfare, Department of Ayurveda, Yoga & Naturopathy, Unani, Siddha and Homeopathy (Order F.No.K-11020/5/97-DCC (AYUSH), 14 October 2005).
42. Marek A. Mikulski and others, "Toxic Metals in Ayurvedic Preparations from a Public Health Lead Poisoning Cluster Investigation" (2017) 23 *International Journal of Occupational and Environmental Health* 187.
43. Laura Breeher and others, "A Cluster of Lead Poisoning among Consumers of Ayurvedic Medicine" (2015) 21 *International Journal of Occupational and Environmental Health* 303.
44. Radha Sharma and Paul John, "Poison in Ayurvedic Drugs" *The Times of India* (31 March 2017) <https://timesofindia.indiatimes.com/life-style/health-fitness/health-news/poison-in-ayurvedic-drugs/articleshow/57934912.cms> accessed 13

September 2021; Haritha John, "Ayurvedic Lead Poisoning: Is Bengaluru Man's Case an Isolated One?" *The News Minute* (15 June 2015) <https://www.thenewsminute.com/article/ayurvedic-lead-poisoning-bengaluru-mans-case-isolated-one-30056> accessed 13 September 2021; Uday Yanamandra and others, "Lead Poisoning Secondary to Unprescribed Ayurvedic 'cures' Intake" (2020) 13 BMJ *Case Reports* e238576; A. Raviraja and others, "Three Cases of Lead Toxicity Associated with Consumption of Ayurvedic 'cures's'" (2010) 25 *Indian Journal of Clinical Biochemistry* 326; Sujay Khandpur and others, "Chronic Arsenic Toxicity from Ayurvedic 'cures's'" (2008) 47 *International Journal of Dermatology* 618; G. Gnanashanmugam and others, "Mercury Toxicity Following Unauthorized Siddha Medicine Intake—A Mimicker of Acquired Neuromyotonia—Report of 32 Cases" (2018) 21 *Annals of Indian Academy of Neurology* 49; Krishna S. Gunturu and others, "Ayurvedic Herbal Medicine and Lead Poisoning" (2011) 4 *Journal of Hematology and Oncology* <http://www.scopus.com/inward/record.url?scp=83655197902&partnerID=8YFLogxK> accessed 13 September 2021.

45. Abhishek Anand, "Surge in Self-Medication Leading to Liver Damage during Covid, Says Dr Abby Philips" *India Today* (New Delhi, 13 April 2022) <https://www.indiatoday.in/coronavirus-outbreak/story/surge-in-self-medication-leading-to-liver-damage-during-covid-says-dr-abby-philips-1936969-2022-04-13> accessed 2 May 2022.
46. Preetu Nair, "Kerala: Doctor Sees Bid to Defame Him Using 'Toolkit'" *The Times of India* (Kochi, 11 June 2021) <https://timesofindia.indiatimes.com/city/kochi/doc-sees-bid-to-defame-him-using-toolkit/articleshow/83411333.cms> accessed 2 May 2022.
47. Cyriac Abby Philips and others, "Ayurvedic treatment induced severe alcoholic hepatitis and non-cirrhotic portal hypertension in a 14 year old girl", 2022 (10) *Oxford Medical Case Reports* 350-356. <https://www.ncbi.nlm.nih.gov/pmc/articles/PMC9589464/> accessed 3 October 2024.

48. Department Related Parliamentary Standing Committee on Health and Family Welfare, *DEMANDS FOR GRANTS 2012-13 (DEMAND NO. 47) OF THE DEPARTMENT OF AYUSH (MINISTRY OF HEALTH AND FAMILY WELFARE)* (Fifty-Fifth Report) (RS 2012) para 13.5-13.6.
49. ibid para 13.6.
50. Department Related Parliamentary Standing Committee on Health and Family Welfare, *Action Taken by Government on the Recommendations/Observations contained in the Ninety-Fifth Report on Demands for Grants 2016-17 (Demand No. 5) of the Ministry of AYUSH* (Ninety-Eighth Report) (RS 2016) para 3.23; Department Related Parliamentary Standing Committee on Health and Family Welfare, *Demands for Grants 2018-19 (Demand No. 5) of the Ministry of AYUSH* (One Hundred Eighth Report) (RS 2018) para 3.13.
51. Reply to RTI application dated 14.11.2017 by the Ministry of Ayush (Application No. AYUSH/R/2017/50378 dated 3.10.2017).
52. The Drugs & Cosmetics (Eleventh Amendment) Rules 2018 published in the *Gazette of India* (21 December 2018).
53. The Drugs and Cosmetics Rules 1945, Rule 170.
54. *Reckitt Benckiser India vs Union of India* W.P. (C) 321 of 2019 before the High Court of Delhi (15 January 2019); *Magnet Labs Pvt Ltd vs Union of India* W.P. (C) 502 of 2019 before the High Court of Delhi (18 January 2019); *Mankind Pharma Ltd vs Union of India* W.P. (C) 505 of 2019 before the High Court of Delhi (18 January 2019); *Association of Manufacturers of Ayurvedic Medicine vs Union of India* W.P. (C) 985 of 2019 before the High Court of Delhi (18 January 2019).
55. *Reckitt Benckiser India vs Union of India* W.P.(C) 321 of 2019, C.M. Appl. No. 1529-1530/2019 before the High Court of Delhi (15 January 2019) <http://delhihighcourt.nic.in/dhcqrydisp_o.asp?pn=6336&yr=2019> accessed 23 September 2021.
56. Anonna Dutt, "Supreme Court pulled up Ayush Industry

over Rule 170 of Drugs Act" *Indian Express* (3 September 2024) <https://indianexpress.com/article/explained/explained-health/supreme-court-pulled-up-ayush-ministey-over-rule-170-of-drugs-act-heres-what-it-says-9545226/> accessed 4 October 2024.

57. *CBI vs Gurbachan Singh* R.C. No. 0282010A0009 before Special Judge CBI, Punjab SAS Nagar, Mohali decided on 31 October 2017.
58. *FDA Maharashtra State vs Velaram Choudhary and others* R.C.C. No. 1500099/SW/16 before the Additional Chief Metropolitan Magistrate Mazagaon, Mumbai filed on 7 June 2016; Test report from government lab generated by the government analyst, FDA Maharashtra (Report No NSQ/MUM/36735/2014, 29 October 2014); Test report from government lab generated by the government analyst, FDA Maharashtra (Report No NSQ/MUM/36736/2014, 29 October 2014).
59. "Nimesulide Must Be Withdrawn Worldwide Due to Serious Liver Damage" (*Therapeutics Initiative*, 4 February 2008) <https://www.ti.ubc.ca/2008/02/04/nimesulide-must-be-withdrawn-worldwide-due-serious-liver-damage/> accessed 14 September 2021.
60. Savita Verma, "Govt Bans Nimesulide Banned over Adverse Effects on Liver" *India Today* (New Delhi, 15 February 2011) <https://www.indiatoday.in/india/north/story/government-bans-nimesulide-128660-2011-02-15> accessed 14 September 2021.
61. *FDA Maharashtra State vs Mahavir Ratilal Kothari and others* R.C.C. No. 01/2016 before the District & Sessions Judge, Shrirampur, District Ahmednagar decided on 19 October 2016; Test report from government lab generated by the government analyst, FDA Maharashtra (Report No NSQ/MUM/48742/2015, 18 March 2015).
62. Test report from government lab generated by the government analyst, FDA Maharashtra (Report No NSQ/MUM/48830/2015, 5 March 2015).

CHAPTER EIGHT

The Chaos of Indian Pharmacies and Their Supply Chains

Since much of the debate on drug regulation tends to be focused on the pharmaceutical industry, the issue of storage conditions of drugs during transportation and at the pharmacies receives little attention from policymakers in India. This is worrying because the lack of proper storage can degrade the quality of drugs. Despite the Supreme Court warning the government of India as far back as 1974 about gaps in the law in this regard, the Ministry of Health has done nothing to fix the issue. Writing for the court in a case involving prosecution of person for storing drugs without the appropriate licence, Justice Krishna Iyer had noted the following gap in Indian law:

> ...it is a glaring deficiency that while the Rules visualise wholesale distribution licences the forms do not spell out licences for mobile vans or distribution depots so essential for a wholesale distribution system. There is no doubt that if a scientific system of over-seeing wholesale distribution and a viable scheme of

> protected distribution is to be devised, licences for large and well-equipped conveyances and storage depots is desirable, nay, necessary. Indeed, storage in transit must also be licensed so that medicines do not suffer in the process. At present, no rules take care of transit by road or rail. Actually, cold storage or air-conditioned facilities for sensitive medicines are scarce in nationalised and private transport services and the drugs legislation winks at it. Likewise, the forms do not provide for storage depots or medical vans for wholesale supplies. Social guilt attaches to legal lacunae, the community being the victim. Arguments in this case have exposed these shortfalls in the law and we state them for legislative attention.[1]

Justice Iyer hit the nail on the head with his diagnosis on the complete silence of the law on conditions in which drugs are to be stored during transit. But what has the Ministry of Health done to address this issue pointed out by the Supreme Court since 1974? The answer is, not very much. As of October 2024, the Drugs & Cosmetics Rules, 1945 remains silent on the issue of mandating cold-chain equipment for the supply chain dealing in pharmaceutical drugs. In fact, even those provisions in the Drugs & Cosmetics Rules, 1945 dealing with retail pharmacies are completely inadequate. Technical requirements for starting a pharmacy are laid out in Schedule N to the Drugs and Cosmetics Rules, 1945 and have remained largely unchanged since 1972 when the requirements were first introduced into the law. It is entirely silent on cold-chain storage requirements, the maintenance of sterility, mechanisms for adverse event reporting, drug recall, etc. At most, Rule 64 requires pharmacies to maintain sales records and for premises to be "equipped with proper storage accommodation for preserving the properties of the drugs to which the licence applies." The law is silent on what exactly qualifies as "proper storage accommodation."

From a scientific and legal standpoint, these are poorly drafted regulations for a country that has climatic conditions varying from Himalayan cold to soaring heat in the rest of the country. In peak summer, the temperature across most parts of India can easily touch 40 degrees Celsius. Since most (not all) drugs manufactured for the Indian market are required by law to be stable only till 30 degrees Celsius, these drugs will degrade in an environment where the temperature exceeds 30 degrees Celsius, unless stored in a controlled environment where temperature is controlled. The law should then mandate that each pharmacy has storage equipment, power backups and temperature alarms to inform the owner when the temperature crosses a certain threshold.

The other truly appalling aspect of the Drugs & Cosmetics Rules, 1945 when it comes to storage conditions is its complete silence on the issue of humidity control. This again is a huge issue in many coastal states where humidity can rise beyond the average, affecting the stability of the drug. WHO recommends humidity sensors and alarms to be installed in storage units for drugs.[2]

These shortcomings in Indian law should truly terrify both the pharmaceutical industry and the medical community in India, since both of them are likely to face legal liability due to drugs that degrade when stored poorly and therefore fail to treat patients or fail to pass quality tests.

The knight in shining armour in this story is once again the 59th report of the Parliamentary Standing Committee on Health, which was tabled in 2012. This now famous and scathing report on the functioning of the national drug regulator asked some pointed questions on the storage of drugs in pharmacies. These questions led to the CDSCO drawing up a set of Guidelines on Good Distribution Practices (GDP) for Pharmaceutical Products.[3] For the most part, these guidelines bore close resemblance to the WHO's guidelines on GDPs for pharmaceutical products. While a good step forward, these guidelines failed to incorporate the more specific WHO model guidance for the storage and transport of time-and-temperature-sensitive pharmaceutical products.[4]

However, even in its limited form, the GDP guidelines proposed by the CDSCO would have been an upgrade if given the force of the law that could be enforced against pharmacies. Unfortunately, these guidelines ran into trouble at the Drugs Consultative Committee (DCC). Originally, the DCC, in its 46th meeting held on 12 and 13 December 2013, was of the opinion that "guidelines on Good Distribution Practices for Pharmaceutical products [are] the need of the hour as India is a vast country having major variations in temperature and climate" and it setup a sub-committee to recommend a path forward.[5] However, the very next year, the DCC rejected the recommendations of the sub-committee to give the GDP guidelines a binding legal status, on the rather absurd grounds that it would be "difficult to implement" across the entire chain of distribution consisting of 600,000 retail outlets.[6]

From a public health perspective, this was an outrageous decision because it meant that the DCC was willing to risk degradation of drugs travelling through poor supply chains merely because the state drug controllers did not want to take upon the responsibility of implementing the more rigorous GDP guidelines.

Four years later, in 2018, the same GDP guidelines mysteriously made its way back onto the DCC Agenda at its 53rd meeting. It is not clear why the GDP guidelines made it back to the agenda of the DCC but one possible reason is a well-publicized raid ordered by the Ministry of Health in 2017 on the infamous wholesale medical trading market at Bhagirath Palace, New Delhi. A retired joint secretary, K.L. Sharma, from the Ministry of Health recounts the raid and its shocking findings in his book on the state of drug regulation in India. This raid, which involved 142 inspectors of the CDSCO, along with police protection, was conducted on 9 June 2017. According to Sharma, the inspection revealed a shocking state of affairs at the wholesale market including the storage of heat sensitive drugs, which should have been stored at a temperature of 8–25 degree Celsius but were stored in a room whose temperature was 40 degrees Celsius. Many of the warehouses inspected during the raid were found lacking in cold storage facilities and even in those where refrigerators were available, they were not always switched on. In one instance, the inspection team discovered a consignment of Tetanus Toxoid vaccines stocked in boxes containing icepacks or kept on open racks and shelves. These vaccines were actually required to be stored at 2–8 degree Celsius and were most likely degraded because of the poor storage conditions. Further, the inspections team discovered that none of the outlets had power backup in case of a failure of electricity.[7]

Sharma also narrates a startling account of premises so cramped that staff had to walk on top of boxes of medicines to reach the other end of the premises. The staff apparently were not trained in the handling or storage of medicine. This is not at all surprising because unlike pharmacies, which are expressly required by the law to be under the charge of a "registered pharmacist" (which requires a degree in pharmacy), the law provides wholesalers with the option of keeping their premises under the charge of either a "registered pharmacist" or a person who has passed the "matriculation examination or its equivalent with four years experience in dealing with drugs." This requirement, which was introduced into the law in 1980 was further diluted in 2000, when the following third category of qualifications was added to the rules: any person "who holds a degree of a recognised University with one year's experience, in dealing with drugs."[8] In other words, even a person with a Bachelor's Degree in Horticulture could be placed in charge of a premises as long as he had a year's experience in handling drugs.

Even more worryingly, Sharma reveals that documentation and record-keeping practices at these facilities were abysmal. The law clearly specifies certain record keeping requirements for wholesalers.[9] However in 17 instances during this raid, wholesale dealers at Bhagirath Palace were unable to produce purchase bills raising doubts about the source of the drugs in question.[10] Summing up the results of the inspections, Sharma concluded:

> Whatever the inspection revealed, speaks very poorly of the storage and distribution practices in vogue and it poses a serious threat to millions of unsuspecting consumers. If this could happen in the capital city that also houses the national regulator, the position in far-flung areas can only be imagined.[11]

The fact that the above statement was made by the top bureaucrat responsible for drug regulatory policy should give us serious cause for worry.

It is possible that the shocking revelations from the inspection of Bhagirath Palace forced the DCC to put the GDP guidelines back on the agenda. At the next meeting in 2019, at the 54th meeting of the DCC, it was reportedly decided to make the GDP guidelines into binding law.[12]

Pressure from individual states may have also played a role in shaping the above recommendation. For example, at the same meeting, states like Punjab specifically asked for a mandatory requirement for all pharmacies to have air-conditioning and power backup especially in the summer months when room temperatures soared above 30 degrees Celsius, which is the outer limit in the stability specification for drugs being sold in India.[13]

But as is the case with many of these recommendations by the DCC, there is many a slip between the cup and the lip. Five years later, as this book goes to print, the Ministry of Health is yet to introduce the required amendments to the Drugs & Cosmetics Rules, 1945 to give legal force to the GDP guidelines. In other words, nothing really changed despite the official acknowledgment that the GDP guidelines require legal status in order to ensure the quality of medicine travelling through the supply chain.

Presumably, private pharmacies and distributors are not particularly keen on the GDP guidelines becoming binding law because they would have to then invest in better storage equipment. A key factor contributing to their nonchalance on this issue is the fact that Section 19 of the Drugs & Cosmetics Act, 1940, gives pharmacies complete legal immunity in cases where a drug purchased or stored at their premises fails quality testing. This immunity is contingent on their having procured the drug from a licensed entity after exercising "reasonable due diligence" and being able to prove that the drug was "properly stored". Removing or even diluting this immunity from prosecution may create pressure on pharmacies and distributors to actively support the enactment of new regulations on storage and distribution of drugs.

Regardless of the indifference on part of the pharmacies and distributors, one would expect sustained public pressure to be applied on the government to reform this sector since a poorly regulated supply chain has significant implications for public health. However, there is barely a squeak in the Indian press or civil society on the delays in enacting these much-needed and long-delayed reforms.

Rather, much of the regulatory discussion on pharmacies in India is concentrated on the following issues: the necessity of mandating the presence of registered pharmacists in pharmacies, unlicenced sale of prescription drugs that can be abused and the resistance against the e-pharmacy juggernaut, which is threatening the existence of the "brick and mortar" pharmacies that form the backbone of the politically powerful All India Organisation of Chemists & Druggists (AIOCD). Each of these debates have implications for public health and are explained in the following pages.

Do pharmacies require pharmacists?

When the Drugs Inquiry Committee submitted its report in 1931, it spent a fair deal of print on the issue of regulating pharmacies. At the time, there was no regulation of the profession of pharmacists and the committee clearly had a poor opinion of the crop of people in charge of pharmacies, complaining that, "Their standard of education is low and not much is expected of them by way of professional training."[14]

Clearly dissatisfied with the functioning of the profession, the committee recommended a radical reorganization of the profession of pharmacy. It called for the enactment of a legislation to prescribe educational qualifications for pharmacists and regulation of the profession through a body that represented pharmacists.[15] Those recommendations translated into law 17 years later when the Pharmacy Act was finally enacted in 1948 by the Constituent Assembly. This law created the Pharmacy Council of India, as a self-regulatory body that could prescribe qualification, educational and registration requirements for pharmacists in India. This legislation, however, did not immediately mandate all pharmacies to be run only under the supervision of this new class of registered pharmacists. This law allowed persons already in the business of compounding, preparing, mixing or dispensing drugs to continue doing so with the caveat in Section 42 of the legislation that individual states could fix cut-off dates, after which only pharmacists registered under the Pharmacy Act, 1948, could engage in the aforementioned acts of compounding or dispensing drugs. Presumably, this power had been delegated to states because each state needed time to invest in the training, education and creation of this new class of professional pharmacists.

The states made slow progress in enforcing Section 42 of the Pharmacy Act. Commenting on the situation in 1954, the Pharmaceutical Enquiry Report, setup by the Government of India, had this to say:

> It is not enough, if the Pharmacy Act is extended on paper to all the States in the country. Excepting for a very few States, the progress made by other States in the enforcement of the Drugs and Pharmacy legislation has been very poor. The State Governments have not realized the urgent need for starting institutions for providing courses of study in pharmacy.[16]

A decade later, the situation vis-à-vis the enforcement of Section 42 by the states was no better as evidenced from a tense discussion in the Rajya Sabha during Question Hour in September 1965, where Arjun Arora, a MP from Uttar Pradesh, accused the Deputy Minister of Health of misleading the House on the status of enforcement of the Pharmacy Act, 1948. In his oral statement, P.S. Naskar, the Deputy Minister for Health, had informed the house that all states and union territories, except for five, had "enforced the Pharmacy Act, 1948 in varying degrees."[17] However, the statement tabled by the Deputy Minister had indicated that only the state of Uttar Pradesh had enforced Section 42 of the Pharmacy Act, 1948, restricting the profession of pharmacy to pharmacists registered as per the Pharmacy Act, 1948. When the government was accused by the MP who raised the question, of "seriously misleading" the House, the Health Minister was quick to explain that "many of the states" lacked qualified pharmacists and hence could not enforce Section 42.[18]

Finally, in 1970, some much-needed legal reforms were executed by the Union Government. To begin with, Rule 65 of the Drugs & Cosmetics Rules, 1945 (under which pharmacies are licensed) was amended to fix 31 December 1969 as the relevant date after which licences for pharmacies would mandatorily require the business of dispensing drugs to be carried out under the supervision of a registered pharmacist. Similarly, a more wide-ranging reform was enacted in 1975 when the Ministry of Health introduced in Parliament a legislation to amend Section 42 of the Pharmacy Act, 1948. This amendment aimed at deleting the earlier wording that allowed state governments to decide the cutoff date beyond which only registered pharmacists could dispense drugs and instead, replaced it with a deadline of five years, after which, all states would have to ensure that only "registered pharmacists" could engage in the business of mixing, dispensing or compounding drugs.

During the debates preceding the vote on the bill in the Rajya Sabha, the Minister of State in the Ministry of Health, Chaudhary Ram Sewak, explained that although the Pharmacy Act, 1948, had been in force for 27 years, only three states and the Union Territory of Delhi had enforced the mandate of Section 42 i.e., restricting the business of pharmacy to "registered pharmacists" who had the qualifications prescribed under the Pharmacy Act and were registered with the Pharmacy Council of India.[19] Given the inaction on the part of the states in notifying cut-off dates under Section 42, the Union Government had moved the bill under discussion to fix a cut-off date of five years for the enforcement of Section 42 across India. The Bill breezed through Parliament in 1976 with little opposition and literally so, since Prime Minister Indira Gandhi had jailed most of the Opposition after declaring an Emergency in 1975. The enactment of this amendment meant that only pharmacists registered with the Pharmacy Council of India could practice the profession of pharmacy from September 1981 onward. Except that there was opposition brewing to this rule.

A few years after the enactment of this amendment, in 1978, the DCC discussed concerns raised by many states that due to a shortage of pharmacists, there was a shortage of pharmacies in rural areas thereby limiting access to medicine. As a result, many states were pressing for some kind of relaxation of the rule which made the presence of a registered pharmacist compulsory for all pharmacies.[20] Only some states like Goa and Tamil Nadu resisted any dilution of standards. The drug controller from Tamil Nadu even disputed the reasoning offered by some state drug controllers regarding the shortage of pharmacies in rural areas. According to him, the real reason for lack of pharmacies in rural areas, was the lack of doctors in these areas because of which there was little interest in opening pharmacies in rural areas. At the end of the meeting, the DCC resolved to drop the "registered pharmacist" requirement for opening and operating a pharmacy for towns with a population of less than 20,000 persons and instead allow anyone who has "passed a matriculate examination with science or any other equivalent examination, and who has also passed a 6 months training course approved by the State Government" to open a pharmacy.[21] It is not clear whether this decision was actually implemented by a rule change. Similarly, the deadline of 31 August 1981 prescribed in the 1976 amendment to the Pharmacy Act, 1948 was proposed to be extended by the Ministry of Health by an additional three years because "representations" had been received from various quarters about the inadequacy of trained pharmacists. This time around, the Minister of Health B. Shankaranand, who described the legislation extending the deadline as a "very simple bill" came under withering criticism from MPs in both the Rajya Sabha and the Lok Sabha. These MPs questioned not just the logic of extending a deadline three months after it had recently expired, but also the guarantee that the supposed shortage of pharmacists would be resolved in a period of three years.[22] Some MPs also strongly resisted pushing the deadline any further on the grounds that allowing untrained persons to dispense medicine posed a serious danger to public health. One MP, who was also a doctor, complained that many of the persons in charge of pharmacies were unable to even read the prescriptions of doctors resulting in errors while dispensing medicines, apart from lacking knowledge about the incompatibility of drugs and storage of drugs.[23]

Notwithstanding this opposition to any more extensions, the Parliament voted in favour of extending the deadline for Section 42 by another three years to 1 September 1984. In the following years, the existing lobby of "chemists and druggists", who qualified for pharmacy licences under the older rules, protested and even went on a strike against the upcoming deadline in 1984, the reverberations of which were felt even in Parliament as at least one MP took up the issue in Parliament.[24] In any event, the deadline of 1 September 1984 was not extended any further, thereby officially closing the door to anybody but "registered pharmacists" to be in charge of dispensing drugs at pharmacies.

Through the entire course of the aforementioned policy-making exercise, the Ministry of Health never once produced any report with empirical evidence stating the number of "registered pharmacists" available in India or the supposed shortage faced in different states. As a result, no measures were instituted to help states that did actually face a shortage of pharmacists. It was therefore not surprising when in the following decades, some states like Bihar repeatedly complained about the lack of "registered pharmacists". The most recent such complaint from Bihar was at the meeting of the DCC held in July 2020, when the drug controller from the state once again asked for a relaxation in the criteria to start a pharmacy. The DCC for its part dismissed the demand on the grounds that there was no shortage of pharmacists in the country.[25] Once again, the DCC did not cite any empirical evidence to back its claim. It is important for the government to tackle such issues with empirical evidence because even the drug controller from a prosperous state like Maharashtra "confessed" at a DCC meeting that 34% of the pharmacies in the state did not have registered pharmacists![26] While accurate figures are not available, we noticed quite a few prosecutions in some states against pharmacies for the offence of dispensing drugs under the supervision of persons who were not registered pharmacists. It is not clear whether this is due to a shortage of pharmacists or because the owners of pharmacies are trying to maximize their profits by hiring unqualified staff in lieu of registered pharmacists who tend to ask for higher salaries.

The Schedule K crisis

One of the peculiar aspects of law making in India is that every law will always have that one provision granting the government the discretion to create exemptions wide enough to render the law toothless. In case of the Drugs & Cosmetics Act, 1940 that provision is Schedule K, which basically exempts certain categories of drugs handled by certain categories of people from different legal requirements that generally apply to pharmacies. For example, government hospitals are exempted from the requirement of applying for sales licences like private pharmacies, although they are still required to ensure that drugs are stored in an appropriate manner. Similarly, registered medical practitioners are allowed to store and dispense drugs for their patients without the requirement for applying for sales licences, provided the drugs are stored properly.

In 1961, an exemption was created in Schedule K, for pharmacies in villages with less than 1,000 people allowing them to stock 15 "household remedies" that included Aspirin, "syrups, lozenges, pills and tablets for cough" and tablets of Quinine Sulphate without being subject to any of the regular licensing requirements that applied to other pharmacies. Along the years, the government continued amending Schedule K to include more categories such as ophthalmic ointments required to be distributed as part of the National Trachoma Control Programme or Chloroquine tablets required to be distributed as part of the National Malaria Eradication Programme. Unlike the earlier conditional exemptions granted to government hospitals or doctors (subject to storage conditions), these were unconditional exemptions with no mention on how the drugs in question were to be stored.

The list of exemptions in Schedule K was expanded in 1980 to the following categories of medical workers for drugs being supplied by either the central or state governments: multipurpose workers attached to primary health centres/sub-centres, community health volunteers under the Rural Health Scheme; nurses, auxiliary nurses, midwives and health visitors attached to urban family welfare centres, PHC and anganwadi workers (added in 1989).[27] All of these workers were given an unconditional exemption from Chapter IV of the Drugs & Cosmetics Act, 1940, which dealt with licensing requirements for pharmacies, meaning that they were not even required to adhere to proper storage conditions (whatever that means in context of Indian law).

This trend of widening Schedule K continues. As late as 2019, the Ministry of Health proposed expanding Schedule K further to include primary healthcare centres and wellness centres in urban areas and Accredited Social Health Activist (ASHA) workers.[28] As originally envisaged under the National Health Mission, the ASHA worker, whose minimum qualification is to be literate or preferably pass 10th grade examinations, was supposed to be a "depot holder" for essential drugs like oral rehydration therapy, Iron Folic Acid tablet, Chloroquine, oral pills and condoms so that they could be made available to people in the community.[29]

These kind of exemptions in Schedule K, prior to 1984, would have allowed these government health workers to dispense medicine despite lacking the qualification of a registered pharmacist. However, these exemptions in Schedule K could not extend to dispensing drugs once Section 42 of the Pharmacy Act, 1948 came into effect in 1984. This is because a provision of the Drugs & Cosmetics Rules cannot create an exemption to the provisions of a completely different law like the Pharmacy Act. This fact, however, appears to have missed the attention of the policymakers in the Ministry of Health and also the state governments, both of whom continue to seek cover under Schedule

K to justify their decisions to allow government health workers to prescribe drugs despite them not being registered pharmacists.

The only pushback to these proposals, including the one made by the Ministry of Health in 2019 to include ASHA workers in Schedule K, was from the Pharmacy Council of India (PCI) and other associations of pharmacists on the grounds that such an exemption would violate Section 42 of the Pharmacy Act and that the government should just hire more registered pharmacists and that there was no shortage of pharmacists in the country.[30]

Ultimately, the government walked back on its proposal to include ASHA workers but it did include Community Health Officers in Schedule K. These health workers, who were a new category of "mid-level health provider" created under a new government health scheme called Ayushman Bharat are not trained doctors but anybody with a Bachelors in Science in Community Health, a Nurse or an Ayurvedic practitioner trained and certified through a university![31] There is a case to argue that none of these "medical" workers can dispense drugs given the bar in Section 42.

State governments are no better when it comes to evading the requirement of hiring registered pharmacies at public hospitals. For example, in 2012, in Rajasthan, nurses went on a strike because the state government tried to put them in charge of dispensing prescription drugs for one particular government scheme.[32] The nurses complained that they would be liable for violation of Section 42 of the Pharmacy Act since they were not registered pharmacists. In Kerala, the All Kerala Pharmacists Unions has litigated extensively against the state government over the involvement of nurses in dispensing of drugs.[33] Similarly in Haryana, pharmacists accused government run hospitals and primary health centres of violating Section 42 of the Pharmacy Act, 1948 by not employing registered pharmacists.[34]

At some point, the Ministry of Health has to tackle this issue of medical professionals other than pharmacists dispensing drugs. This should be done through a rigorous, well-planned survey aimed at capturing the extent to which pharmacies and hospitals in India in both the private and public sector are staffed with pharmacists, the extent of the alleged shortage of registered pharmacists and the reasons for such shortage. Such an exercise is essential to protect public health in India. Poorly qualified personnel in charge of pharmacies are bound to make mistakes in filling prescriptions or substituting drugs based on their generic names or even playing the role of first medical provider, as is often the case with most pharmacies in India. If there is indeed a shortage of pharmacists, the Ministry of Health must come up with a plan to address the shortage, preferably by investing more in pharmacy colleges and training people. The current haphazard approach which is centred on tinkering with Schedule K is unacceptable.

Cracking the whip on illegal pharmacies, drug peddlers and fake doctors

Despite the skeletal regulatory requirements for pharmacies in India, state drug controllers in India are very actively instituting prosecutions for violation of these skeletal requirements in pursuit of goals that have little to do with quality of drugs. The principal categories of prosecutions launched against pharmacies include the stocking or sale of drugs without the required licences (these include instances of moving premises without changing the address on the licence), flouting licence conditions by not having a registered pharmacist at the pharmacy during working hours, the failure to maintain necessary documentation of purchases or sales and lastly, dispensing drugs without a prescription. The most serious offence, however, from a public health perspective is the first category i.e., stocking or selling drugs without a licence. In a good percentage of such cases, the drugs in question are "habit forming" drugs, as addictive drugs are often described in judgements delivered by Indian courts.

In the state of Punjab, which has been in the middle of a drug addiction crisis for the last decade, drug inspectors have been very active in raiding and prosecuting establishments storing and selling drugs without having the relevant pharmacy licences under the Drugs & Cosmetics Rules, 1945. Unlike many other states, the accused in these cases actually spend time in jail until the trials for these offences are concluded. Through the e-courts website, we were able to find at least 230 cases that were prosecuted by drug inspectors across Punjab over the last decade for violation of the provisions relating to stocking and selling drugs. In 124 of these cases, the drug inspectors managed to secure convictions against the persons accused of violating the law related to the stocking and selling of drugs. Most of these cases pertained to stocking and selling of drugs without the required licences. The punishments handed out by judges in these cases were surprisingly tough. In several cases, the accused were actually given the statutory minimum punishment of three years, along with the minimum fine of 1 lakh rupees.[35] In most of these cases, though the accused had either already served time in prison awaiting their trial or alternatively, if they were first-time offenders, the court would release them on probation, meaning that they could find their way back to jail to complete the sentence if they were found breaching the terms of their probation. In some cases, judges rejected the request for probation "because of the fact that in the State of Punjab, there is hue and cry regarding the youth becoming addicts day by day and if the unauthorised persons are allowed to keep and sell the drugs, more and more persons will be becoming users and addicts of the drugs."[36]

We were also able to access approximately 95 cases in West Bengal through the e-courts system for the time period between 2015 and 2019. In 61 of these cases, the state was prosecuting persons found to be "stocking", without a licence, large quantities of habit-forming, addictive drugs including fixed-dose-combinations that contained Tramadol (an opiate prone to abuse), sleeping medication that contained Benzodiazepam (a psychoactive drug) and an assortment of cough syrups that contained Codeine, which is an opiate and known to be heavily abused in India. The problem, however, was that in all these cases, it was the police that was conducting raids, arresting persons and prosecuting them before Sessions Judges. The Drugs & Cosmetics Act, 1940 is very clear that only drug inspectors notified by the state in the official gazette can institute prosecutions for offences under this legislation. As a result, in all 61 cases, the Sessions Judge acquitted the accused on the grounds that the police had no jurisdiction to prosecute cases under the Drugs & Cosmetics Act, 1940. In another 22 cases that were prosecuted by drug inspectors who had the jurisdiction under the law to do so, the courts acquitted the accused due to poor investigations or procedural irregularities.

Far away in Maharashtra, we were able to access 62 judgements delivered in prosecutions filed between 1990 and 2017 against unlicenced pharmacies for "stocking" drugs or pharmacies breaching the terms of their licences (maintenance of records and having a registered pharmacist). Unlike in West Bengal, these prosecutions were at least filed by the correct authorities and before the correct courts, resulting in 26 convictions and 36 acquittals. Unlike in West Bengal and Punjab, the prosecutions in Maharashtra did not appear to be targeted at persons stocking "habit forming" drugs. Also, unlike in Punjab where prosecutions are quite speedy, the successful convictions in Maharashtra were achieved in a time frame ranging from three years to 18 years. Even then, the sentencing was exceptionally lenient. Of the 26 cases that ended in conviction, in 19 cases, the Judicial Magistrates awarded a sentence of "Simple imprisonment till the rising of the court", meaning that the convicted persons could leave the court soon as the judge rose for the day. This virtual non-punishment was accompanied by small fines ranging from ₹5,000 to ₹30,000.

In neighbouring Andhra Pradesh, we were able to access 55 prosecutions pertaining to the violations of laws that apply to pharmacies. Convictions were secured in only 14 cases, while there were acquittals in the remaining 41 cases. A small number of these cases involved "habit forming" drugs. In most of the other cases, a large variety of modern drugs were seized, indicating that the persons in question were running unlicenced pharmacies. For example, in one case, a total of 249 different drugs were seized.[37] In the 14 cases where convictions were secured, courts in Andhra Pradesh delivered sentences of up to three years imprisonment in six cases, along with fines ranging from ₹1,000 to ₹1,20,000.

The last state that warrants a discussion is Haryana, where the state government has been using the Drugs & Cosmetics Act to crack down on fake doctors and unregistered medical practitioners who were storing and selling drugs. While practicing medicine without being registered is an offence under the laws regulating the practice of modern medicine and traditional Indian medicine, we suspect that the state finds it quite difficult to prove beyond reasonable doubt, that these unlicensed medical practitioners were actually practicing medicine. In such cases, it may be easier to successfully prosecute them on the grounds that they were storing drugs illegally. We came across at least 27 such prosecutions in Haryana, 17 of which ended in convictions for unlawfully stocking drugs without a licence. In most cases, the court awarded imprisonment of three to four years accompanied with fines of ₹1 lakh.

Take for example, the case of *State of Haryana vs. Dr. Mohinder Kumar*[38] who was supposedly running a clinic in Panipat. A raid by a drug inspector found him to be stocking at least 20 different types of "allopathic drugs". When asked to produce proof of his registration, the accused was unable to do so. If he was a registered medical practitioner, he could have taken benefit of Schedule K which allows such practitioners of medicine to store drugs without the requirement of a pharmacy licence. He was unable to provide such evidence and was hence found guilty of violating the provisions of the Drugs & Cosmetics Act that require licences to be procured for stocking or selling drugs and was hence, sentenced to three years in prison along with a fine of ₹1 lakh.

Together, these prosecutions across these various states reveal a severely compromised supply chain with wholesale distributors of drugs not verifying the credentials of those to whom they are selling drugs.

The common thread running through the above discussion is that the provisions related to regulation of pharmacies under the Drugs & Cosmetics Act are used primarily to prosecute illegal pharmacies, drug peddlers and fake doctors. Little attention is being paid to the issue of how exactly drugs are stored by licensed pharmacies, especially in India's hot and humid climate. The lack of prosecutions on the issue of improper storage conditions is because of the original sin of the Drugs & Cosmetics Rules not prescribing regulations that mandatorily require pharmacies to maintain cold storage equipment, power-backups and alarms that can warn of humidity and heat crossing certain limits. If there is no law regulating these issues, it cannot be broken. From a public health perspective, the silence on storage requirements across the supply chain is a disaster.

The policy paralysis on regulating online pharmacies and a chance to reform the regulation of pharmacies and supply chains

The Indian drug market is currently witnessing an epic clash between the traditional "brick and mortar" pharmacies (mostly small businesses) and new online pharmacies, which sell drugs through the internet; i.e., they accept orders and payments through apps on smart phones and deliver the drugs ordered directly to the consumer. Most online pharmacies are owned by big corporations and are currently attracting billions of dollars in investment from foreign funds. The populist tendency in such battles is to side with small businesses, except that in the case of "brick and mortar" pharmacies, there have been several findings by the Competition Commission of India (CCI) that these businesses regularly colluded with each other, under the umbrella of trade associations, in order to raise the prices of drugs instead of competing with each to provide the consumer with medicines at the lowest possible price.[39] On occasion, pharmacists have also required pharmaceutical manufacturers to take "no object certificates" from their trade associations before appointing "stockists", failing which all pharmacists in an area would refuse to buy from the "stockist". Such carterlization is illegal under the Competition Act and over the years the CCI has repeatedly ruled against different trade associations comprising pharmacists for engaging in anti-competitive behaviour that hurts consumer interests. The hope of many, including the CCI, is that online pharmacies with their venture-capital backing and eagerness to capture market share through deep discounts, can disrupt these old cartels in the pharmacy sector and lower prices of drugs for consumers.[40]

As a part of their advocacy campaigns against online pharmacies, trade associations of "brick and mortar" pharmacies have adopted fear as their primary tactic, claiming that online pharmacies will open the door to drug abuse and sale of substandard and counterfeit medicine. They have also exploited the lack of a specific legal framework for online pharmacies to litigate before the courts seeking injunctions against online pharmacies.[41] However these tactics have not worked to deter investors as can be witnessed by the massive investments being made by private capital in online pharmacies.[42] The COVID-19 pandemic further gave a boost to this sector when the Ministry of Health invoked its special powers under Section 26B of the Drugs & Cosmetics Act, 1940, to allow all pharmacies to accept prescriptions through email and also deliver the drugs to the doorstep of the consumer.[43]

Apart from the above notification, the government for its part is doing precious little to lay down regulations specifically for online pharmacies. At most, in 2017 it did publish a set of draft rules to regulate online pharmacies but never notified them into law.[44] In any case, these draft rules were completely inadequate to deal with the issue of possible prescription abuse. Under the Drugs & Cosmetics Rules, 1945, a prescription once filled, has to be physically marked by the pharmacist to prevent its reuse.[45] Since online pharmacies typically deal with photographed prescriptions, it is not possible for pharmacists to physically mark the prescription. The solution as devised in other countries like the USA is to create a system of electronic prescriptions that can be electronically verified by pharmacies. Apart from reducing the possibility of abuse, electronic prescribing in the USA has also increased the efficiency and accuracy of pharmacies.[46] The Indian government needs to seriously consider a similar initiative before prescription abuse becomes a significant problem with online pharmacies.

But more importantly, apart from tackling the issue of prescription abuse, the Ministry of Health must seriously consider using this opportunity to dramatically upgrade the current bare-boned licensing requirements to open and run a pharmacy or engage in the whole-sale trading of drugs. The entire supply chain is in the middle of a churn with big capital investing in online pharmacies. These changes are eventually going to reorder the manner in which drugs reach consumers from pharmaceutical manufacturers. These new businesses have the capital to invest in far better storage systems for drugs and also human resources like registered pharmacists to manage the storage and sale of drugs. There could be no better time for the Ministry of Health to completely overhaul the regulation of pharmacies in a manner that guarantees better storage of drugs during transit and distribution while protecting against prescription abuse and guaranteeing supply chain integrity. More importantly, law making in the Ministry must move to a data and evidence driven process.

Notes

1. *Swantraj vs State of Maharashtra* 1974 SCR (3) 287 (5 February 1974).
2. World Health Organization (WHO), *WHO good distribution practices for pharmaceutical products* (WHO Technical Report Series, No. 957, 2010).

3. Government of India, Drugs Controller General (India), *Notice: Draft Guidelines on Good Distribution Practices for pharmaceutical products-Reg.* (File No: 15-14/2018-DC, 25 September 2018).
4. World Health Organization (WHO), *Model guidance for the storage and transport of time- and temperature-sensitive pharmaceutical products* (WHO Technical Report Series, No. 961, 2011).
5. Drugs Consultative Committee (DCC), "*REPORT OF THE 46TH MEETING OF THE DRUGS CONSULTATIVE COMMITTEE HELD ON 12TH AND 13TH NOVEMBER, 2013 AT THE HOTEL METROPOLITAN NEW DELHI-110001*" (2013) 15 <https://cdsco.gov.in/opencms/opencms/system/modules/CDSCO.WEB/elements/common_download.jsp?num_id_pk=ODA4> accessed 8 April 2022.
6. Drugs Consultative Committee (DCC), "*REPORT OF THE 47TH MEETING OF THE DRUGS CONSULTATIVE COMMITTEE HELD ON 30TH AND 31ST JULY, 2014 AT NEW DELHI*" (2014) 28 <https://cdsco.gov.in/opencms/opencms/system/modules/CDSCO.WEB/elements/common_download.jsp?num_id_pk=ODA5> accessed 8 April 2022.
7. K.L. Sharma, *Healing the Pharmacy of the World: An Inside Story of Medical Products Manufacturing and Regulation in India* (Notion Press 2021) 109-111.
8. Government of India, Ministry of Health & Family Welfare, *GSR 681(E)* (*Gazette of India Extraordinary*, Part II–s 3(i), 5 December 1980)—Rule 64 of the Drugs & Cosmetics Rules, 1945; Government of India, Ministry of Health & Family Welfare, *GSR 351(E)* (*Gazette of India Extraordinary*, Part II–s 3(i), 26 April 2000)—Drugs & Cosmetics (Third Amendment) Rules, 2000.
9. The Drugs & Cosmetics Rules 1945, Rule 65(5)(1).
10. Sharma (n 7).
11. ibid 111.
12. Drugs Consultative Committee (DCC), "*REPORT OF 54TH MEETING OF DRUGS CONSULTATIVE*

COMMITTEE HELD ON 30TH JULY, 2018 AT NEW DELHI" (2018) 5 <https://cdsco.gov.in/opencms/opencms/system/modules/CDSCO.WEB/elements/common_download.jsp?num_id_pk=ODE2> accessed 8 April 2022.

13. Drugs Consultative Committee (DCC), *"REPORT OF 54TH MEETING OF DRUGS CONSULTATIVE COMMITTEE HELD ON 30TH JULY, 2018 AT NEW DELHI"* (2018) 19 <https://cdsco.gov.in/opencms/opencms/system/modules/CDSCO.WEB/elements/common_download.jsp?num_id_pk=ODE2> accessed 8 April 2022. Pages 19–56 DCC.
14. Government of India, *Report of the Drugs Enquiry Committee* (1931) 73.
15. ibid 102.
16. Government of India, Ministry of Commerce & Industry, *Report of the Pharmaceutical Enquiry Committee* (1954) 212, para 6.1.8.
17. The Deputy Minister in the Ministry of Health, Rajya Sabha Deb 15 September 1965, 4036.
18. ibid 4037, 4040.
19. The Minister of State in the Ministry of Health and Family Planning on The Pharmacy (Amendment) Bill 1975, Rajya Sabha Deb 12 May 1976, 162.
20. Drugs Consultative Committee (DCC), *"MINUTES OF THE 20TH MEETING OF THE DRUGS CONSULTATIVE COMMITTEE HELD AT NEW DELHI ON THE 4th & 5th JULY. 1978"* (1978) 11-12 <https://cdsco.gov.in/opencms/opencms/system/modules/CDSCO.WEB/elements/common_download.jsp?num_id_pk=ODUz> accessed 8 April 2022.
21. ibid 27.
22. Discussion on Pharmacy (Amendment) Bill, Lok Sabha Deb 29 April 1982, 388-89; Discussion on Pharmacy (Amendment) Bill, Rajya Sabha Deb 1 December 1981, 242-243.
23. Dr M.M.S. Siddhu (MP, Uttar Pradesh), Rajya Sabha Deb 1 December 1981, 245.
24. Shri Ratansinh Rajda (MP, Bombay South), Rajya Sabha Deb 7 August 1984, 480-81.

25. Drugs Consultative Committee (DCC), "*MINUTES OF 58TH MEETING (VIRTUAL) OF DRUGS CONSULTATIVE COMMITTEE HELD THROUGH WEB CONFERENCE ON 14TH JULY, 2020 AT CDSCO (HQ)*" (2020) 3 <https://cdsco.gov.in/opencms/opencms/system/modules/CDSCO.WEB/elements/common_download.jsp?num_id_pk=MTI1NQ==> accessed 8 April 2022.
26. Drugs Consultative Committee (DCC) (n 6) 5.
27. Government of India, Ministry of Health & Family Welfare, *GSR 540(E)* (*Gazette of India Extraordinary*, Part II–s 3(i), 22 September 1980); Government of India, Ministry of Health & Family Welfare, *GSR 784(E) (Gazette of India Extraordinary*, Part II–s 3(i), 28 August 1989).
28. Government of India, Ministry of Health & Family Welfare, *GSR 827(E)* (*Gazette of India Extraordinary*, Part II–s 3(i), 6 November 2019)—Drugs & Cosmetics (Amendment) Rules, 2019.
29. Government of India, National Rural Health Mission (NRHM), *Guidelines on Accredited Social Health Activists (ASHA)*.
30. Pharmacy Council of India, *Objections of Pharmacy Council of India to proposed amendment in Schedule K against serial number 23 of the Drugs and Cosmetic Rules, 1945* (Ref No: 14-150/2015-PCI/6703-08, 27 November 2019); Peethaambaran Kunnathoor, "OPIF Urges Health Ministry Not to Proceed with Its Plan to Amend Schedule K of D&C Rules" (*Pharmabiz*, 17 December 2019) <http://www.pharmabiz.com/NewsDetails.aspx?aid=119983&sid=1> accessed 9 April 2022; Peethaambaran Kunnathoor, "Legalising Nurses and Community Health Workers to Dispense Drugs an Open Challenge against Pharmaceutical Care: TGPA" (*Pharmabiz*, 27 November 2019) <http://pharmabiz.com/NewsDetails.aspx?aid=119607&sid=1> accessed 9 April 2022.
31. Government of India, National Health Systems Resource Centre, *AYUSHMAN BHARAT: Comprehensive Primary*

Health Care through Health and Wellness Centers—Operational Guidelines (2018) 39, s4.1.

32. Syed Intishab Ali, "Over 400 SMS Nurses Strike Work" *The Times of India* (Jaipur, 3 March 2012) <https://timesofindia.indiatimes.com/city/jaipur/over-400-sms-nurses-strike-work/articleshow/12118805.cms> accessed 9 April 2022.
33. *All Kerala Pharmacists Union & Ors vs State of Kerala* WP(C).No.33715 OF 2019(L) before the Kerala High Court decided on 25 February 2021.; *All Kerala Pharmacists Union & Ors vs State of Kerala* W.A. No. 495/2021 before the Kerala HC decided on 13 January 2022).
34. Peethaambaran Kunnathoor, "Legal Notice Served to Health, FDA Authorities in Haryana for Breach of Section 42 of Pharmacy Act" (*Pharmabiz*, 3 September 2019) <http://www.pharmabiz.com/NewsDetails.aspx?aid=117908&sid=1> accessed 9 April 2022.
35. Drugs & Cosmetics Act, 1940 Section 27(b)(ii).
36. *State through Drug Inspector vs Inderjit Singh* S.C. No.2 of 2015 before the Special Court, Ludhiana decided on 17 February 2016.
37. *State of Andhra Pradesh vs Jaggurothu Rambabu* CC No. 146 of 2009 before the Court of the Judicial Magistrate of I Class, Palakol decided on 27 April 2016.
38. Case No. 5 of 2018 before the Court of the Additional Sessions Judge, Panipat decided on 6 June 2018. An appeal against the conviction and sentencing is pending before the High Court.
39. Ajay Bhaskarabhatla et. al., "Hit Where It Hurts: Cartel Policing Using Targeted Sales and Supply Embargoes" (2016) 59 *The Journal of Law and Economics* 80; Ajay Bhaskarabhatla et. al., "Mitigating Regulatory Impact: The Case of Partial Price Controls on Metformin in India" (2017) 32 *Health Policy and Planning* 194.
40. Competition Commission of India, *Policy Note: Making Markets Work for Affordable Healthcare* (October 2018); Prashant Reddy T., "The Correct Prescription" *The Hindu*

(26 February 2019) <https://www.thehindu.com/opinion/op-ed/the-correct-prescription/article26368011.ece> accessed 10 April 2022.

41. *Dr Zaheer Ahmed vs The Union of India* W.P.(C) 11711/2018 & CM APPL. 45307/2018 (Delhi HC, 12 December 2018); *The Tamil Nadu Chemists and Druggists Association vs The Union of India* W.P.No.28716 of 2018 (Madras HC, 17 December 2018); *Practo Technologies (P) Ltd vs Tamil Nadu Chemists and Druggists Assn* 2018 SCC OnLine Mad 3577 (Madras HC, 20 December 2018).
42. Saritha Rai, "India's E-Pharmacy Segment Mints Its First Unicorn, Raises $350 Million" *Business Standard India* (7 April 2021) <https://www.business-standard.com/article/companies/india-s-e-pharmacy-segment-mints-its-first-unicorn-raises-350-million-121040700228_1.html> accessed 10 April 2022; Gireesh Babu, "Online Pharmacies See Record Funding in 2019, Investments Double to $321 Mn" *Business Standard India* (18 January 2020) <https://www.business-standard.com/article/companies/online-pharmacies-see-record-funding-in-2019-investments-double-to-321-mn-120011800340_1.html> accessed 10 April 2022.
43. Government of India, Ministry of Health & Family Welfare, *GSR 220(E)* (*Gazette of India Extraordinary*, Part II–s 3(i), 26 March 2020).
44. Government of India, Ministry of Health & Family Welfare, *GSR 817(E)* (*Gazette of India Extraordinary*, Part II–s 3(i), 28 August 2018).
45. The Drugs & Cosmetics Rules 1945, Rule 65(11)(c).
46. Amber Porterfield, Kate Engelbert and Alberto Coustasse, "Electronic Prescribing: Improving the Efficiency and Accuracy of Prescribing in the Ambulatory Care Setting" (2014) 11 *Perspectives in Health Information Management* 1g.

CHAPTER NINE

Of Drug Advertisements, Promotions and Trademarks

In 2008, Indian television witnessed the launch of an unprecedented advertising campaign for "i-Pill", an emergency contraceptive pill (ECPs) for women looking to avoid pregnancies after unprotected sex. The advertisements featured women of differing ages and marital status worrying about a possible pregnancy before they are reassured by a companion or the voiceover that they could avert a pregnancy by consuming ECPs.[1]

While ECPs had already been available over the counter in India for a few years, the advertising campaign in 2009 was justified by pharmaceutical companies as a way to empower women to take decisions about their sexual health by educating them about the existence of ECPs.[2] Sure enough, the sales of ECPs reportedly shot through the roof after that advertising campaign—increasing four times from 2008 to 2013![3] Clearly, the pharmaceutical industry had tapped into an unmet need amongst Indian women.

However, not everyone was happy with this advertising campaign. There was an outcry from doctors, who were the traditional information intermediaries between the pharmaceutical industry and patients. Many of them worried about the tone and tenor of the advertisements, which they felt could mislead young women into thinking that ECPs could be used as substitutes for regular contraceptives leading to the improper use of these pills and possible side-effects.[4] There is some evidence from surveys to justify this argument made by doctors about a significant number of women mistaking ECPs as a regular contraceptive without understanding the possible side-effects of long-term use.[5] These advertisements also ran into legal trouble because of an ancient law called the Drugs & Magic Remedies (Objectionable Advertisements) Act, 1954.[6]

This string of controversies over advertisements for ECPs provoked a rare public conversation in India on the many issues surrounding the advertisement and promotion of drugs by pharmaceutical companies. Since then, there have been multiple occasions on which the issue of pharmaceutical companies funding medical conferences for doctors has made the headlines. Yet, the regulatory framework for advertisements by the pharmaceutical industry has remained largely unchanged since 1954, despite the nature of medicine, the Indian pharmaceutical industry and the mode of advertisements undergoing a revolution of sorts in the last seven decades.

The early debates on regulating drug labelling and advertising

Historically, drug advertising has been one of the focal points of governments looking to regulate the pharmaceutical industry because it is through these advertisements that the general public, doctors and their elected representatives noticed the extravagant claims made by the pharmaceutical industry. In India, the issue was debated in the Council of States in 1927, especially in context of advertisements for "patent and proprietary" medicine, which at the time were basically secret remedies whose ingredients were not publicly disclosed and known only to the manufacturer.[7]

In 1931, when the Drugs Inquiry Committee under Lt. Col. Ramnath Chopra submitted its final report to the government, it documented in detail over five whole pages, numerous examples of astonishingly absurd advertisements made by manufacturers of various cures.[8] Here are a few examples:

> "Cures snake bites on inhalation only."
>
> "It cleans the blood, purifies it and infuses strength-giving properties into it. To those who had left youth behind and feel its want, this tonic will bring back good health quickly, positively and permanently."
>
> "Cures menstrual disorders of every kind, hysteria, rheumatism, sterility, etc., improves the general state of the blood. Most effective in bringing the reproductive functions of women into perfect order."
>
> "Sure remedy for helping expectant ladies to give birth to male children only. Male offspring guaranteed."

> "To increase sex power. Stands unique. A dose or two invigorate and rejuvenate the weak and the impotent."
>
> "Become young again. Sensational discovery by German scientist. It gives youthful freshness, energy and appearance once more, puts an end to sexual trouble, mental fatigue, nervous breakdown and neurasthenia in man and they can be retained for years in certain circumstances."
>
> "Latest wonderful discovery for unyielding urinary diseases. Specific for gonorrhea."
>
> "Diabetes cured at last. Amazing cure endorsed by thousands of eminent doctors."

All of these advertisements were clearly fraudulent for that era. In fact, most of them would be fraudulent even today despite the progress of modern science.

Apart from advertising in the mass media, the purveyors of drugs in that era also advertised in medical journals such as the *Indian Medical Gazette* whose main readership comprised the medical community. Yet another marketing tactic was for salespersons to visit the offices of doctors and provide them with promotional literature featuring fantastical claims and patient testimonials about individual drugs.

Given the nature and volume of these advertisements, it was no surprise that the Drugs Inquiry Committee received significant feedback on the issue leading it to conclude that, "Rigid control over advertisements is a point over which there is unanimity."[9] The committee looked at these advertisements as not just a public health issue that could mislead citizens but also as an issue of vulgarity and obscenity that offended public morals. The committee stated, "The disgust and annoyance aroused by the advertisements is nothing compared to the untold harm they inflict on the people."[10]

The Committee received suggestions ranging from an outright ban to prior censorship by the government, to prior vetting of the claims made in these advertisements by doctors with expertise in the area. Surprisingly, the Committee took a very restrained view on the issue of regulating drug advertisements, most likely because of its view that "control over advertisements" could lead to "undue interference in legitimate trade in certain cases."[11] As a result, the committee made only two recommendations with regard to regulation of advertisements of patent and proprietary medicine.

The *first* recommendation was a complete prohibition on any advertisements relating to "aphrodisiacs, venereal diseases, remedies for the diseases of women, cures for cancer, leprosy and tuberculosis." The first three categories appear to be inspired by a need to regulate "obscene" advertisements. The latter three categories of diseases in the committee's recommendation—cancer, leprosy and tuberculosis—were most likely included out of concern for public health, since it was well-known that there existed no cures or treatment, at that point in time, for these diseases.

The *second* recommendation made by the committee was a prohibition on "false, misleading or exaggerated claims...on the labels, wrappers or advertisements".[12]

The committee was entirely silent on how such a determination would be made. Unlike today, in 1931, there was no requirement for pharmaceutical companies to submit clinical data regarding the safety and efficacy of new drugs. So how then was anybody, whether government or the courts, to determine the accuracy or lack thereof of a certain claim made in an advertisement? This major policy issue was left unanswered by the Drugs Inquiry Committee in its final report submitted in 1931.

Nine years later, after one failed attempt in 1937, the Government of India introduced a new Drugs Bill in the Federal Legislature in 1940. In the intervening years, stakeholders like the All India Medical Conference had continued to pressure the government to enact legislation prohibiting the "publication of obscene literature and advertisements advocating the claims of the efficacy of various drugs and appliances", "controlling and regulating the public advertisements of patent and proprietary medicines", etc.[13]

When the Drugs Bill, 1940 was introduced in the legislature, more than one legislator raised the issue of regulating drug advertising.

For its part, the government explained to legislators, that it incorporated two clauses to tackle the extravagant claims made by the pharmaceutical industry.[14] The first was a provision on misbranding, which made it an offence for a drug to feature on its labelling any "statement, design or device which makes any false claim for the drug or which is false or misleading in any particular."[15] A second provision in the Bill delegated to the Federal Government (for import) and Provincial Governments (for domestic manufacture) the power to make rules specifying "the diseases or ailments which a drug may not purport or claim to cure or mitigate and such other effects which a drug may not purport or claim to have."[16] This power eventually translated into Rule 106 of the Drugs & Cosmetics Rules, 1945 which forbade any drug from claiming to cure any of the 34 categories of diseases/ailments mentioned in Schedule J to the Drugs Rules, 1945.

The fact of the matter, however, was that the Drugs Act, 1940 did not create an effective enough framework to regulate drug advertisements. To begin with, a large loophole in the Drugs Act, 1940 was that it entirely excluded Ayurvedic and Unani cures from the definition of "drug". This meant that purveyors of Ayurvedic and Unani cures could make all kinds of unsubstantiated claims without attracting any penalties under the law.

The second problem with the Drugs Act, 1940 was that the "misbranding" provision was limited to only the labelling of the drug and would technically not cover advertisements in the press. Even with respect to inflated claims on the labelling of drugs, it would have been quite difficult for drug inspectors to prosecute such cases before criminal courts because they would have to present scientific evidence to prove, beyond a reasonable doubt that the claims in question were exaggerated.

Third, the wording of Rule 106 was strange in that it did not specifically prohibit advertisements. Rather it prohibited a "drug" from purporting or claiming to cure the 34 listed diseases/ailments. To further complicate matters, given the scheme of the Drugs Act 1940 (prior to 1955) each province was free to draft its own version of Rule 106 (which applied only to imports) meaning that India did not have a uniform scheme that was applicable across the country despite being a common market through which goods could move easily.

The failure of the Drugs Act, 1940 to create an effective framework to govern advertisements became obvious when a few years after its enactment, the DTAB, which was a newly created statutory board under the Drugs Act, conveyed to the government, "the necessity for legislation to prevent advertising" of secret remedies including Ayurvedic and Unani medicine in the press and cinema.[17]

Even medical journals, like the prestigious *Indian Medical Gazette,* lamented about the quality of advertisements that it was receiving from the pharmaceutical industry during the war years. It complained as follows:

> We will quote a few examples of advertisements which have recently been rejected by this journal. Some have been "infallible cures" of malaria but containing "no quinine or arsenic". One remedy was guaranteed "to cure every case of dysentery" within a few days. One remedy was an arrowroot preparation said to be an excellent food for infants. Others have been "sovereign

> remedies" for "all respiratory diseases" including, one supposes, tuberculosis. One advertisement stated that the product cured most fevers, but if the fever had not subsided after a few weeks' treatment, a doctor should be consulted! Some advertisements have been rejected, not because the remedy appeared to be useless, but because the claims made for it were grossly exaggerated and un-scientific.[18]

The editorial ended with a plea to advertisers, asking them to send for publication only "good, simple, straightforward, informative and attractive advertisements" but refrained from asking the government to enact any legislative measures in this regard.[19]

It would take another decade for India to enact a new law regulating drug advertisements—this time under a new Constitution adopted by a newly independent India in 1950.

A new law and a constitutional challenge

In 1953, responding to the increasing complaints about the kind of advertisements being published by the pharmaceutical industry, the government , introduced in the Rajya Sabha a new legislation called the Drugs and Magic Remedies (Objectionable Advertisements) Bill to regulate drug advertisements.

In her introductory remarks before the Rajya Sabha the Minister of Health Amrita Kaur explained the reason for introducing such a Bill in Parliament in the following words:

> In recent years there has been a great increase in the number of objectionable advertisements relating to certain diseases and these advertisements border on the obscene—in fact they are obscene—and in addition they cause the ignorant and the unwary to resort to self-medication with very harmful drugs and appliances and even to resort to quacks who indulge in such advertisements and offer treatment which causes very great harm.[20]

As evident from the Minister's introduction, the primary purpose of the legislation was to deal with obscene advertisements while protecting public health and preventing self-medication remained a secondary objective. Except, the issue of obscenity could have easily been dealt under the Indian Penal Code, 1860 (which had long since made obscenity an offence) rather than through a law whose primary concern should have been protecting public health. The nature of the proposed prohibitions gives a clearer picture of the priorities of the government of the day. The Bill specifically prohibited three categories of advertisements.

The first category of prohibited advertisements included those making false or misleading claims about any drug and its effects.

A second category of prohibited advertisements were those publicising "magic remedies", which was defined in the law as any "talisman, mantra, kavacha and any other kind of charm" claiming to "possess miraculous powers".

The third category of prohibited advertisements

were for those drugs promising "the procurement of miscarriage in women or prevention of conception in women," "the maintenance or improvement of the capacity of human beings for sexual pleasure," "the correction of menstrual disorder in women" and "the diagnosis, cure, mitigation, treatment or prevention of any venereal diseases or any other disease or condition which may be specified in rules made under this Act."[21] This prohibition was likely motivated by complaints of obscenity in advertisements for drugs related to these diseases.

During the course of the parliamentary debates, most MPs expressed their support for the bill, often recounting instances of both bizarre advertisements and instances of quackery that they had witnessed across the country. One MP spoke of a boy in Travancore who offered magic cures, of a man who offered "cure-all" medical powder to treat children's diseases, of an advertisement for *kumari* pills offering assistance to *kumaris* who missed their menses and lastly, an advertisement for a stimulant that would provide for gradual and complete rejuvenation for old people.[22] Other MPs described advertisements of tonics that promised old people that they would become young and that the ugly would become beautiful, oils that would turn white hair into black, etc.[23] A few MPs were skeptical about the bill. Some questioned the government on how it would establish whether a claim was misleading and others wondered whether the bill gave the government draconian powers over the press, which also fell under the purview of this law.

In any event, the Bill was passed by the Lok Sabha and received presidential assent, thereby giving India a second law on drug regulation after the Drugs & Cosmetics Act, 1940. Most notably however, unlike the former, the Drugs & Magic Remedies (Objectionable Advertisements) Act, 1954 applied to even Ayurvedic and Unani medicines since the definition of "drug" in this law (unlike the one in the Drugs & Cosmetics Act, 1940) did not specifically exclude traditional medicine. This was perhaps the most significant aspect of this bill because it brought in for the first time some form of regulation of a previously unregulated sector that had so far been allowed to make all kinds of unsubstantiated claims without facing any legal liability.

After the law was enacted and enforcement actions picked up, two entities—Hamdard Dawakhana, a manufacturer of Unani remedies and Sadhana Ausadhalaya, a manufacturer of Ayurvedic medicine—were the first to challenge the constitutionality of the Drugs & Magic Remedies (Objectionable Advertisements) Act, 1954 before the Supreme Court.[24]

Both the petitioners argued that the Drugs & Magic Remedies (Objectionable Advertisements) Act, 1954 curtailed their right to advertise their products and infringed on their fundamental right to free speech, enshrined in Article 19(1)(a) of the Constitution of India. They also argued that it was unconstitutional for Parliament to delegate to the government the power to decide the list of diseases for which advertisements could be banned, without laying down any parameters to guide the exercise of this power by the government.[25] This latter provision prohibited advertisements for drugs aimed at the treatment of any venereal diseases and also "any other disease or condition which may be specified in rules made under this Act."[26] The last leg of the challenge was directed at Section 8 of the Act which gave the government wide and untrammeled search and seizure powers while enforcing the law.

In its defence, the government argued that that this law was meant "to prevent people from self-medicating with regard to various serious diseases" since self-medication had "a deleterious effect on the health of the community" and that it was in the "interest of public health" to regulate drug advertisements.[27]

In a typical case involving a constitutional challenge, the court will have to determine the "reasonableness" of the restriction imposed by the state. The Supreme Court however did not get into the "reasonableness" of the restrictions imposed by the Drugs & Magic Remedies (Objectionable Advertisement) Act, 1954 because it concluded that commercial advertisements did not qualify as the type of "speech" that was protected in Article 19(1)(a) of the Constitution. The court did, however, strike down the provisions giving the government the power to notify any other diseases for which advertisements would be prohibited and also, the provisions which gave the government wide powers to conduct search and seizures. Four years later, Parliament passed amendments to this law and addressed the defects pointed out by Parliament. The amending legislation introduced a list of 54 specific medical conditions for which no advertisements could be published while also delegating power to the government to expand on these conditions in consultation with the DTAB.

The enforcement of the Drugs & Magic Remedies (Objectionable Advertisements) Act, 1954

Since its enactment, the Drugs & Magic Remedies (Objectionable Advertisements) Act, 1954 has been enforced against a range of bizarre advertisements for bewildering products. For instance, in 1975, the Supreme Court heard a case involving an advertisement in the Hindi newspaper *Sanmarg* in West Bengal, for a "machine of science and electric treatment" to treat amongst other conditions weakness, laziness, aging etc. The conviction and penalty of ₹100 imposed by the lower courts was upheld by the Supreme Court.[28]

In 1982, the Bombay High Court heard an appeal against the conviction of the proprietor of a store called "Breast Beauty Stores" because he had advertised a device called "Bust Developer" for the "proper development of breasts of a woman". This was in violation of Sr. 21 of prohibited diseases/conditions contained in the schedule to the Drugs & Magic Remedies (Objectionable Advertisements) Act, which read as follows: "Form and structure of the female bust". Surprisingly, the Bombay High Court set aside the conviction by the lower court on the grounds that the very concept of objectionable advertisement had changed from 1954 when the law was enacted and that courts had to keep in mind the "new environment of permissive culture emerging around us."[29]

In a case heard by the Madras High Court in 1990 involving an advertisement in the Tamil weekly *Kalkandu* for a "Durka Ayurveda Tumbler", it was claimed that water drunk from the tumbler was capable of controlling diabetes, blood pressure, weakness, etc.[30] The court refused to stay the investigation by the drug inspector in this case.

In states like Kerala, this legislation has served as a useful, though not always successful, handle for public-spirited NGOs and individuals to campaign against the sale of products like "Musli Power Xtra" which was marketed as having the capacity to increase sexual pleasure.[31] For example, in 2017 a public interest litigation was filed before the Kerala High Court, impleading the Drug Controllers of Kerala along with many popular print and broadcast media organizations, asking the court to issue orders for rigorous enforcement of the law against unscientific and misleading advertisements. The government responded by informing the court that it was enforcing the law and that 137 actions under the Drugs & Magic Remedies (Objectionable Advertisements) Act were pending before various trial courts in Kerala.[32]

There have, however, been cases where courts have stayed prosecutions under this law. In one such case in Delhi, the Delhi High Court simply refused to allow the prosecution of an advertisement in the

Hindustan Times for a new technology developed by Bosch and Lomb to treat "cataract", which is Sr. No. 7 in the schedule to the Drugs & Magic Remedies (Objectionable Advertisements) Act, 1954 containing a list of conditions for which advertisements are not permitted. The court reasoned that the law was meant to prevent self-medication and that it was impossible for prospective patients to self-medicate with the technology being advertised.[33]

All of the above examples are mostly judgements rendered by High Courts hearing appeals or petitions to stay prosecutions. It is much more difficult tracking prosecutions before trial courts as these orders unlike High Court orders are not reported in private law journals and databases. To complicate matters further, various drug controllers do not proactively disclose their prosecutions on their websites. However, we did manage to get our hands on a set of approximately 85 judgements from trials courts, through the e-courts database, mainly in Andhra Pradesh, Kerala and Maharashtra, delivered in prosecutions under the Drugs & Magic Remedies (Objectionable Advertisements) Act. These judgements were mostly delivered over the last decade.

Of the 24 judgements from Maharashtra that we could access, in 15 cases, the accused pled guilty to the charges and were fined between ₹1,000 to ₹50,000. None were sentenced to imprisonment. This was true even for a case where the seized products had labels claiming to be able to treat cancer, cardiac conditions, blood pressure, malaria, typhoid and improve the central nervous system. The accused in this case, who was the proprietor of Cura Pharmaceuticals, voluntarily pled guilty to the charges but was let off with a fine of ₹5,000 per product seized, totaling ₹40,000.[34] This, despite the law allowing for an imprisonment of up to six months for first time offenders and up to one year for repeat offenders.

In another case, where two firms were charged with violating the Drugs & Magic Remedies (Objectionable Advertisement) Act, 1954 because they were advertising and selling a tablet for the cure of AIDS, a syrup to improve memory in children and an oil for sexual pleasure, the accused declined to plead guilty and faced a criminal trial before the Chief Judicial Magistrate, Pune. The court found both firms guilty of the offences.[35] As with the cases where the accused voluntarily pled guilty, the court in this case too imposed a paltry fine of ₹40,000 without sentencing anybody to prison.

In another judgement against Lupin Laboratories, the company was being prosecuted for a product called "U-Sedate", which was marketed by its Natural Product Division as useful treatment for the "Management of Menorrhagia, Metrorrhagia and dysfunctional uterine bleeding." The Judicial Magistrate at Aurangabad found the company guilty in 2009, 12 years after the case was first filed. In particular, the labelling was found to violate the prohibitions in Sr. 12 (disease of the uterus), 13 (disease of menstrual flow) and 18 (female diseases) of the Schedule to the Drugs & Magic

Remedies (Objectionable Advertisement) Act, 1954. Despite concluding that the guilty company deserved the maximum punishment permissible under the law, the Judicial Magistrate imposed only a monetary fine of ₹50,000, refusing to sentence anybody in the management to imprisonment.[36]

We noticed similar trends in cases that were prosecuted in Andhra Pradesh. Of the 33 randomly selected judgements from this state, there were 12 convictions after trial, while in the remaining 21 cases the accused pled guilty. In all of these cases the courts only fined the accused between ₹3,000 to ₹60,000 without sending a single offender to prison. This was true even in cases involving products claiming to treat serious conditions like diabetes, ulcers, kidney stones and asthma.[37]

In one set of cases, the court of the Judicial Magistrate in Atmakur, in Nellore District of Andhra Pradesh found the same firm—Ayurgen Herbals—guilty of violating the Drugs & Magic Remedies (Objectionable Advertisements) Act, 1954 in 11 cases that were simultaneously filed against it by a drug inspector for selling an assortment of tonics, extracts and capsules for a range of conditions that included diabetes, asthma, menstrual disorders, rheumatism, ulcers, fever, weight loss and impotence. Despite this gross violation of the law including clearly false advertising for serious conditions like diabetes and asthama, the magistrate only imposed a fine of ₹5,000 in each case.[38]

Things were no different in Kerala. In all 15

judgements that we were able to access, the courts found the accused guilty of the offences charged under the Drugs & Magic Remedies (Objectionable Advertisements) Act, 1954 but the only penalty slapped on the accused were minor fines. In only one case did the judicial magistrate sentence a person to serve three months in prison (in addition to a fine of ₹10,000) for stocking and selling a drug "Musli Power Xtra" which described itself on the label as an "aphrodisiac" capable of solving "erectile problems".[39] On appeal, however, the Sessions Judge set aside the sentence of imprisonment on the grounds that the fine was sufficient.[40]

There are four aspects that really stand out from a reading of these judgments. *First* that almost all the cases involve Ayurvedic or "natural" drugs, some of which were even licensed by drug controllers in different states, *second* that the management and editors of newspapers in which advertisements are published are almost never prosecuted and *third* that almost nobody is sentenced to imprisonment under this law, despite being found guilty of gross violations of the law—including in cases where false claims were made of treating serious life-threatening diseases such as cancer, AIDs etc. A *fourth* observation is that in the absence of legislative guidance on the issue of fines, judges are imposing arbitrary and inconsequential fines, without providing any reasoning. As obvious from the cases being discussed above, the Drugs & Magic Remedies (Objectionable Advertisements) Act,

1954 is not enforced very strictly by the courts. It is unlikely that this law has a serious deterrent effect since potential offenders are aware that they will escape serious punishment. The complete impotence of this law was on display when in a brazen violation of the law, Patanjali Ayurved, the company founded by Baba Ramdev, published advertisements on the front pages of most influential English-language newspapers, for Ayurvedic products that claimed to treat diabetes, cardiac diseases and liver disorders in 2022.[41] These advertisements caused a huge controversy and the matter eventually landed up before the courts in long-drawn proceedings. The brazenness of the entire exercise was a sign that neither the newspapers nor Patanjali had any fear of facing serious punishment under the law.

The loophole for drug advertisements in promotional literature directed at the medical practitioners

When the Drugs & Magic Remedies (Objectionable Advertisement) Act, 1954 was enacted, it contained a large carve out for drug advertisements that were published in medical journals or drug promotional literature that is sent directly to medical practitioners in a confidential manner. These two categories of advertisements are excluded from the purview of the Drugs & Magic Remedies (Objectionable Advertisement) Act, 1954.[42] The rationale for this exclusion appears to have been that doctors cannot be fooled by pharmaceutical companies.

These advertisements in journals and drug promotional literature supplied directly to doctors are critical cogs in the marketing efforts of pharmaceutical companies since it is doctors at the end of the day who prescribe drugs to patients. If a pharmaceutical company can convince a doctor of the efficacy and safety of its new drug, it will result in additional sales because the doctor is likely to prescribe the drug to more patients.

A consistent problem, however, with drug advertisements in medical journals and drug promotional literature in India is the fact that much of the information in these publications is either incomplete or inaccurate. According to the WHO's guidelines for ethical drug promotion, all advertisements targeted at doctors should contain the following information: the name of the active ingredient or the International Non-Proprietary Name (INN), the approved generic name of the drug, the brand name, the content of active ingredient per dosage form, name of other ingredients known to cause problems, approved therapeutic uses, dosage forms, side-effects and major adverse drug reactions, precautions, warnings and contraindications, major interactions, name and address of manufacturer or distributor and reference to scientific literature as appropriate.[43] A significant portion of drug advertising and promotional literature in India fails to meet this criteria and there is no shortage of studies documenting this problem.

In 1992, in a small study published in the *Indian*

Journal of Physiology and Pharmacology by researchers from the Mahatma Gandhi Institute of Medical Sciences, the authors studied 903 drug advertisements published in Indian medical journals to discover that only 8.86% of the advertisements referenced the possible side-effects and major adverse reactions; while only 9.63% of the advertisements mentioned the "precaution, contra-indications and warnings" and only a pitiful 2.77% mentioned the "major interactions".[44]

In 1997, a group of researchers from the renowned Jawaharlal Institute of Postgraduate Medical Education and Research conducted another small study on drug advertisements published in the Indian edition of the *British Medical Journal.* The study was then published in the *British Medical Journal.* It demonstrated how advertisements in the Indian edition of the *BMJ* were likely to be more misleading and make more unsubstantiated claims, when compared to the British edition of the *BMJ.*[45] The researchers also picked 10 advertisements at random and sent them to international experts for a review. The response of these experts revealed the serious magnitude of misleading advertisements even in reputed journals like the *BMJ.* For example, for a drug called Pentoxifylline, an advertisement in the Indian edition made therapeutic claims that the manufacturer did not dare make in America or Britain. For another drug called Diclofenac, the manufacturer claimed the drug was gentle on the gastrointestinal tract despite it being well-known that the drug had a high incidence of gastrointestinal side-effects. In another advertisement for Ciprofloxacin, the advertisement claimed "super power in your hands" without providing basic information like contra-indications or side-effects.[46]

In their response, the editors of the Indian edition of the *BMJ*, outlined the three-fold challenge they faced while dealing with advertisements from the Indian pharmaceutical industry. The first was the lack of laws in India as they existed in the USA where the accuracy of drug advertisements is regulated; the second was the lack of effective consumer watchdog groups and third, the large presence of ayurvedic and other traditional medicines which are widely used despite the lack of adequate scientific data supporting the claims they make. The editors also explained their efforts to instruct advertisers on the editorial policy of the *BMJ* and how internal review committees were setup to vet advertisements leading to rejections of advertisements. Ultimately, they simply passed the buck to doctors who were the final consumers of such advertisements by making a case for doctors and medical students to be better educated so as to increase their ability to recognize misleading advertisements.[47]

The situation appears to be significantly worse in the case of drug promotional literature provided directly to doctors by pharmaceutical salespersons.

In a study on drug promotional literature that was published in the *Indian Journal of Pharmacology* in 2010, researchers studied 134 promotional leaflets that were given to medical practitioners. An analysis of the claims made in the drug promotional literature found that 20% of the claims were exaggerated, 32% were inconclusive, 17% were false and only 21% were authentic. The study concluded that its findings were similar to other studies in developing countries and that there was a dire need for the supply of unbiased information to medical practitioners.[48] Other studies have reported similar findings.[49]

To be certain, the issue of providing unbiased information to medical practitioners is not unique to India. It is a global problem. Pharmaceutical companies often devise deceptive "promotional literature" under the guise of providing medical education to doctors. Common transgressions are to highlight marginal improvements in outcomes based on a small or a limited clinical study without disclosing the study design. The problem is exacerbated in India due to lack of strict laws, regulatory oversight and lax editorial standards followed by domestic publications.

Despite the fact that these advertisements in journals and promotional literature are widely published, it hardly features on the reform agenda of the government which is yet to commission a single official study on the issue. In 2014, a voluntary marketing code called the Uniform Code for Pharmaceutical Marketing Practices (UCPMP) was brought in by the Department of Pharmaceutical, Ministry of Chemicals & Fertilizers for the pharmaceutical industry. The Department is entirely silent on the law which gives it this power to introduce such a voluntary code. That said, this Code includes the WHO's criteria for ethical advertising. But given that it is voluntary, it is also toothless and has little effect on the ground.

The regulatory vacuum around confusing pharmaceutical brand names in India

One of the key components of any marketing campaign by a pharmaceutical company for a new drug is the trademark/brand name adopted by a pharmaceutical company. An easy-to-remember brand name is all the more important in the case of the pharmaceutical industry since the chemical name or even the "International Non-Proprietary Name" (INN) chosen by WHO is often too complicated for the general public to remember.

Patients are more likely to remember the brand name "Crocin" coined by Glaxosmithkline, rather than "Paracetamol" which is the INN. The INN will always be complex because it has to reflect certain chemical characteristics of the drug as per the naming conventions adopted by WHO. For example, all drugs of a certain class may share the same "stem" as a suffix. All, cancer drugs that are Tyrosine Kinase inhibitors will have "tinib" as a suffix and all anti-virals will have "vir" as a suffix. Marketing departments of pharmaceutical companies are not bound by similar naming conventions and can pick and choose fancy brand names that work better from a marketing perspective. All these brand names will generally be protected as registered trademarks and depending on the commercial success of the drug and the marketing campaign around it, the trademark in itself can become a valuable asset for a pharmaceutical company.

Given the centrality of the brand name in the marketing process, most developed countries have very strict regulations on the type of names that can be chosen by pharmaceutical companies to brand their products. The USFDA has two divisions to carry out this analysis: the Division of Medication Error, Prevention & Analysis (DMEPA) which conducts a safety review to prevent possible confusion with other drug names and the Office of Prescription Drug Promotion (OPDP) which evaluates proposed proprietary names to determine "if they are overly fanciful, so as to misleadingly imply unique effectiveness or composition".[50] The USFDA also releases detailed guidance documents for the industry explaining the factors that must be kept in mind while choosing a brand name.[51] The EMA has a "name review group" to perform reviews of brand names submitted by pharmaceutical companies from a safety and promotional aspect.[52] Both regulators take this issue of brand names very seriously. At one point, the EMA was rejecting more brand names than it was accepting.[53] Similarly, the USFDA at one point was rejecting around 50% of the brand names submitted to it.[54]

The reason that the Americans and Europeans take this issue so seriously is the fact that errors in medications due to confusion between brand names could have dire consequences for patients.

Unlike in the USA and Europe, the Indian drug regulator does not perform any review of the brand names/trademarks of pharmaceutical products being sold in India. This is because the Ministry of Health has not put in place any regulations requiring the Indian drug regulator to conduct such a review. This, despite thousands of pharmaceutical trademarks being registered in India every year by the Trade Mark Registry under the Trade Marks Act, 1999. The annual reports of the Intellectual Property Office reveal that the annual number of trademarks registered under Class 5, which pertains to pharmaceuticals, increased from 2,634 in 2002–2003 to 41,351 in 2020! The total number of pharmaceutical trademarks registered under the Trade Marks Act, 1999 between 2002 and 2020 stands at an incredible 327,681! In addition, it is possible that some pharmaceutical companies do not register their brand names under the Trade Marks Act, 1999 because there is no legal necessity to do so under the law. The above numbers should be understood in context of the National List of Essential Medicines (NLEM) announced by the Government of India in 2011 which contains only 348 medicines.

The sheer volume of registered trademarks for pharmaceuticals are an indication of intense competition in the Indian pharmaceutical market but who exactly is reviewing these trademarks from a medical perspective? It is no secret that the review performed by the Trade Mark Registry is very limited and not thorough since the Registry has been understaffed with a huge backlog. Even in theory, the review by the Trade Mark Registry is limited to similarity of the proposed mark to existing marks in the Registry's database and the likelihood of confusion caused by the similarity to the average consumer. Such a review is unlike the medical review conducted by regulators in Europe and the USA of every brand name from a perspective of public health.

It should then be no surprise when different Indian pharmaceutical companies end up using the same or similar brand names for marketing different drugs. Our research assistant managed to compile the following list of identical brand names being used by pharmaceutical companies for entirely different medications:

Brand Name	*Indication*
Zita Vital	Zita Vitamin (Premium nutrition for 28–40 week pregnancy).
Zita-100 mg	Treats type 2 diabetes mellitus in adults.
AZ (10 mg)	An antihistamine, used for allergic reactions.
AZ Plus Suspension (10ml)	It is used to treat infections caused by worms.
AZ (500 mg)	Antibiotic for treating bacterial infections such as the infections of the middle ear, typhoid and chancroid etc.
Visol eye drops	Used to relieve dry, irritated eyes.
Vizole capsules	Prescribed for Cancer treatment.
Ofloren eye drops	It is used in treating infections of the urinary tract, nose, throat, skin and soft tissues, and lungs (pneumonia).

Ofloren 200 mg tablets	Use is the same as that of Ofloren Eye drops, however, the dosage is very different.
Clomine 25mg tablet	It is used in adults to treat obsessive-compulsive disorder (OCD).
Clomin Drops	To treat stomach pain, bloating, and abdominal cramps, and pain associated with excessive acidity, gas, infections, and gastrointestinal tract diseases.
Medzole 400 tablets	Used to treat infections caused by worms.
Medzole 40	Gas relief tablets.
Medzol 1 mg injection	Used for sedation in intensive care units and to obtain anesthesia in elderly people before undergoing any surgical procedure.

The above list of examples is not exhaustive and covers only cases where the brand names are identical. The list of cases where the brand names are only similar and not identical likely runs into hundreds. The King Edward Memorial Hospital in Mumbai has compiled a helpful list of few of the similar sounding brand names for different drugs, which is reproduced below.[55]

Brand name	*Generic drug*	*Clinical use*
Tab. Aldactone Inj. Aldarone	Spironolactone Amiodarone	Diuretic Anti-arrhythmic
Inj. Amicom Inj. Amicor	Amikacin Amrinone	Anti-microbial Congestive heart failure

Bactroban cream Batrafen cream	Mupirocin (2%) Ciclopirox oleamine	Topical anti-microbial Topical anti-fungal
Tab. Cadolac Tab. Carloc	Ketorolac Carvedilol	NSAID Non-selective beta blocker
Tab. Cetrine Inj. Cytarine	Cetrizine Cytarabine	Anti-histaminic Anti-neoplastic
Tab. Combutol Tab. Carbatol	Ethambutol Carbamazepine	Anti-tubercular Anti-convulsant
Cap. Dilantin Tab. Dilcontin	Phenytoin Diltiazem	Anti-convulsant Anti-hypertensive
Tab. Epitril Tab. Enapril	Clonazepam Enalapril	Anti-convulsant Angiotensin converting enzyme inhibitor
Cap. Moclox Cap. Macox	Amoxacillin + cloxacillin Rifampicin	Anti-microbial Anti-leprotic
Cap. Neurontin Tab. Nitrocontin	Gabapentin Glyceryl trinitrate	Anti-convulsant Anti-anginal
Tab. Opam Cap. Opaz	Pioglitazone Omeprazole	Oral anti-diabetic Proton pump inhibitor
Inj. Oframax Inj. Okavax	Ceftriaxone Live attenuated vaccine of varicella zoster	Anti-microbial Vaccine
Tab. Rapilin Tab. Ranitin	Repaglinide Ranitidine	Anti-diabetic Histamine receptor 2 antagonist

Tab. Rokcin Tab. Roxin	Roxithromycin Thyroxine	Anti-microbial Hormone
Tab. Tricort Tab. Tricox	Triamcinolone Rifampicin + Isoniazid + Pyrazinamide	Corticosteroid Anti-tubercular
Inj. Vasopin Tab. Vasoprin	Vasopressin Isosorbide mononitrate + Aspirin	Bleeding esophageal varices Vasodilator + platelet inhibitor
Tab. Zetop Inj. Zyrop	Cetrizine Erythropoietin	Anti-histaminic Haemopoietic

Even worse is when the same pharmaceutical company uses the same brand name for different drugs. Take for example, the case of I-Pill, which was initially marketed as an ECP to prevent conception. After the thumping success of the advertising campaign around I-Pill, the same company began to use the brand name "I-Pill Daily" to market a daily birth control pill. An ECP is completely different from a daily birth control in that it is taken after unprotected sex in order to prevent pregnancy, while a daily birth control pill stops ovulation. Confusing these two drugs could result in unwanted pregnancies.

As a result of the entire Indian pharmaceutical industry using similar brand names, the industry endlessly litigates against each other on the issue of trademark infringement. The obvious problem with using identical or similar sounding brand names for different drugs that contain different active ingredients is that it increases the possibility of errors in dispensing drugs at pharmacies. In a country like India where self-medication is rampant and most of the population is not familiar with the English language (which is the most commonly used language for pharmaceutical brand names in India), the consequences of using similar sounding brand names can be dire.

Despite being alerted to this issue by both the Supreme Court and the Parliamentary Standing Committee on Health & Family Welfare, the Ministry of Health has been dragging its feet on regulating the use of brand names by pharmaceutical companies in India.

In 2001, the Supreme Court, in a judgement on—*Cadila Healthcare Ltd. vs. Cadila Pharmaceuticals Ltd.*[56]—deciding a case about infringement of a pharmaceutical trademark, had urged the government to put in place a mechanism to ensure that the drug regulator evaluated brand names for drugs before granting manufacturing licences.

In 2012, the Parliamentary Standing Committee on Health & Family Welfare in its scathing review of the functioning of the CDSCO flagged the problem of similar sounding brand names for entirely different drugs, warning the government that, "...this is a highly dangerous situation where wrong medicine can be sold and consumed leading to serious injury."[57] Despite the urging of the committee, the Ministry of Health did little to address the problem.

This inaction by the government continued till 2018 when the government received a gentle judicial nudge from the Delhi High Court. The court reminded the government that:[58]

> The issue of pharmaceutical preparations and medicines being sold under identical brand names has been a concern in a large number of disputes. The said issue is not just one which concerns statutory rights or trademark rights of a particular IP owner, but has a larger impact on the health of the patients.[59]

This time around, after the judicial nudge from the Delhi High Court, the DTAB made a recommendation to implement the Supreme Court's recommendation in the *Cadila* case and the DCC agreed with the recommendation.[60]

On 6 November 2019, the Ministry of Health notified a mutilated version of the Supreme Court's recommendation into law via the Drugs & Cosmetics (Thirteenth Amendment) Rules, 2019.[61] As per these new rules, pharmaceutical companies would now have to submit an undertaking to the state drug controller issuing the manufacturing licence, informing them of the brand/trade name they intended to use to market the drug and that their chosen brand name to the best of their knowledge, was not similar to the name of any existing drug being sold in India, as per a search that they had conducted in databases maintained by the trademark registry, the CDSCO and also in existing literature, reference books and the internet.

The problem with this reform measure is two-fold. *First,* the CDSCO never created the "central database" of pharmaceutical tradenames mentioned in the amendments introduced in 2019. We asked them in a RTI application filed in December 2021 to provide us a weblink to this database. We received a one-line answer from the CDSCO stating "No such information is maintained presently."[62]

The *second* problem with this reform measure is that it failed to impose any obligation on the CDSCO or state drug controller to conduct a review of the brand name from a safety and promotional perspective and reject the use of specific names on the grounds of confusion or safety. There is nothing stopping a pharmaceutical company from submitting an undertaking that it is of the opinion that its chosen brand name is not confusing when compared to existing brand names since the question of similarity is a question of law not fact. Two different people can have different opinions on the similarity of a name, which is why we see so much litigation on trademark infringement around the world. This is exactly why an impartial sovereign authority like a drug regulator must be made responsible for conducting a review of proposed pharmaceutical brand names from a safety and promotional perspective instead of leaving it to the pharmaceutical industry to self-regulate itself.

The reluctance of the Ministry of Health to tackle the situation with well thought out reforms, despite being alerted to the problem by Parliament and the

Supreme Court is telling of its weak commitment to protect public health.

Inter-ministerial chaos on India's drug advertising policy

The Government of India is well aware of the problems with drug advertising in the country but instead of developing and enforcing an integrated policy on the issues of misleading advertisements, promotional literature, labelling and confusing brand names, three different ministries have been announcing different policy initiatives on these issues, often in a piecemeal manner.

The first initiative was announced by the Department of Pharmaceuticals, Ministry of Chemical & Fertilizers in the form of the UCPMP in 2014.[63] The UCPMP was supposed to be a voluntary self-regulating code to regulate advertising by the pharmaceutical industry. It is not clear why the Department of Pharmaceuticals, which is responsible for the growth of the pharmaceutical industry, took up a public health issue like advertising by the pharmaceutical industry, which is within the purview of the Ministry of Health. In fact, the notification by the Department of Pharmaceuticals does not even mention the law under which it is ordering the pharmaceutical industry to adopt the UCPMP.

Then in 2015, the Ministry of Health amended the Drugs & Cosmetics Rules, 1945 to introduce a prohibition on advertising any prescription drugs mentioned in Schedule H, H1 and X without the "previous sanction of the Central Government", except, the rules are entirely silent on the procedure to secure such prior sanction and the grounds on which such sanction may be granted or denied.[64] Six years after this amendment was notified, when we asked the Ministry of Health, in an application under the RTI Act, the procedure to seek its prior sanction for such advertisements, it informed us that it had "no information available" with it and transferred the application to the CDSCO to respond to us.[65] This, despite the fact that it is the Ministry and not the CDSCO that has the power to make rules. The CDSCO then replied informing us that it had no "additional information" to provide.[66] So basically, nobody in the government knows how exactly to grant sanction for the advertisement of a prescription drug despite the law allowing for advertisement after receipt of previous sanction from the government.

The third measure was brought in by the Ministry of Ayush in 2018 when it introduced a provision called Rule 170 to regulate the advertisement of Ayush drugs. That rule was subsequently deleted from the law, by the Ministry, in July 2024 without ever being enforced.[67]

The fourth measure taken by the Ministry of Health was in 2019 when it amended the Drugs & Cosmetics Rules, 1945 (as discussed in the previous section), requiring pharmaceutical companies to self-certify the fact that their own brand names were not similar or causing confusion. This was a pointless measure, as explained earlier.

Apart from these four policy initiatives, the

Ministry of Health in 2020 introduced a draft bill to amend the Drugs & Magic Remedies (Objectionable Advertisements) Act, 1954 to expand the application of the law to the internet, expand the list of diseases covered by the law and to increase the penalties that can be levied on offenders. This Bill is yet to be introduced in Parliament.

This fragmented approach by different ministries is reflective of a chaotic approach towards policy making in India. It is clear that the government is simply tying itself up in knots on a crucial issue that deserves an integrated approach through a single legislation.

The path to future reform and the fundamental right to speech

As is obvious from this chapter, the Government of India needs a consolidated policy and an integrated law that covers all aspects of advertising by the pharmaceutical industry, whether it is targeted at doctors or consumers.

The current system of regulating advertisement and promotions of drugs under the Drugs & Cosmetics Act, 1945 or the Drugs & Magic Remedies (Objectionable Advertisements) Act, 1954 is wholly inadequate, not only because it does not cover many aspects of advertising such as brand names and promotional literature for doctors, but also because it applies ex-post after the advertisements, etc. have already been published and the damage has been caused. A new efficient system should be put in place with a prepublication screening mechanism, where the drug regulator certifies advertisements, brand names and promotional literature before the same are published or used by the pharmaceutical industry publicly. The basis of approving claims made in these advertisements and promotional literature should be the data generated from clinical trials, which are the basis of the drug being approved by the regulator. In particular, attention should be paid to adequate disclosure in all advertisements or promotional literature of the potential and actual side-effects of the drug. Similarly, the brand names of drugs should be closely scrutinised to prevent not just confusion amongst brand names but also the possibility of misleading names from a public health perspective.

Presuming the Parliament enacts a regulatory regime that requires the pharmaceutical industry to secure ex-ante approvals for advertisements, promotional literature and brand names, it would also have to ensure that the drug regulator is provided with the resources to screen all such material thoroughly from a public health perspective. This is a task that can easily drown any regulator unless it is given adequate resources to conduct the job in an efficient manner. Executing such reforms will require immense political will on part of the government given that it is likely to face an exceptional pushback from not just the pharmaceutical industry, but also the newspapers and publishers who currently gain monetarily from such advertisements.

Apart from creating a new ex-ante regulatory regime to regulate advertising, India will also need to tighten existing laws like the Drugs and Magic Remedies (Objectionable Advertisements) Act, 1954 to significantly increase monetary and penal punishments for those making misleading therapeutic claims about their products. The existing law is very lenient and barely enforced by the courts even when drug inspectors prosecute cases of gross violations. At the very least, the law should be sharpened to deter brazen violations. Of course, any such reforms will staunchly be opposed by the Ayurved industry. Whether there is the political will to lock horns with the Ayurved industry, remains to be seen.

Notes

1. Vishakha Talreja, "Morning after, Men Try to Find What's i-Pill" *The Economic Times* (29 September 2007) <https://economictimes.indiatimes.com/industry/healthcare/biotech/pharmaceuticals/morning-after-men-try-to-find-whats-i-pill/articleshow/2413553.cms?from=mdr> accessed 1 December 2021; "i-pill emergency contraceptive pill", Youtube (16 October 2008) <https://www.youtube.com/watch?v=9m1-xAiGC8Y> accessed 1 December 2021.
2. Radhieka Pandeya and Priyanka Mehra, "Morning after Pill Ads Come under Drug Regulator Lens" *Mint* (23 September 2009) <https://www.livemint.com/Consumer/FnjyYJnbO8d6aC0C4qaVmO/Morning-after-pill-ads-come-under-drug-regulator8217s-len.html> accessed 2 December 2021.
3. Anvita Dixit, M.E. Khan and Isha Bhatnagar, "Mainstreaming of Emergency Contraception Pill in India: Challenges and Opportunities" (2015) 40 *Indian Journal of Community*

Medicine: Official Publication of Indian Association of Preventive & Social Medicine 49.

4. Pandeya and Mehra (n 2).
5. Maria Thomas, "A Shocking Proportion of Indians Have Got Morning-after Pills All Wrong" *Quartz* <https://qz.com/india/1408192/indias-overuse-of-i-pill-reveals-a-crisis-of-sex-education/> accessed 1 December 2021.
6. Kounteya Sinha, "Ban on Morning-after Pills' Ads Lifted" *The Times of India* (15 October 2011) <https://timesofindia.indiatimes.com/india/ban-on-morning-after-pills-ads-lifted/articleshow/10360543.cms> accessed 1 December 2021.
7. Council of State Debates 9 March 1927, vol I, 520-522.
8. Government of India, *Report of The Drugs Enquiry Committee* (1930-31) 378-382.
9. ibid 114.
10. ibid 116.
11. ibid.
12. *Report of The Drugs Enquiry Committee* (n 8) 116-117.
13. "Medical News" (1939) 74 *The Indian Medical Gazette* 172, 173.
14. ibid 2235.
15. The Drugs Act 1940, s 9(f) and s 17(f).
16. The Drugs Act 1940, s 12(2)(d) and s 33(2)(f).
17. Drugs Technical Advisory Board (DTAB), "*Minutes of the 3rd Drugs Technical Advisory Board meeting held in the office of the Director General, Indian Medical Service, New Delhi from 23 January 1945 to 26 January, 1945*" (1945) 20.
18. "Advertisements" (1943) 78 *The Indian Medical Gazette* 347.
19. ibid 348.
20. Amrita Kaur, Minister of Health on the Drugs and Magic Remedies (Objectionable Advertisements) Bill 1953, Rajya Sabha Deb 16 February 1954, 75-76.
21. The Drugs & Magic Remedies (Objectionable Advertisements) Act 1954, s 3.

22. Debate on the Drugs and Magic Remedies (Objectionable Advertisements) Bill 1953, Lok Sabha Deb 26 April 1954, 5737, 5740.
23. ibid 5744.
24. *Hamdard Dawakhana (Wakf) Lal Kuan, Delhi & Anr vs Union of India and Others* (1960) 2 SCR 671 (18 December 1959) <https://indiankanoon.org/doc/591481/> accessed 22 December 2021.
25. ibid para 3, 5.
26. The Drugs & Magic Remedies (Objectionable Advertisements) Act 1954, s 3(d) (as originally enacted and before its amendment in 1963).
27. *Hamdard Dawakhana* (n 24) para 4.
28. *Zaffar Mohammed vs State of West Bengal* [1976] 2 SCR 782 <https://indiankanoon.org/doc/1148857/> accessed 23 December 2021.
29. *Smt Kantirani Jayanarayan Mangal vs State of Maharashtra* 1982 Cri LJ 1454 <https://indiankanoon.org/doc/1705154/> accessed 23 December 2021, para 20.
30. *T.K. Kuppuswamy vs Union of India* AIR 1991 Mad 17 (6 April 1990) <https://indiankanoon.org/doc/1385012/> accessed 23 December 2021.
31. *A.S.P. Kurup vs Union of India & Ors* AIR 1983 Ker 259 (15 February 1983) <https://indiankanoon.org/doc/740590/> accessed 23 December 2021; *K.C. Abraham vs State of Kerala* WP(C) No 11410 of 2011 (Kerala HC, 27 June 2011) <https://indiankanoon.org/doc/117903436/> accessed 23 December 2021.
32. *G. Jayaprakash vs State of Kerala* WP(C) No 5740 of 2017 before the Kerala High Court decided on 15 January 2021 <https://indiankanoon.org/doc/70232357/> accessed 23 December 2021.
33. *Amit Singh vs The State* MANU/DE/2191/201.
34. *State of Maharashtra vs Mr Hemant Kumar Sharma, Proprietor of Cura Pharmaceuticals* R.C.C. No. 267/2017 before the Court of Judicial Magistrate First Class at Vashi, District Thane, Maharashtra decided on 9 April 2018).

35. *State of Maharashtra vs Pramod Sakharam Arolkar, Anandi Pharmaceuticals* R.C.C. No. 770 of 2007 before the Court of the Chief Judicial Magistrate at Pune, Maharashtra decided on 29 April 2014).
36. *State of Maharashtra vs Lupin Laboratories* S.C.C. No. 36 of 1997 before the Court of Judicial Magistrate First Class, Aurangabad, Maharashtra decided on 9 September 2009.
37. *State of Andhra Pradesh vs S Vijaya, Proprietor of Balaji Natural Remedies, Apollo Medicare Agencies & Ors* C.C. No. 243 of 2012 before the Court of the IV Addl. Judicial Magistrate of 1st Class, Chittoor, decided on 20 September 2014. (the case involved the advertisement and sale of ASTHMA-ex capsules to give relief for Asthma); *State of Andhra Pradesh vs Shived Herbals, Vign Aayurceuticals & Ors* C.C. No. 902 of 2016 before the Court of Metropolitan Magistrate, Vijaywada, decided on 14 February 2017, (the case involved the advertisement and sale of Pramehnil Liquid for the treatment of diabetes).
38. *State of Andhra Pradesh vs Ayurgen Herbals & Anr* CC. No. 339, 340, 341, 342, 343, 345, 346, 347, 348, 349 & 350 of 2017 before the Court of the Judicial Magistrate of First Class at Atmakur, Nellore District decided on 12 December 2017.
39. *State represented by Drug Inspector vs Kunnath Pharmaceuticals* C.C. No. 640 of 2007 before the Court of the Judicial First Class Magistrate–II, Ernakulam decided on 1 August 2016.
40. *Kunnath Pharmaceuticals vs State represented by Drug Inspector* Crl. Appeal No. 241 of 2016 before the Court of the IInd Addl. District & Sessions Judge, Ernakulam decided on 18 January 2018.
41. Dinesh Thakur & Prashant Reddy T., "When violations aren't penalized: The legality of the Patanjali advertising tsunami" *Newslaundry* (12 February 2022) <https://www.newslaundry.com/2022/02/12/when-violations-arent-penalised-the-legality-of-the-patanjali-advertising-tsunami>.

42. The Drugs & Magic Remedies (Objectionable Advertisement) Act 1954, s 14.
43. World Health Organization, *Ethical criteria for medicinal drug promotion* (1988), 7-8.
44. A. Lal and M.L. Sharma, "Drug Advertisements in Indian Medical Journals" (1992) 36 *Indian Journal of Physiology and Pharmacology* 139.
45. B. Gitanjali et al., "Are Drug Advertisements in Indian Edition of BMJ Unethical?" (1997) 315 *BMJ* 459.
46. ibid.
47. G.G. Christo and R. Balasubramaniam, "Commentary: Advertising Adversities" (1997) 315 *BMJ* (Clinical research ed.) 460.
48. Mangala Bhaskar Murthy and Bhaskar Krishnamurthy, "Authenticity of Claims Made in Drug Promotional Literature" (2010) 42 *Indian Journal of Pharmacology* 59.
49. Gurpreet Kaur Randhawa and others, "A Critical Analysis of Claims and Their Authenticity in Indian Drug Promotional Advertisements" (2015) 2015 *Advances in Medicine* 469147; Puttaswamy Ganashree, Krishnaswamy Bhuvana and Narayana Sarala, "Critical Review of Drug Promotional Literature Using the World Health Organization Guidelines" (2016) 5 *Journal of Research in Pharmacy Practice* 162.
50. The United States Food and Drug Administration (USFDA), *How FDA Reviews Proposed Drug Names.* < https://www.fda.gov/files/drugs/published/How-FDA-reviews-drug-names.pdf> accessed 23 December, 2021.
51. The United States Food and Drug Administration (USFDA), *Best Practices in Developing Proprietary Names for Human Prescription Drug Products: Guidance for Industry* (December 2020).
52. European Medicines Agency, *Mandate, objectives and rules of procedure for the Name Review Group (NRG)* (EMA/411943/2014, 7 October 2019).
53. Ian Schofield, "High Rejection Rate of Proposed Brand Names On EMA Radar" (*Pink Sheet*, 19 May 2017) <https://

pink.pharmaintelligence.informa.com/PS120676/High-Rejection-Rate-of-Proposed-Brand-Names-On-EMA-Radar> accessed 23 December 2021.

54. Laura Helbling, "FDA Rejecting Fewer Proprietary Names" (*Pink Sheet*, 2 January 2015) <https://pink.pharmaintelligence.informa.com/PS079808/FDA-Rejecting-Fewer-Proprietary-Names> accessed 23 December 2021.
55. "Sound Alike Drug Names in the Indian Market" (*King Edward Memorial Hospital*) <https://www.kem.edu/sound-alike-drug-names-in-the-indian-market/> accessed 23 December 2021.
56. *Cadila Healthcare Limited vs Cadila Pharmaceuticals Limited* 2001 PTC 541 (SC).
57. Department Related Parliamentary Standing Committee on Health and Family Welfare, *The Functioning of The Central Drugs Standard Control Organisation (CDCSO)* (Fifty-Ninth Report) (RS 2012) para 11.1.
58. *Curewell Drugs & Pharmaceuticals vs Ridley Life Science Private* CS (COMM) 1071/2018 (Delhi HC, 6 February 2019) <https://indiankanoon.org/doc/188331718/> accessed 23 December 2021.
59. ibid. para 11.
60. Drugs Technical Advisory Board (DTAB), "*MINUTES OF THE 81ST MEETING OF DRUGS TECHNICAL ADVISORY BOARD HELD ON 29TH NOVEMBER, 2018 AT DGHS, NIRMAN BHAWAN, NEW DELHI*" (2018) 6 <https://cdsco.gov.in/opencms/resources/UploadCDSCOWeb/2018/UploadCommitteeFiles/dtab29nov18.pdf> accessed 23 December 2021; Drugs Consultative Committee (DCC), "*MINUTES OF 55TH MEETING OF DRUGS CONSULTATIVE COMMITTEE HELD ON 31ST JANUARY & 01ST FEBRUARY, 2019 AT NEW DELHI*" (2019) 21, Agenda No 15 <https://cdsco.gov.in/opencms/opencms/system/modules/CDSCO.WEB/elements/common_download.jsp?num_id_pk=ODMz> accessed 23 December 2021.

61. The Drugs and Cosmetics (Thirteenth Amendment) Rules 2019.
62. Reply to RTI application dated 12 January 2022, CDSCO (Application No. CDSCO/R/E/21/00594, 13 December 2021).
63. Government of India, Ministry of Chemicals & Fertilizers, *Uniform Code of Pharmaceuticals Marketing Practices (UCPMP)* (F No 5/3/2009-PI-I/PI-II (Vol. III), 12 December 2014).
64. Government of India, Ministry of Health & Family Welfare, *GSR 289(E)* (*Gazette of India Extraordinary*, Part II–s 3(i), 15 April 2015), 2.
65. Reply to RTI application dated 10 December 2021, Ministry of Health and Family Welfare (Application No MOHFW/R/E/21/06748, 19 November 2021).
66. Reply to RTI application dated 12 December 2021, Central Drug Standard Control Organization (Application No MOHFW/R/E/21/06748, 19 November 2021).
67. Refer Chapter 7 for a more detailed discussion around Rule 170.

CHAPTER TEN

The Politics and Levers of Reforming India's Drug Regulatory Framework

The path to reforming India's drug regulatory framework is a minefield of competing interests. It includes not just the obvious stakeholders like the powerful Indian pharmaceutical industry but also the state and union governments, the bureaucracy and public health activists. The first and foremost challenge in the journey towards reform is for India to accept that its pharmaceutical industry has a quality problem, which its regulator is unable to address. This would require the country to accept that every complaint regarding the quality of drugs manufactured by the Indian pharmaceutical industry is not a "conspiracy theory" against the country by foreigners or "anti-national" elements. Once it accepts this problem, India has to consciously choose to protect the public health of its people over the growth, employment and export dollars provided by the Indian pharmaceutical industry.

Presuming the country places public health over and above the commercial interests of the industry, it will have to resolve intense politics on the issue of federalism between the union and state governments, as well as inter-ministerial politics that is opposed to the idea of creating an independent regulator. Then there is intra-bureaucracy politics wherein the cadre of drug inspectors made primarily of pharmacists will do everything in their power to resist surrendering their position and significant powers to more qualified medical professionals. There also exist other levers of reforms, such as increased transparency, guaranteed public participation and an overhaul of public procurement procedures for drugs.

While this journey towards reform may appear overwhelming if not impossible, we are confident that when citizen advocacy is combined with intrepid journalism and watchful parliamentarians, Indian democracy will triumph in forcing the interests of pharmaceutical companies to surrender before the needs of public health of the country. In this chapter, we explain some of these politics of reform along with the levers through which India can hopefully overhaul its drug regulatory framework.

Conspiracy theories and the "victim card"

13 May 2013 was one of the most important days in the history of the Indian pharmaceutical industry. It was on this day that Ranbaxy Laboratories, the "crown jewel" in the growth story of the Indian pharmaceutical industry, pled guilty before an American court to seven felony counts, also agreeing to pay penalties of

$500 million for manufacturing violations at two of its facilities located at Paonta Sahib and Dewas, both in India.[1]

In most countries, a scandal such as the guilty plea entered by one of the country's largest pharmaceutical companies before an American court would have prompted some national soul-searching with citizens and political parties questioning the effectiveness of their own national regulator. Not so in India. This, despite the fact that all of Ranbaxy's manufacturing facilities that were at the center of the scandal were located in India and subject to the scrutiny of Indian law and its regulators. Save for a few individual hospitals and pharmacy chains that expressed concern in the press about the continued consumption of Ranbaxy's drugs by Indian patients, there was little outrage or calls for accountability in the Indian media.[2] In fact, some prominent members of the medical community like Dr Devi Prasad Shetty actively defended the company on television.[3] This muted criticism of Ranbaxy or the country's drug regulator was because the Government of India, the Indian pharmaceutical industry and public health activists all worked in tandem to paint the case against Ranbaxy as a conspiracy to defame the Indian pharmaceutical industry despite the fact that Ranbaxy pled guilty to all the charges!

Here is an account of the events that followed the news about Ranbaxy's guilty plea. The Ministry of Commerce, which has nothing to do with drug regulation in India, published a boisterous press release, on 3 June 2013, mere weeks after Ranbaxy's guilty plea propagating this conspiracy theory. An extract of the press release is reproduced below:

> There are reasons to believe that vested interests are raking up isolated issues reported regarding technical deficiencies on manufacturing and GMP. India is enjoying a unique position of low cost manufacturing and highest quality medicine, best of both the worlds. Government has strong reason to believe that some of the spurious drugs detected in the international markets, alleged to be exported from India, are desperate attempts by other countries getting affected by the strength of Indian pharma industry.[4]

So, who according to the Government of India, were these "vested interests" raking up "isolated issues"? The answer to that question can be found in an earlier statement by the Health Secretary Naresh Dayal in 2008 when the USFDA first announced an import ban on drugs from Ranbaxy into the USA after an inspection revealed serious issues at their manufacturing plant. Dayal was quoted in the Indian press, blaming the ban on Ranbaxy on both the American government and the American pharmaceutical industry. He had said:

> The FDA never had problems with the same drugs earlier. The moment the House (US Congress) committee on trade, commerce and energy created a ruckus, FDA started having problems. All these are non-tariff barriers. There is a huge and growing market for Indian generic drugs in the US and drug lobbies there never want this to happen. Clearly, they

> are putting pressure on FDA. You have to understand there is a vested commercial interest in this.[5]

In effect, Dayal was accusing the USFDA of dancing to the tune of the American pharmaceutical industry; a serious accusation of corruption against a foreign regulator despite there being no evidence to substantiate it. While the Commerce Ministry in 2013 stopped short of naming the American government, the timing of its statement, close on the heels of the Ranbaxy scandal, was a clear indication that it was continuing the same strategy of blaming all of Ranbaxy's woes on the "foreign hand".

Indian public health activists were not very far behind the government when it came to deflecting the blame towards the "foreign hand". The *Hindu Business Line* ran a report titled "Public Health Activists smell conspiracy against Indian pharma" stating:

> the convenor of Jan Swasthya Abhiyan, B. Ekbal, said attempts were being made by multinational drug companies to belittle Indian drug-makers engaged in generic drug trade. Calling India the pharmacy of Third World countries, he said, "Though Ranbaxy is no more an Indian company, the targeting of Indian companies is part of a strategy".[6]

An influential public health activist, the late Amit Sengupta who worked with the Jan Swasthya Abhiyan and other NGOs, while accepting that Ranbaxy was guilty of falsifying regulatory data, dismissed the magnitude of the plea on the grounds that the definition of "Adulteration" in American law included not just drugs that failed quality tests but also drugs manufactured without following proper documentation procedures as required by the code of "Good Manufacturing Practices". According to Sengupta, "The fact that Ranbaxy provided false documents does not prove that its drugs were of bad quality, and by extension it is definitely not evidence that Indian generic drugs are generally of poor quality."[7] He then concluded that the Ranbaxy episode was being used unfairly by "Big Pharma" and "its supporters in the corporate controlled media" to unfairly "demonize" the entire generic pharmaceutical industry in India.[8]

This argument that Ranbaxy was only guilty of not maintaining proper documentation was a common excuse being trotted out at the time by Ranbaxy and the Government to explain the fine of $500 million penalty and the guilty plea. Arun Sawhney, who was Ranbaxy's CEO at the time, had given similar interviews stating that:

> An incomplete understanding of the word 'adulteration' would have caused some to believe that the drugs are not safe, when in fact it was (simply) a question of (improper) documentation.[9]

Minister of Health Ghulam Nabi Azad too gave a similar answer in Parliament when questioned by anxious MPs to explain the implications of Ranbaxy's guilty plea for Indian patients. When asked whether the Health Ministry could assure the country that

Ranbaxy was not selling any adulterated drugs in India, the Health Minister chose to respond by outlining the differing legal definition of adulteration in India and in the USA:

> As per the US Law, any drug is considered adulterated, if it is not manufactured, processed, packed, etc. in conformity with the Current Good Manufacturing Practice (GCMP) regulations of the USFDA. However, as per Drugs & Cosmetics Act and Rules, in India, manufacturing of drugs not in conformity with Good Manufacturing Practices (GMP) is viewed as non-compliance to GMP under the said Act and Rules.[10]

In all three statements, by the noted public health activist, the CEO of the guilty pharmaceutical company and the Union Health Minister, the aim was to portray the Ranbaxy plea as a "documentation issue" wherein the company failed to maintain proper records of its manufacturing process rather than a case where the company actually sold drugs of questionable quality to unsuspecting patients. These assertions were, however, completely factually incorrect because Ranbaxy had pled guilty to selling drugs in the American market even after it had knowledge that the drugs had failed certain quality tests. As explained by the Department of Justice press release outlining the guilty plea by Ranbaxy:

> Ranbaxy USA further admitted to failing to timely file required reports known to FDA as "field alerts" for batches of Sotret and gabapentin that had failed

> certain tests. With respect to Sotret, Ranbaxy USA was aware in January 2003 that a batch of Sotret failed an accelerated dissolution stability test but continued to distribute the batch into the United States for another 13 months. With respect to gabapentin, Ranbaxy USA was aware at various times between June and August 2007 that certain batches of gabapentin were testing out-of-specification, had unknown impurities, and would not maintain their expected shelf life. Nevertheless, Ranbaxy USA did not notify FDA and institute a voluntary recall until October 2007.[11]

By pleading guilty, Ranbaxy admitted to the charge of selling adulterated medicine in the USA. But even the issues dismissed as so called "documentation issues" were actually of a very serious magnitude since Ranbaxy had basically pled guilty to fabricating data with respect to crucial quality tests and making false statements in this regard to the USFDA. Two of the accusations to which Ranbaxy pled guilty as explained in the Department of Justice press release:

> Ranbaxy USA also admitted to making false, fictitious, and fraudulent statements to the FDA in Annual Reports filed in 2006 and 2007 regarding the dates of stability tests conducted on certain batches of Cefaclor, Cefadroxil, Amoxicillin, and Amoxicillin and Clavulanate Potassium, which were manufactured at the Dewas facility. Ranbaxy USA was found to have conducted stability testing of certain batches of these drugs weeks or months after the dates reported to FDA. In addition, instead of conducting some of the stability tests at prescribed intervals months apart,

> the tests were conducted on the same day or within a few days of each other. This practice resulted in unreliable test results regarding the shelf life of the drugs. Ranbaxy USA also acknowledged that drug samples waiting to be tested were stored for unknown periods of time in a refrigerator, which did not meet specified temperature and humidity ranges for an approved stability chamber, and that this was not disclosed to the FDA.[12]

These false statements and the inconsistencies in conducting the required tests at the prescribed time to ensure quality of its drugs is a cause for serious concern since stability testing is crucial in order to guarantee the therapeutic efficacy of a drug, which is why such testing is mandated in the GMP code of most countries. A drug that is stable at the six months mark post manufacturing may begin to degrade at the eight months mark if it is not formulated properly which is why such regular testing is mandated. Without such testing, no company can guarantee the quality of their product until its labelled expiration date and hence the presumption in American law that drugs not tested as required by the GMPs are adulterated. Thus, the tendency to dismiss the failure to conduct quality tests as a mere "documentation issue", equivalent to the misfiling of documents in the wrong folder is a dangerously misconceived and a misleading exercise. Yet, that is exactly how the CEO of Ranbaxy, the Minister of Health and the public health activist chose to dismiss the magnitude of Ranbaxy's guilty plea.

As the USFDA ramped up scrutiny of pharmaceutical manufacturing facilities in the years following the Ranbaxy scandal by issuing a number of warning letters to the Indian pharmaceutical industry, Indian public health activists doubled down on conspiracy theories centred around the "foreign hand". One such activist from the All India Drug Action Network (AIDAN), an influential collective of public health activists, directly imputed in an opinion editorial in a national newspaper that the USFDA was acting as a proxy for the western pharmaceutical industry:

> The USFDA's warning letters are no doubt the handiwork of the MNC. This is more a political battle than just the quality of few medicines and so it needs a political stand and solution. The Indian government should acknowledge the unique contribution and should not bend to the forces and strategies of the MNCs. This is not the first time that this lobby has tried this. Eternal vigilance and lobbying against such vested threats are the only way out.[13]

Rarely did the Indian government or Indian public health activists attempt to get into the weeds of the allegations made by foreign regulators despite regulators like the USFDA publishing all of its regulatory observations on its website, in a document called Form 483.

Less than two years after the controversy over Ranbaxy's guilty plea, came a new scandal at GVK Bio, a clinical research organization (CRO). The scandal at GVK Bio, as discussed elsewhere in this book began after the French drug regulator ANSM was contacted by a whistleblower, who was a former employee of GVK Bio, and turned over evidence of data fabrication at the company. A detailed investigation by ANSM, resulting in a long investigation report, accused GVK Bio of fabricating certain patient data as a result of which the regulator declared that it had no faith in any of the data generated by the CRO. On the basis of ANSM's findings, the EMA cancelled the marketing approvals it had granted to 700 drugs because the drugs in question were approved on the basis of regulatory data generated at GVK Bio.

Despite both Indian and foreign drug companies being affected by this decision of the EMA, the Indian government once again played the victim card. The DCGI G.N. Singh told *The Hindu* "...one must understand that there is a bigger game being played out here. I have repeatedly stated that multinational pharmaceutical companies constantly use incidents like this to bring disrepute to Indian generic drug makers."[14] The generic industry's top lobbyist, the late Mr D.G. Shah, who spoke for the Indian Pharmaceutical Alliance (IPA) was not far behind, telling *The Hindu* that the manner in which the European regulator went about the ban "... only leaves doubt about its intention".[15] Neither the drug regulator nor the industry lobbyist provided any factual evidence to substantiate their claims that the EMA was acting on behalf of foreign pharmaceutical companies.

The Ministry of Commerce then got into the fray by not just threatening to sue the European Union before the WTO for unfair trade practices but also cancelling pending trade talks with the European Union on a possible free-trade agreement with India. The Minister for Commerce, Nirmala Sitharaman, claimed that the decision had been taken at the highest level of government, implying that it had the blessings of the Prime Minister's Office.[16] The top rungs of the government appeared to be convinced that there was a conspiracy against India. Quoting the then Commerce Secretary Rajiv Kher, the *Hindu Business Line* reported: "The Secretary said that there were just a few big multinationals that were driving an agenda against the generic (off-patent drug) industry, affecting India's annual drug exports of $15 billion."[17] Once again, a senior government official was basically accusing the EMA of acting on behalf of a "few big multinational(s)" without any evidence of the same. Once tempers cooled and the issue fell off the front pages, India quietly restarted the trade talks and never approached the WTO. All the bluster somehow vanished into thin air.

These conspiracy theories are not limited to instances where foreign regulators take action against Indian pharmaceutical companies but also extend to instances where foreign academics have published studies on the quality of Indian drugs. One such study, in 2014, funded by the National Bureau of Economic Research (NBER) and authored by a team of American and Canadian academics had collected 1470 samples of "Made in India" drugs from Indian cities and also from cities in middle income countries and Africa for the purpose of testing the drugs.[18] Amongst other conclusions, the study also concluded that the samples drawn from poorly regulated countries in Africa were more likely to fail quality testing thereby implying that Indian pharmaceutical companies were exporting poorer quality drugs to Africa.[19] This is not completely unbelievable; the Government of India's own survey report of drug quality published in 2017 pegs the quantity of NSQ drugs in government hospitals at 10.02%, which is three times the 3.16% detected by the survey in the open market.[20] The likely reason for this is because the Indian pharmaceutical industry knows that the public procurement system in India is inefficient, meaning that they are more likely to get away with cutting corners when selling to government agencies. It is therefore not unbelievable that the Indian pharmaceutical industry would apply less rigorous quality standards to drugs exported to poorly regulated markets in Africa, as concluded by the NBER study, when compared to better regulated markets in other countries like the USA and Europe.

The NBER report provoked a huge backlash from the Indian government, industry lobbyists and Indian public health activists. A public health activist belonging to AIDAN condemned the report as "an attempt by Western pharmaceutical companies to malign the reputation of Indian generic drug makers."[21] The India Brand Equity Foundation (IBEF), which is a trust setup by the Government of India to promote the "Made in India" brand and headed by the Commerce Secretary, asked the government to sue the academics![22]

The late D.G. Shah, who at the time was the top lobbyist for the IPA made similar noises, alleging that, "[The research paper] tarnishes the image of the Indian pharmaceutical industry. It would be to the advantage of our adversaries as they can then sell more expensive drugs to the poor countries."[23]

The fact of the matter however is that a number of developing countries in Africa and Asia, such as Ghana, Mozambique, Vietnam and Sri Lanka have officially complained to the Government of India about the quality of drugs being exported to their respective countries by Indian pharmaceutical companies. In 2014, the same year as the NBER study, Vietnam blacklisted a record 45 Indian companies and prohibited them from exporting to Vietnam because of quality concerns.[24] These complaints by African and Asian countries have been quietly acknowledged in government meetings.[25] Ultimately the Government of India never sued the authors of the NBER study for defamation, the study was published in a peer-review publication and the controversy faded away.

The conspiracy theories and ad hominem attacks, however, continued to be used against critics of the Indian pharmaceutical industry. In 2016 when one of us, Dinesh Thakur, filed a public interest petition before the Supreme Court asking for regulatory reform, the DCGI had this to say: "We welcome whistleblowers, we have got great respect, but their intentions should be genuine, should be nationalistic...I don't have any comment on this guy."[26] The imputation being that

Dinesh was anti-national for questioning, before the highest court of the land, the functioning of the CDSCO which is headed by the DCGI.

Similarly, when Katherine Eban's best-selling book, *Bottles of Lies: The Inside Story of the Generic Pharmaceutical Boom* was published in 2019, exposing the details of the scandals at Ranbaxy and other generic pharmaceutical companies in India, the CDSCO reportedly sent a note to the Ministry of Health recommending that the Government of India take "appropriate action to counter the allegations made in the book."[27]

According to *The Print*, which broke the story, the CDSCO's note stated that, "A brief perusal of the book reveals that there is no co-relating data available in the representing story and statements have been made based on the assumptions," and that the author's allegations were "fiction-filled stories" and that such allegations have been made "time to time attempting to malign Indian pharmaceutical industries due to their strong presence globally".[28] This, despite the fact that Eban had extensively substantiated her reporting by citing primary sources. Ultimately *Bottle of Lies* became a bestseller in both the USA and India.

This pattern of ad hominem attacks and conspiracy theories which blamed all regulatory woes of Indian pharmaceutical industry on foreign regulators and foreign companies is reflective of a governance culture in India that is used to blaming domestic problems on a "foreign hand" or "anti-national" forces". That many prominent public health activists in India have sided with the government's position has only lent credibility to these conspiracy theories. All of this has happened despite the Parliamentary Standing Committee on Health and Family Welfare roasting the CDSCO, in its report tabled in 2012, for doing an abysmal job in ensuring drug quality in India just a year before the guilty plea by Ranbaxy.[29]

A similar event played out in December 2022 when the WHO blamed the deaths of 70 children in Gambia on cough syrup exported from India. At the time, the then DCGI, V.S. Somani, in a widely publicized letter to the WHO, accused the international body of contributing to a "narrative being built internationally targeting the quality of Indian pharmaceutical products" and causing "irreparable damage to the supply chain of pharmaceutical products, as well as repute of the national drug regulatory framework" by making "unsubstantiated" claims. This, despite the fact that there was a mountain of evidence to back the WHO's claim that the cough syrups were responsible for the deaths of the children in Gambia.

For any serious attempt at drug regulation to succeed in India, the government must first accept that the Indian pharmaceutical industry and the Indian regulator have serious problems when it comes to ensuring quality of "Made in India" drugs. Only then can India have an honest conversation on reforming its drug regulator.

Growth of the pharmaceutical industry vs public health: What is the job of the drug regulator?

In the race for economic growth, countries like India tend to put "development" and "economic growth" front and centre of the national agenda. In the context of the pharmaceutical industry, this often means promoting growth of the industry at the cost of public health. In India, the key stakeholders in the regulatory framework are quite transparent about diluting regulatory standards that stand in the way of the growth and profitability of the domestic pharmaceutical industry. Take, for example, the decision taken by the Government of India in 2004, to dilute GMP standards that had been introduced in Indian law merely three years ago in 2001. The Minister of Health admitted in Parliament that the government was diluting the GMP standards because it had received a memorandum from 34 MPs asking the government to delay enforcement of the new GMP standards on the grounds that "thousands of small scale pharmaceutical units" would shut down if the new GMP standards were enforced.[30] This, despite the fact that enforcement of the new standards introduced in 2001 had already been delayed by three years.

This attitude at the highest level of the government is reflected down the chain of command. For example, the CDSCO for the longest time had a mission statement that seemed to indicate it was more interested in the growth of the pharmaceutical industry than it was in protection of public health. This was pointed out by no less an authority than the Parliamentary Standing Committee on Health & Family Welfare in its 59th report. The committee noted with shock that the status report submitted by the CDSCO to Parliament defined the regulator's mission as meeting "the aspirations... demands and requirements of the pharmaceutical industry."[31] As rightly noted by the Parliamentary Committee, most national drug regulators put the interests of public health, not the pharmaceutical industry, at the front and centre of their mission statement.

After this indictment, the CDSCO did redefine its "mission" statement. The new statement is as follows: "To safeguard and enhance the public health by assuring the safety, efficacy and quality of drugs, cosmetics and medical devices." Unfortunately, changing bureaucratic attitudes is not as easy as changing mission statements.

At some point, there has to be a shift in these attitudes within government to recognize that public health should be at the front and centre of regulatory policies. Other departments, like the Department of Pharmaceutical which operates under the Ministry of Chemicals can be responsible for the growth of the industry but the policy matrix of the Ministry of Health or the CDSCO should always be focused on protecting the public health of the people. These bureaucratic attitudes will change only when an elected Minister forces such a change. Until then, we are only likely to witness new slogans rather than new attitudes towards public health.

The politics of federalism in the context of drug regulation

One of the central issues of drug regulation in India over the last century has been the issue of whether drug regulation should be the responsibility of the Union Government or the State Governments. This issue has been at the centre of debates on regulatory reform since 1927. As discussed in Chapter 2, the colonial government in the pre-independence days often passed the buck on enacting a national drug regulatory law on the grounds that it fell under the legislative purview of the provinces under the Government of India Act, 1935. Eventually the Drugs Act, 1940 was enacted by the Federal Legislature only when provincial legislatures passed resolutions empowering it to enact a law on their behalf. Although the Drugs Act, 1940 was a single legislation, it created a federated regulatory mechanism delegating to each province the right to enact its own rules, set its own standards and appoint its own drug inspectors to regulate domestic manufacture. Similar powers were delegated to the Federal Government to enact its own rules, set standards and prosecute cases related to the import of drugs.

The post-independence debate in this regard has concentrated on whether drug regulation should be further centralized. The first serious recommendation in this regard was made a few years post-independence in the report of the Pharmaceutical Enquiry Committee, 1954. This committee had "strongly recommend[ed] that the administration of Drug Control should be centralised by bringing control on manufacture, sale and distribution, which is, at present exercised by the State Drug Controller, under the control of the Drugs Controller (India)."[32]

The main reason for this recommendation by the Committee was its finding that state drug controllers were doing a woefully poor job of enforcing the Drugs Act, 1940, partly because they lacked resources and partly due to a reluctance to act against industries that provided employment and tax revenue.[33]

Since the Constitution adopted in 1950 vested the power to regulate "drugs" with both the union and the states, Parliament was able to amend the Drugs Act, 1940 and centralize a number of functions that previously existed with state governments. This included licensing powers for manufacturing facilities for the pharmaceutical industry.

In order to achieve this goal, this legislation replaced the phrase "provincial government" in Section 33 of the Drugs Act, 1940 with "Central Government" (aka Union Government). By doing so, Parliament basically stripped the state governments of their right to enact their own rules with respect to creation of standards, issuance of manufacturing licences, qualification of drug inspectors, etc. leaving them only with the right to test drugs and prosecute manufacturers of NSQ drugs. Post the enactment of this law in 1955, the Union Government had control over the setting of uniform standards across India and more importantly, the power to appoint licensing authorities.

Surprisingly, however, after having moved the

Parliament to appropriate these powers for itself, the Union Government in 1960 once again delegated the power of appointing the licensing authority to the state governments via an amendment to Rule 69 of the Drugs & Cosmetics, Rules, 1945! This meant that state governments continued to exercise the power to appoint licensing authorities, thereby going against the very rationale of the amending law introduced in 1954 on the recommendations of the Pharmaceutical Enquiry Committee to centralize drug licensing.

This delegation of power by the Government of India to the State Governments was in fact illegal. According to the administrative law principle captured in the Latin maxim *delegatus non potest delegare*, power once delegated to an authority cannot be further delegated. Therefore, if Parliament delegated to the Union Government the power to appoint a licensing authority the Union Government cannot give away this power to state governments. Such further delegation would go against the Parliamentary mandate and could be struck down by a court of law. It is not clear as to why the Union Government gave away these powers.

Surprisingly, the sleight of hand with regard to Rule 69 was not noticed by subsequent expert committees setup by the Union Government to advise it on drug regulation. The first of these committees was the Hathi Committee, which submitted its report in 1975. This committee acknowledged the varying standard of enforcement of the Drugs & Cosmetics Act, 1940 across the country, but did not recommend any centralization of powers. It instead made recommendations to beef up the resources available to state drug controllers and for better coordination between different state and union authorities responsible for drug regulation.[34] The second report prepared many decades later was by a committee headed by Dr Mashelkar. This committee which submitted its report in 2003, focused extensively on the issue of centralizing licensing powers with a strengthened drug regulator called the Central Drug Administration (CDA).[35] The Mashelkar committee noted that state drug controllers and the Indian Drug Manufacturers Association (IDMA) opposed switching over to a centralized licensing system.[36] Opposition from state drug controllers was predictable since they would be losing their licensing powers over manufacturing units, which was their main source of power.

Since the Mashelkar Committee's recommendation in 2003, there have been two legislative attempts, in 2007 and 2013, which sought to centralize licensing powers with the central drug regulator. Neither of these legislations were put to vote in Parliament.

In reality, if the Government of India had sought and received competent legal advice, it would have realized that it did not have to move a legislative amendment in Parliament to centralize licensing powers since, as mentioned earlier, the Drugs (Amendment) Act, 1955 had already given the Government of India the power to appoint licensing authorities for the country via the amendment to Section 33. Given this position of law, one of us, Dinesh Thakur, filed a constitutional challenge against Rule 69 before the Supreme Court via the route of a public interest litigation (PIL).

It was our case that Rule 69 should be struck down on the grounds that it offended the principle of *delegatus non podest delegare* and that the Union Government could not further delegate powers that had been delegated to it by Parliament Since the law enacted by Parliament in 1955 delegated the power to appoint licensing authorities to the Union Government, we argued that this power could not be further delegated to the State Governments. Unfortunately, despite the strength of our argument, the court was reluctant to hear the matter; as a result of which we withdrew the petition with liberty to petition the government.[37]

Even though the court did not hear our argument, it appears that someone in the Ministry of Health realized that the government did not have to go to Parliament to seek the power to regulate manufacturing facilities. We say this because in 2017, the Ministry of Health notified the Drugs and Cosmetics (Tenth Amendment) Rules, 2017 to create a requirement for joint inspections by both central and state drug inspectors once in three years or before the issuance of a new manufacturing licence or a new pharmacy licence. The rules are silent on how differences between state and central drugs inspectors are to be resolved.

This new arrangement had the potential to disrupt the cozy arrangements between the state drug inspectors and the pharmaceutical industry, which had long been used to dealing with only state level officials. Not surprisingly, an association of state drug controllers called the All India Drugs Control Officers Confederation, along with the Pharmaceutical Manufacturers Association of Tamil Nadu, filed a constitutional challenge against the new rules on a variety of grounds, including that the said rules were against the federal scheme of the Constitution of India.[38] The Madras High Court rejected this challenge by the drug control officers and the pharmaceutical industry on the grounds that the Union Government had the power to mandate joint inspections.[39]

The larger question to ask is whether further centralization of various aspects of drug regulation is required?

Our own research indicates that the findings of the Pharmaceutical Enquiry Committee, 1954 continue to be true even in 2022. Not all state governments are enforcing the Drugs & Cosmetics Act, 1940 with equal vigour and this is true across various indicators ranging from the volume of testing to the rate of prosecution of pharmaceutical companies found to be manufacturing NSQ drugs. States like Tamil Nadu do a far better job at testing drug samples than states like Bihar or Himachal Pradesh which lack well-equipped laboratories.

Similarly, there is also a lot of data available to indicate that states like Himachal Pradesh and Uttarakhand are the fountainhead of the NSQ problem in India, partly because these states are also home to a large number of pharmaceutical companies who setup shop to take advantage of tax incentives available in those states.

We suspect this is because neither state has an incentive to improve the quality of drug regulation lest it adversely affect local investment in the state by the pharmaceutical industry and local employment.

However, since India is a common market where goods manufactured in one state can travel across the country, the abysmal state of drug regulation in Himachal Pradesh and Uttarakhand has a deleterious effect on public health across the country. States like Karnataka and Tamil Nadu, with relatively better drug regulators, have to allow entry to drugs manufactured from all states. In the best-case scenario, where drug inspectors in these better regulated states detect substandard drugs manufactured in other states, they can only initiate a criminal prosecution against the out-of-state manufacturers but these prosecutions can take years before Indian courts. These better regulated states lack the powers to cancel manufacturing licences of out-of-state companies because of which they cannot stop these companies from continuing to manufacture and ship poor quality drugs into their territories.

But will greater centralization under a single authority necessarily improve the quality of drug supply especially when the functioning of the CDSCO itself has been excoriated by no less of an authority than the Parliamentary Standing Committee on Health & Family Welfare? There is every possibility that an incompetent central regulator can make things worse. There is then also the question of democratic accountability. How responsive will a central regulator be to the local demands of states? To what extent will a central regulator head quartered in New Delhi respond to the needs and demands of citizens in states like Nagaland or Tamil Nadu?

From a strictly theoretical viewpoint, we believe that drugs subject to inter-state trade and commerce across India should be subject to oversight by a centralized regulator not just because it is likely to ensure a more uniform application of the law across a country that is a common market but also because drug regulation is a "national public good" for the entire country. In such a scenario, where the entire country is affected by poor regulation, the burden of that regulation should not fall on individual states. It is only fair that resources for such an exercise be funded from the union's pool of taxes which will then naturally have to be controlled by an authority answerable to the Union Government. The Union Government in turn is answerable to Parliament that comprises of elected representative from across the country. An additional advantage of centralization is that the Union Government has far deeper pockets than states, meaning that it will be in a better position to finance the operation of a central regulator and invest in new well-equipped laboratories.

On the point of accountability, there is certainly merit in the argument that greater centralization will likely impact accountability of the regulator to individual states and their citizens but then again, the situation is much worse under the present system when neither citizens nor their elected representatives from states like Karnataka or Tamil Nadu have any possibility of influencing politics or regulators of Himachal Pradesh and Uttarakhand. At least a central regulator could be subject to some kind of accountability from Members of Parliament across all states. In any event, one way to mitigate this problem of accountability of the central regulator to localized concerns is by creating councils in each state, with representatives from both the central regulators and state government, so that there is a constant feedback loop informing the central regulator about local concerns in different states and requiring the central regulator to respond to these concerns.

An alternate model of reform is to centralize only the licensing function with a central regulator but retain the current split in the law with regard to prosecution powers; wherein both the union government and state governments can appoint drug inspectors to draw market samples, test the same and conduct prosecutions of manufacturers of NSQ drugs. Additionally, state governments should be given the power to block certain companies from selling their drugs in their respective states if they had concerns about the track record of the company based on test reports, etc. Such a model will ensure that state governments act as a check on the central regulator since the former's sampling of drugs will act as a form of a quality audit of the central regulator's licensing and inspection function. If state regulators detect larger amounts of NSQ drugs during their sampling surveys, it would necessarily mean that the central regulator is doing a poorer job at guaranteeing GMP compliance. This split of powers may also be more palatable for the large lobby of incumbent state drug inspectors. The pharmaceutical industry may however be reluctant to deal with two sets of regulators.

Who makes for a good DCGI?

A key stakeholder in the quest to improving the quality of drug regulation is the bureaucracy, which constitutes the backbone of the CDSCO and state drug regulators. Traditionally, the qualification criteria for the leadership position in both the DCGI as well as the rank and file consisting of drug inspectors (employed by the State drug regulators) has been skewed in favour of pharmacy graduates despite the qualification criteria for these positions recognizing a wide pool of educational degrees such as medicine, microbiology, etc. Pharmacy graduates, however, enjoy an advantage despite this wide pool of recognized educational degrees because the qualification criteria for the post of drug inspector also includes an "experience" component that requires those applying for the post to either have experience working in pharmaceutical manufacturing for 18 months or experience working in a testing laboratory for 18 months.[40] Only pharmacists are likely to have such work experience since doctors are unlikely to ever work in pharmaceutical manufacturing or testing laboratories.

Similarly, to be appointed as the DCGI or the state drug controller, there is a compulsory "experience" requirement of having worked in the manufacture or testing of drugs or having worked in the enforcement of the Drugs & Cosmetics Act for a period of at least five years.[41] Once again, medical doctors are unlikely to have this experience. Only drug inspectors (who once again are pharmacists) with 15 years of experience in enforcing the drugs law are likely to meet the qualification criteria for DCGI or state drug controllers. Since the qualification criteria for drug inspectors favour pharmacists, it is almost certain that only a pharmacist will wind up in the post of either the DCGI or state drug controller.

Such qualification criterion that leans heavily in favour of pharmacists is completely outdated because drug regulation in the 21st century is not just about manufacturing but about public health and requires an understanding of bioethics, clinical trials and clinical research.

This existing qualification criterion in the Drugs & Cosmetics Rules, 1945 especially for the post of DCGI has been the subject of harsh criticism by the Parliamentary Standing Committee of Health & Family Welfare in its 59th report, tabled in 2012. The committee pointed out that the qualification criteria "excludes even highly qualified medical doctors from occupying the post of DCGI."[42] The committee pointed out that most developed countries like the USA and the UK have a practice of appointing highly qualified doctors or scientists with a deep understanding of pharmaceutical research and development and/or public health as heads of their national drug regulators.[43] This criticism by the Standing Committee was on point. Manufacturing is only one aspect of the pharmaceutical industry that has a huge impact on public health. The far more complicated aspects of this industry include clinical trials, bioethics and the launch of new drugs. In such a scenario, it is absolutely necessary that the leadership of a drug regulator be vested in persons who have a broader understanding of clinical research, pharmacology of drugs, bioethics and the impact of the pharmaceutical industry on public health.

Post the criticism by the Parliamentary Standing Committee in 2012, the Ministry of Health & Family Welfare did setup a supposed "expert" committee to revise the qualification criteria for the post of the DCGI. The final report of the committee did recommend widening the experience requirement to persons who had experience in clinical research or clinical trials or any research in any related disciplines but was silent on deleting the existing criteria that allowed pharmacists to be appointed to this post.[44] This recommendation to allow persons with experience in clinical research to be appointed as the DCGI was promptly opposed by professional associations of pharmacists like the Delhi Pharmaceutical Trust (DPT).[45]

In any event, the Ministry of Health and Family Welfare has not taken any measure to change the recruitment criteria as per the recommendations of the Parliamentary Standing Committee or its own expert committee.

Upgrading the CDSCO's administrative status and the turf war with the DGHS

One of the truly strange aspects of the CDSCO is its relatively low position in the overall pecking order of government hierarchy. Unlike other sectoral regulators like the Securities Exchange Board of India (SEBI) and Telecom Regulatory Authority of India (TRAI), the CDSCO is not a creation of a statute that has an existence independent of the Government of India. Rather, it is a subordinate office of the Directorate General of Health Services (DGHS) which is one of the many departments operating under the Ministry of Health & Family Welfare. The DCGI, who heads the CDSCO, is answerable to the Director General of Health Services (DG-DGHS), who in turn is answerable to the Secretary of Health, who in turn is accountable to the Minister of Health & Family Welfare, an elected politician.

As a consequence of this arrangement, the DG-DGHS, who heads the DGHS has significant operational control over the functioning of the CDSCO. This in itself would not be a problem if it were not for the fact that the DGHS is a massive department with multiple areas of responsibilities ranging from the execution of national disease control programmes for leprosy, vector borne diseases, tuberculosis to looking after infrastructure of hospitals owned by the central government to collecting health statistics from across the country to setting up public health standards. These are only few examples of the vast responsibilities vested in the DG-DGHS. In such a scenario it is unlikely that a DGHS can give sufficient attention to the functioning of the CDSCO. Since the DCGI is rather far from the Secretary or the Minister, it is unlikely that the DCGI has a direct line to these important power centres in the Ministry.

Further, unlike TRAI or SEBI, which have the powers to "make law" via rules and regulations, the CDSCO has no law-making powers. All the rules under the Drugs & Cosmetics Act, 1940 or the Drugs & Magic Remedies (Objectionable Advertisements) Act, 1954 are actually formulated by the Drug Regulation Section of the Ministry of Health & Family Welfare, which itself operates under a Joint Secretary (who is generally a bureaucrat with no experience in drug regulation) answerable to the Secretary of Health & Family Welfare. This is unlike the situation in other countries like the USA, where the USFDA itself has been given some rule-making power by the US Congress. The advantage of such delegation of power is that it makes the regulator more flexible and powerful, enabling it to deal with emerging issues without having to cut through multiple layers of red-tape.

There have been several calls to upgrade the administrative status of the CDSCO. For example, the Mashelkar Committee that submitted its report on reforms required to India's drug regulatory framework in 2003, had recommended that the CDSCO be renamed the Central Drug Administration (CDA) and made "into an independent office under the Ministry of Health and Family Welfare as is the case in most of the countries."[46] Subsequent to that recommendation, the Ministry of Health made two legislative attempts, one in 2007 and another in 2013, to give statutory backing and an independent corporate identity to a CDSCO that was to be renamed as the CDA. Neither legislative attempt was put to vote in Parliament.

In 2015, an expert committee setup by the government recommended that the CDSCO "be upgraded from the status of a Subordinate Office of the DGHS to an Attached Office of the Department of Health and Family Welfare and given substantial functional freedom."[47] But none of these recommendations have been acted upon.

Our recommendation in this regard would be to recast the CDSCO as a modern regulator, by giving it legislative sanctity through a law enacted by Parliament. As any other modern regulator in India or other countries, the CDSCO in its new avatar should have an independent corporate identity along with the power to manage its own finances and enact its own regulations, subject to safeguards such as prior mandatory public consultation. This should include the power to conduct its own recruitment of professionals from the private sector. Such delegation of power will hopefully create a nimble regulator that has the flexibility and expertise to meet emerging challenges from an innovative industry.

Democratizing regulation: Empowering citizens with information and the right to participate

The most important lever for reforming the drug regulatory system in India, in our opinion, is the Indian citizen's fundamental right to information, which in theory forces the state to be transparent in its functioning.

Unfortunately, neither the CDSCO nor the state drug controllers have taken it upon themselves to proactively disclose any of their records. On the contrary, as demonstrated by the Parliamentary Standing Committee on Health & Family Welfare, the CDSCO struggles to maintain critical files regarding drug approvals in storage without losing them.[48] Even a crucial inquiry report like the Mohapatra Committee report that we requested a copy of went missing from the CDSCO's office.[49] It is unlikely that all of these disappearances were accidental. Missing files are the easiest route to escape accountability despite the fact that the Public Records Act, 1993 requires an investigation into all missing public records.

Even when records are maintained, it can be very difficult for the common citizen to access them even under the RTI Act, 2005. For example, when we tried sourcing data on prosecutions from state drug controllers, many states responded by transferring our request to each district in the state. Each district officer would then either send the information or request us to visit their office to inspect the files on the grounds that we asked for voluminous information. This is the reason we could not get consolidated aggregated statistics from most states on the rates of criminal prosecutions under the Drugs & Cosmetics Act, 1940.

Similarly, the typical response from the CDSCO to our requests for statistical information was to transfer them to its Zonal Offices, which in turn, after a considerable delay, either plead ignorance or transferred the request back to the CDSCO. The entire process exists to frustrate the citizen and deny them anything that can be used to hold the regulator accountable to the people of the country.

One way to resolve the above problems and truly operationalize the "right to information" is by imposing upon the drug regulator, the duty to proactively disclose information for the convenience of the general public.

For example, critical documentation regarding the approval of a new drug is not proactively published by the DCGI's office. Similarly, inspection reports of manufacturing facilities are not publicly available because of which procurement agencies of the Government or those in the private sector do not have complete information while taking the decision to procure drugs from particular pharmaceutical companies.

Unlike in India, regulatory authorities in other jurisdictions like the USA or the European Union proactively publish their internal reviews of all new drug applications on their respective websites. The USFDA also proactively publishes on its websites, its inspection reports of manufacturing facilities and CROs. These practices contribute immensely in building public confidence and trust in the regulator. Further, the functioning of the American regulator itself is subject to performance reviews by statutory bodies like the Government Accountability Office (GAO) in the USA.[50] There is an urgent need for Indian law to be rewritten in a manner that proactively identifies all the information required by a common citizen to conduct a "social audit" of the functioning of the regulator so as to inform themselves of the regulator's effectiveness in enforcing the law.

Transparency in the context of a drug regulator, apart from facilitating accountability of the regulator to common citizens, also has direct implication for public health. For doctors prescribing new drugs, the primary source of information currently, is the promotional material given to them by salespersons from pharmaceutical companies, which as we have explained in this book can often be misleading since pharmaceutical companies tend to downplay unfavourable information about their own drugs. A secondary source of information about new drugs for doctors can be clinical trial studies published in peer-reviewed journals but many of these journals are behind paywalls and incredibly expensive to access for most Indian doctors. In such a scenario, proactive publication of regulatory information by the regulator that can be accessed for free by all doctors can be an important source of information for health professionals looking to make treatment decisions.

Similarly, greater regulatory transparency can facilitate the procurement of quality drugs. Currently, drug procurement agencies in the public and private sector do not have access to either inspection reports of drug inspectors or a consolidated database of all NSQ drugs across the country while making decisions on bulk purchases. As a result, some organizations like the Indian Railways end up conducting their own "inspections", which apart from being wasteful public expenditure is also quite inadequate. Other procurement agencies simply go by "self-declarations" made by pharmaceutical companies since there are no consolidated databases that can be used to verify the "self-declaration" made by the pharmaceutical company. This is not particularly efficient. If the CDSCO and state drug controllers made available such information from across the country in well designed, searchable databases it would dramatically improve the efficiency of both public and private procurement of drugs.

Of all the reforms discussed in this chapter, measures to improve transparency will have a disproportionately large impact on the quality of regulation. But the right to information is in itself not useful unless it is accompanied with a right to participate in regulatory decisions. Given the nature of power delegated to the bureaucracy in the course of drug regulation it is impossible to rely only on parliamentary oversight to ensure the democratic accountability of regulators to the people. Any comprehensive regulatory reform must therefore create pathways for common citizens to participate and challenge regulatory decisions. This is not as ambitious as it sounds. Environmental law and land acquisition law already require the government to conduct public hearings and note public oppositions. In context of drug regulation, the law must have similar safeguards allowing citizens to question drug approvals, petition for specific regulatory action and comment on rules and regulations before they are finalized. In short, the people being affected by bureaucratic decisions must have legal pathways to question and contribute to those decisions.

Increasing accountability of public procurement

Another potentially powerful lever of reform that exists outside the drug regulatory system is the system of public procurement. While no consolidated figures regarding the volume of public procurement of drugs are available, we estimate that between the Government of India and the state governments, a significant sum of public funds are spent on procuring drugs for the public health system. This includes procurements by the Central Medical Service Society (CMSS) for central government hospitals, the Bureau of Pharma PSUs of India (BPPI) which procures for programs like the government's Jan Aushadhi program (aimed at funding generics only pharmacies across the country) and state level agencies like the Tamil Nadu Medical

Services Corporation (TNMSC) which conduct bulk procurement for their respective state governments.

The major problem with the public procurement process is that it has a shockingly high percentage of NSQ drugs. This is obvious from the government's own survey data from 2017, which reported the percentage of NSQ drugs in government hospitals at 10.02%; three times the 3.16% in the general market.[51] Apart from this survey data, there is also anecdotal evidence to suggest serious quality issues with drug supply in the public sector. For example, a report of the Comptroller & Auditor General (CAG) after an audit of the Armed Forces Medical Services Depot (AFMSD) which procures drugs for the Armed Forces reported that the rate of rejection of "locally procured" drugs by the AFMSD over a period of four years due to quality issues averaged at 24%![52] There are several other reports by CAG of other public procurement agencies, which report similar problems with drug quality.[53]

The high percentage of NSQ drugs detected in government hospitals is indicative of not just a threat to persons being treated in these public hospitals but also conclusive proof of the waste of precious public funds on dubious manufacturers who have likely won bids for contracts by cutting corners and bribing public servants. There is no shortage of reports of corruption in procurement of drugs. A simple search for such reports will throw up allegations from across the country of mindboggling corruption during the public procurement process.[54]

One of the reasons for this abysmal state of affairs as pointed out by CAG in successive reports, is the lack of well thought out codified procedures and manuals to guide the procurement process. Even on the issue of blacklisting of manufacturers who supply substandard drugs, academics have pointed out the lack of transparent criteria informing all participants of the grounds on which they can be blacklisted from supplying for future bids.[55] Moreover, as we discovered to our amazement, large purchasers like the Indian Railways do not have a consolidated blacklist for the entire organization. When we asked the headquarters of the Indian Railways for a list of pharmaceutical companies blacklisted from participating in its procurement process for drugs, our application was transferred to each railway zone, each of whom provided us their own blacklist.[56] The Government of India also does not have a single blacklist covering all of the various procurement agencies operating under its auspices.

One simple solution to this problem is for the Parliament to enact an over-arching public procurement law specifically governing the purchase of drugs by the Government of India or any other agency receiving funds from Parliament. Such a procurement law should lay down specific procurement criteria and mandate testing of each batch of drugs purchased before the drugs are released to patients. Drugs that fail such quality testing should result in blacklisting of the manufacturers. Once a pharmaceutical company is blacklisted by one procurement agency, it should automatically be prohibited from supplying to any government entity for the duration it is on the blacklist. This blacklist maintained by the Government of India will likely also be relied upon by state government agencies and large procurement agencies in the private sector such as pharmacy chains and hospital chains.

Thus, even if the Government of India is unable to overhaul the Drugs & Cosmetics Act, 1940 due to opposition from state governments, it can still rely on its enormous purchasing power to inflict significant punishment on pharmaceutical companies that are found to be supplying NSQ drugs by blocking them from lucrative markets. Last but not the least, such a procurement law should mandate the creation of resources that can aid government agencies in assessing the quality track record of pharmaceutical companies across the country by forcing all relevant stakeholders to share information such as quality testing reports and inspection reports into a consolidated database that acts as a single source of truth for procurement officers in both the public and private sector.

Of drug regulation and public health activism

As a country, India is fortunate to have a very active civil society movement comprising of academics and activists who are willing to hold the government accountable. In the context of drugs, most of this activism is directed towards the issue of "access to medicine", price control for drugs or broader public health issues. Little to no attention is paid towards quality of drugs.

A part of the reason that there is little activism on drug regulatory issues, is the fact that "access to medicine" activism in India was premised on building bridges with the Indian pharmaceutical industry to oppose the new patent regime imposed by the Agreement on Trade Related Intellectual Property Right (TRIPs) and also individual patents on crucial drugs. In fact, one of the first meetings, in the 1990s, between the generic pharmaceutical industry and public health activists in India to oppose TRIPs was held at the corporate offices of Ranbaxy.[57] To take up issues related to drug quality in this context would have roiled a partnership that was otherwise very successful in achieving its goals of improving access to medicine.

The only group that has dedicated some space to the issue of drug regulation is the AIDAN, which describes itself as "an independent network of several non-government organizations working to increase access and improve the rational use of essential medicines."[58] This includes mainly Indian NGOs and some international NGOs like the *Médecins Sans Frontières* (MSF). This group has been active in public advocacy against untested, possibly dangerous Fixed Dose Combinations (FDC), against the arbitrary decision of the Ministry of Health to restrict the manufacture of Oxytocin in India and has also advocated for urgent measures to regulate drug advertising and promotion in India.[59]

However, AIDAN rarely dedicates similar bandwidth to issues that goes to the core of drug quality in India, such as the importance of bioequivalence and stability testing. One reason for this could be the fact that AIDAN as a voluntary activist group lacks the resources to advocate multiple causes. The other possibility is that AIDAN suffers from a severe conflict of interest given that one of its founding members is a public charitable trust called "Low Cost Standard Therapeutics", better known as LOCOST. By itself, LOCOST presents an interesting model of pharmaceutical manufacturing since it has been formed as a not-for-profit public charitable trust focused on making low-cost essential drugs. As a manufacturer of drugs, LOCOST and its trustees like S. Srinivasan and Dr Anant Phadke, who are also members of AIDAN, have little incentive to push for stricter enforcement of the Drugs & Cosmetics Act, 1940 because it would directly impact them in their capacity as persons responsible for running a pharmaceutical manufacturing facility. This is not even a hypothetical scenario. In 2009, the Chief Judicial Magistrate, Pune convicted LOCOST, S. Srinivasan and two other managerial personnel, under Section 18(a)(i) read with Section 27 of the Drugs & Cosmetics Act, 1940 for manufacturing and selling a drug that failed quality testing in a government laboratory. The drug in question was Enalapril Maleate and is used to treat hyper-tension. The version manufactured by LOCOST was found to contain only 45.8% of the quantity advertised on the label. As a result, the drug was declared to be NSQ by the government analyst. After a trial, the Chief Judicial Magistrate found LOCOST, Srinivasan and others guilty of manufacturing and selling NSQ drugs. The court sentenced them to pay a fine of ₹10,000 and suffer simple imprisonment till the rising of the court. Given the fact that its members have been convicted of manufacturing substandard drugs, we doubt AIDAN will ever lobby for a stronger regulatory framework which could end up being used against its members like Srinivasan and others at LOCOST.

In fact, quite to the contrary, AIDAN has actively supported legislation like the Jan Vishwas Act, 2023 which decriminalized the manufacture of substandard drugs. Both S. Srinivasan and Dr Anant Phadke appeared on national media, representing themselves as public health activists, voicing their support for this bill, without disclosing to their audience that they are part of LOCOST which had been convicted of violating the very same offence that was being decriminalized under the Jan Vishwas Act, 2023.[60] Their colleagues at AIDAN maintained complete silence about this unethical conduct and made no effort to distance themselves from either S. Srinivasan or Dr Phadke.

There is a real need for the activist community to rethink its stand on the issue of drug regulation. Access to medicines is important but what good is access to a drug that does not work?

Citizen advocacy and political lobbying not the judiciary is the road to reform

Demands by the middle class for governance reform in India generally begin with the filing of "public interest litigation" (PIL) before the Supreme Court. In theory, PILs present the theoretical possibility of achieving radical, albeit undemocratic, reform through the judicial route.

In reality, the Supreme Court's track record on PILs borders on completely arbitrariness as witnessed by the court's approach to two PILs filed by one of us, Dinesh Thakur, in 2016. A bench of the Supreme Court headed by the then Chief Justice of India, T.S. Thakur, expressed its reluctance to hear the PILs, citing amongst other grounds, the allegedly "academic nature" of the petition. In reality the PILs referenced the reports of the government's own committees, pointing out to a litany of unenforced regulatory decisions, their consequences for public health. One PIL challenged the constitutionality of a specific rule that created a federated drug regulatory structure despite the law being clear on the fact that Indian was to have a unified drug regulatory structure. What made the court's reluctance more baffling was the fact that the then Chief Justice of India T.S. Thakur in the months preceding this petition, had admitted absurd PILs to ban jokes about Sardars, to bring back the Kohinoor diamond from the UK and to reform the sports body in charge of the Indian cricket team![61]

In any event, with the benefit of hindsight, we do not think this was a significant setback because the Supreme Court's track record on PILs pertaining to regulatory issues with clinical trials, biotechnology and nuclear technology is quite dismal. At most, the court grants temporary relief and has been unable to achieve systemic reform and understandably so. There is a separation of powers between the judiciary, legislature and the executive. Unelected judges should be careful about the extent to which they take over the functions of the other two branches. The problem however with the Indian Supreme Court is that it is exceptionally inconsistent on this front, choosing to interfere in some cases, while refusing to intervene in others.

In any event, effective reform, as we have learnt over the course of the last several years can be achieved only through sustained advocacy that educates not just parliamentarians and bureaucrats about the shortcomings with the regulator but also educating civil society and convincing them for the need of change. Building a political consensus is a long and messy job but it is the only route to sustainable reform in a democracy. Luckily for India, there are a handful of individuals from the medical community, journalism, government and Parliament who are doing their bit on this front. A few of them deserve a mention before we conclude this book.

First on the list is Dr Chander Gulati, the editor of the *Monthly Index of Medical Specialties* (MIMS) who has blown the whistle on a number of half-baked approvals granted by the DCGI for drugs. For his comments on one particular drug called Deanxit, Dr Gulati has been prosecuted for criminal defamation by a company called Lundbeck.[62]

Second on the list is an outspoken doctor by the name Dr Abby Philips who runs a popular Twitter handle (@theliverdr) regularly exposing the pseudoscience propagated by the influential Ayush industry. As a hepatologist, Dr Philips in the course of his practice often comes across patients suffering from serious ailments, especially liver diseases, after having consumed traditional medicine. He presents many of these case studies on Twitter for common citizens and doctors. The effectiveness of his advocacy is obvious from the fact that practitioners of traditional medicine have complained against Dr Philips to the Government of India on the ground that he is defaming their profession. Acting on these complaints, the Ministry of Ayush has actually threatened defamation proceedings against Dr Philips.[63] He has also faced lawsuits by companies like Himalaya Wellness Corporation and at least one frivolous criminal complaint by a practitioner of Ayush in Uttar Pradesh. These threats have so far had no effect on Dr Philips and he continues to be relentless in his advocacy against the dangers of untested products marketed by the Ayush industry.

Amongst the community of journalists is Priyanka Pulla, a freelance journalist who has reported some of the most detailed and complicated issues pertaining to the state of drug regulation in India. These include stories on the state of investigations into the deaths of the 12 children in Jammu that we mentioned in the prologue, a shocking story about the contamination of generic Remdesivir manufactured by an Indian pharmaceutical company during the COVID-19 pandemic and the controversial approval of COVID vaccines. For her reportage on a Covid vaccine called Covaxin, Pulla has been sued for defamation by the vaccine's manufacturer, Bharat Biotech, along with the publication *Wire* and eight others. A court in Hyderabad passed a temporary injunction against Pulla, *Wire* and others in February 2022, without so much as granting them a hearing.[64]

While much of this book is critical about Indian bureaucrats, we must point out that one particular bureaucrat, Mr K.L. Sharma, the former Joint Secretary of the Drugs Regulation Section of the Ministry of Health & Family Welfare deserves a special mention. After the Supreme Court declined to hear our PIL, one of us, Dinesh Thakur, met Sharma to present him with a report containing our recommendations. To his credit, Sharma heard all our concerns and began reforms based on not just our report but also other sources. During his time, the government finally acted on the prickly issues of illegal FDCs, the issue of mandatory bioequivalence, advertising, etc. The government "rewarded" Sharma by transferring him out to the post of Joint Secretary, National Commission for Women (NCW), from where he retired in October 2018 after an illustrious career in the Central Secretariat

Services. Such transfers in the last year of service to institutions such as the NCW are generally considered to be "punishment" postings. In this case, Sharma's likely "crime" was to have the "temerity" to push through reforms that were unpopular with the Indian pharmaceutical industry but absolutely necessary from a public health perspective. Upon retirement Sharma penned a book, *Healing the Pharmacy of the World*, which is well worth a read for anybody interested in how the government machinery deals with policy making in the field of drug regulation.

This list of outstanding individuals contributing to the debate on drug regulatory reform would not be complete without a reference to the outstanding Parliamentarians sitting on the Parliamentary Standing Committee on Health and Family Welfare, especially those who authored the famous 59th report on the functioning of the CDSCO that has been cited throughout this book.[65] These MPs displayed the glory, brilliance and courage of Indian democracy with that one report hauling up the CDSCO for the shoddy job that it was doing with regard to drug regulation. Three MPs on the sub-committee that drafted the reports, deserve a special mention: Dr Jyoti Mirdha, Balbir Punj and Dr Sanjay Jaiswal. Together with the Chairperson of the Committee Brajesh Pathak, these MPs demonstrated the power of parliamentary standing committees in holding the government accountable for their action and inaction. If only they did so more frequently.

Notes

1. The United States Department of Justice, Office of Public Affairs, *Generic Drug Manufacturer Ranbaxy Pleads Guilty and Agrees to Pay $500 Million to Resolve False Claims Allegations, cGMP Violations and False Statements to the FDA* (Press Release No 13-542, 13 May 2013).
2. TNN, "Ranbaxy Drugs: Apollo Pharmacy Issues Advisory" *The Times of India* (Chennai, 8 June 2013) <https://timesofindia.indiatimes.com/business/india-business/Ranbaxy-drugs-Apollo-Pharmacy-issues-advisory/articleshow/20487741.cms> accessed 23 May 2022.
3. NDTV, *Ranbaxy under Fire: Will India's Pharma Industry Be Hit?* (2013) <https://www.youtube.com/watch?v=MwmXXWwUSMs> accessed 23 May 2022.
4. Government of India, Ministry of Commerce & Industry, Press Information Bureau, "Clarifications on Reports of Malpractices of Pharma Manufacturing in India" (3 June 2013) <https://pib.gov.in/newsite/PrintRelease.aspx?relid=96366> accessed 22 May 2022.
5. Vikas Bhardwaj and Khomba Singh, "India Sees US Lobbies behind FDA Ban on Ranbaxy Drugs" *The Economic Times* (New Delhi, 16 October 2008) <https://economictimes.indiatimes.com/industry/healthcare/biotech/pharmaceuticals/india-sees-us-lobbies-behind-fda-ban-on-ranbaxy-drugs/articleshow/3600276.cms?from=mdr> accessed 23 May 2022.
6. "Public Health Activists Smell Conspiracy against Indian Pharma" *The Hindu Business Line* (New Delhi, 24 May 2013) <https://www.thehindubusinessline.com/companies/public-health-activists-smell-conspiracy-against-indian-pharma/article20617469.ece1> accessed 23 May 2022.
7. Amit Sengupta, "Who Manufactures Dirty Medicines?" *NewsClick* (15 June 2013) <https://www.newsclick.in/who-manufactures-dirty-medicines> accessed 23 May 2022.
8. ibid.
9. Interview with Arun Sawhney (CEO & MD, Ranbaxy), "It's Just Improper Documentation" *Outlook* (5 February

2022) <https://www.outlookindia.com/magazine/story/its-just-improper-documentation/286855> accessed 23 May 2022.

10. Reply by the Minister of Health and Family Welfare Shri Ghulam Nabi Azad to question raised by Shri Anil Desai, Rajya Sabha Deb 6 August 2013, Question No 232, 138-139.
11. The United States Department of Justice (n 1).
12. ibid.
13. Dr Gopal Dabade, "MNCs Play Proxy War against Indian Generics" *Deccan Herald* (9 January 2016) <https://www.deccanherald.com/content/522212/mncs-play-proxy-war-against.html> accessed 23 May 2022.
14. Vidya Krishnan, "A Love Story That Cost GVK Its International Reputation" *The Hindu* (New Delhi:, 8 October 2015) <https://www.thehindu.com/news/national/A-love-story-that-cost-GVK-its-international-reputation/article60296519.ece> accessed 23 May 2022.
15. ibid.
16. P. Vaidyanathan Iyer, "Suspending EU Trade Talks 'Unilateral', but Not 'Unconsidered': Nirmala Sitharaman" *The Indian Express* (New Delhi, 8 September 2015) <https://indianexpress.com/article/business/business-others/suspending-eu-trade-talks-unilateral-but-not-unconsidered-nirmala-sitharaman/> accessed 23 May 2022.
17. Amiti Sen, "Data Manipulation: India Contests EU Charges against GVK Bio" *The Hindu Business Line* (New Delhi, 5 April 2015) <https://www.thehindubusinessline.com/companies/data-manipulation-india-contests-eu-charges-against-gvk-bio/article21016776.ece1> accessed 23 May 2022.
18. Roger Bate et. al., "Poor-Quality Drugs and Global Trade: A Pilot Study" (2016) 2 *American Journal of Health Economics* 373.
19. ibid 394.
20. Government of India, Ministry of Health & Family Welfare, "National Drug Survey 2014-2016: SUMMARY

& RECOMMENDATIONS On Possible Strategies and Implementation Plan to Address the Problems Identified" (Chapter 11, 2017) 215.

21. Dinsa Sachan, "Indian Manufacturers Hit Back over Quality Claims" (*Chemistry World*, 17 October 2014) <https://www.chemistryworld.com/news/indian-manufacturers-hit-back-over-quality-claims/7869.article> accessed 23 May 2022.
22. Sanjeet Bagcchi, "Indian Generic Drugs Debate Heats Up" (2014) 384 *The Lancet* 1334.
23. ibid.
24. Maitri Porecha, "Vietnam Shows the Door to 45 Indian Pharma Companies" *DNA* (Mumbai, 21 April 2014) <https://www.dnaindia.com/mumbai/report-vietnam-shows-the-door-to-45-indian-pharma-companies-1980761> accessed 23 May 2022.
25. Drugs Consultative Committee (DCC), *"REPORT OF THE 47th MEETING OF THE DRUGS CONSULTATIVE COMMITTEE HELD ON 30TH AND 31ST JULY, 2014 AT NEW DELHI"* (2014) 19 <https://cdsco.gov.in/opencms/opencms/system/modules/CDSCO.WEB/elements/common_download.jsp?num_id_pk=ODA5> accessed 23 May 2022; Drugs Consultative Committee (DCC), *"REPORT OF 50TH MEETING OF DRUGS CONSULTATIVE COMMITTEE HELD ON 04 & 05TH NOVEMBER, 2016 AT NEW DELHI"* (2016) 2 <https://cdsco.gov.in/opencms/opencms/system/modules/CDSCO.WEB/elements/common_download.jsp?num_id_pk=ODEy> accessed 23 May 2023.
26. Zeba Siddiqui, "Pharma Crusader Dinesh Thakur Takes India's Drug Regulators to Court" *Reuters* (New Delhi, 7 March 2016) <https://www.reuters.com/article/india-pharma-whistleblower-idUSKCN0W90C8> accessed 23 May 2022.
27. Himani Chandna, "Modi Govt Plans Action against US Writer Who Said Indian Drugs Are 'Flea-Market Quality'" (*ThePrint*, 10 January 2020) <https://theprint.in/health/modi-govt-plans-action-against-us-writer-who-said-indian-drugs-are-flea-market-quality/347189/> accessed 23 May 2022.

28. ibid.
29. Department Related Parliamentary Standing Committee on Health and Family Welfare, *The Functioning of The Central Drugs Standard Control Organisation (CDCSO)* (Fifty-Ninth Report) (RS 2012).
30. Chittabratta Mazumdar and Dipankar Mukherjee on the "Revision of Schedule M of Drugs and Cosmetics Act", Rajya Sabha Deb 10 December 2004, Question No 874.
31. *The Functioning of The Central Drugs Standard Control Organisation* (n 29) at para 2.1.
32. Government of India, Ministry of Commerce & Industry, *Report of The Pharmaceutical Enquiry Committee* (1954) 153, para 3.7.
33. ibid. 164-165, para 6.4.2.
34. Government of India, Ministry of Petroleum & Chemicals, *Report of The Committee on Drugs and Pharmaceutical Industry (Hathi Committee Report)* (1975) 190-201.
35. Government of India, Ministry of Health and Family Welfare, *Report of The Expert Committee on a Comprehensive Examination of Drug Regulatory Issues, including the problem of Spurious Drugs (Mashelkar Committee Report)* (No Z.28015/112/2002-D/DMS&PFA, 2003) 36, para 5.7.3.
36. ibid. 44, para 6.1.8.
37. *Dinesh Thakur vs Union of India* WP(C) No. 137 of 2016 before the Supreme Court of India.
38. Special Correspondent, "Drug Control Officers Challenge Amendment to Statutory Rules" *The Hindu* (Chennai, 6 January 2018) <https://www.thehindu.com/news/national/tamil-nadu/drug-control-officers-challenge-amendment-to-statutory-rules/article22388587.ece> accessed 24 May 2022.
39. *All India Drugs Control Officers Confederation vs The Government of India* WP.No.33924/2017 before the High Court of Madras (28 February 2020) <https://indiankanoon.org/doc/191958036/> accessed 24 May 2022.
40. The Drugs and Cosmetics Rules 1945, Rule 49.
41. The Drugs and Cosmetics Rules 1945, Rule 50A.

42. *The Functioning of The Central Drugs Standard Control Organisation* (n 29) at para 2.23.
43. ibid. 7, para 3.2-3.3.
44. Government of India, Department of Health and Family Welfare, *Report of The Expert Committee Set Up to Suggest Recruitment Rules/Job Description for Senior Level Posts in Central Drugs Standard Control Organisation* (2015).
45. Nandita Vijay, "DPT Urges Ministry of Health Not to Make Changes in Recruitment Rules for DCGI Post, Other Tops Jobs in CDSCO" *Pharmabiz* (Bengaluru, 19 January 2015) <http://www.pharmabiz.com/NewsDetails.aspx?aid=86219&sid=1> accessed 24 May 2022.
46. Government of India, Ministry of Health and Family Welfare, *Report of The Expert Committee on a Comprehensive Examination of Drug Regulatory Issues, including the problem of Spurious Drugs (Mashelkar Committee Report)* (No Z.28015/112/2002-D/DMS&PFA, 2003) 41, para 5.9.4.
47. *Report of The Expert Committee* (n 46) 6.
48. *The Functioning of The Central Drugs Standard Control Organisation* (n 29) at para 7.12.
49. *Prashant Reddy vs Ministry of Health & Family Welfare* Second Appeal No. CIC/MH&FW/A/2018/159460-BJ before the Central Information Commission (26 May 2020) <https://indiankanoon.org/doc/115080764/> accessed 24 May 2022.
50. United States Government Accountability Office, "Drug Safety: FDA's Future Inspection Plans Need to Address Issues Presented by COVID-19 Backlog" (GAO-21-409T, 4 March 2021).
51. Government of India, Ministry of Health & Family Welfare, "National Drug Survey 2014-2016" (Chapter 11, 2017) 215.
52. Comptroller and Auditor General of India, *Report on Performance of Medical Establishments in Defence Services* (Report No 18 of 2012-13, ch 5: Procurement of drugs and quality inspection, 14 December 2013).
53. Comptroller and Auditor General of India, *Performance audit of Procurement of medicines and medical equipment in the Ministry of Health and Family Welfare* (Report No

20 of 2007, 27 November 2007); Comptroller and Auditor General of India, *Performance Audit of National Rural Health Mission of Union Government, Ministry of Health & Family Welfare* (Report No 8 of 2009, ch 7: Procurement and supply of medicine and equipment, 18 December 2009); Comptroller and Auditor General of India, *Report of the Comptroller and Auditor General of India State Finances Audit Report for the year ended March 2021* (Report No 2 of 2022, ch II: Compliance Audit, 31 March 2022) 33; PTI, "Expired Vaccines, Unutilised Funds: CAG Report Exposes Jharkhand's Health Infrastructure" *The New Indian Express* (Ranchi, 17 March 2022).

54. U. Sudhakar Reddy, "Telangana: Vigilance Unearths Drug Purchase Scam in ESI Hospitals" *The Times of India* (Hyderabad, 17 July 2019) <https://timesofindia.indiatimes.com/city/hyderabad/vigilance-unearths-drug-purchase-scam/articleshow/70252212.cms> accessed 24 May 2022.
55. Harleen Kaur, Ajay Shah and Siddhartha Srivastava, "How Elements of the Indian State Purchase Drugs" (xKDR 2021) 5 <https://ideas.repec.org/p/anf/wpaper/5.html> accessed 24 May 2022.
56. RTI case no.G.542/1/2015-16/HQ/14718 dated 03.2.2016 filed with Railways HQ and received on 09.3.2016.
57. Amiti Sen Gupta, "B.K. Keayla: A Personal Reminiscence" (2010) 45 *Economic and Political Weekly* 7.
58. "About Us" (*All India Drug Action Network (AIDAN)*, 1 September 2008) <https://aidanindia.wordpress.com/about-us/> accessed 24 May 2022.
59. PTI, "Government Approves Public Procurement Bill" *The Hindu* (New Delhi, 12 April 2012) <https://www.thehindu.com/news/national/government-approves-public-procurement-bill/article3306949.ece> accessed 24 May 2022.
60. Dinesh Thakur, "NDTV's Jan Vishwas Act debate: Viewers should know if panelists have conflict of interest" *Newslaundry* (17 August, 2023) <https://www.newslaundry.com/2023/08/17/ndtvs-jan-vishwas-act-debate-viewers-should-know-if-panelists-have-conflict-of-interest> accessed 3 October 2023.

61. "SC Agrees to Hear PIL Seeking Ban on Websites Spreading 'Sardar Jokes'" (*LiveLaw*, 30 October 2015) <https://www.livelaw.in/sc-agrees-to-hear-pil-seeking-ban-on-websites-spreading-sardar-jokes/> accessed 24 May 2022; Bhadra Sinha, "Kohinoor Our Property, Govt Tells Supreme Court" *Hindustan Times* (New Delhi, 20 September 2016) <https://www.hindustantimes.com/india-news/kohinoor-our-property-govt-tells-supreme-court/story-j1jqu8qSukJcyHBvDFLt0N.html> accessed 24 May 2022; Nagraj Gollapudi, "Supreme Court Admits BCCI Petition" *ESPN* (7 August 2013) <https://www.espncricinfo.com/story/_/id/21871852/supreme-court-admits-bcci-petition> accessed 24 May 2022.
62. *M/s Lundbeck India Private Limited vs Dr Chandra M. Gulhati* Criminal Petition No. 4683/2011 before the Karnataka High Court decided on 26 July 2012 <https://indiankanoon.org/doc/183428285/> accessed 24 May 2022.
63. Staff Reporter, "Union AYUSH Ministry Threatens Defamation against Kerala Doctor" *The Hindu* (Kozhikode, 27 September 2021) <https://www.thehindu.com/news/national/kerala/union-ayush-ministry-threatens-defamation-against-kerala-doctor/article36696410.ece> accessed 24 May 2022; Sheryl Sebastian, "Bengaluru Court orders suspension of X account of 'The Liver Doctor' in defamation suit filed by Himalaya Wellness Corporation", *LiveLaw* (28 Sept. 2023) <https://www.livelaw.in/top-stories/bengaluru-civil-court-orders-suspension-of-x-account-of-dr-cyriac-abby-philips-popularly-known-as-the-liver-doctor-in-defamation-suit-filed-by-himalaya-wellness-corporation-238916> accessed 3 Oct 2024.
64. Ayush Tiwari, "Bharat Biotech Defamation Case: A Day after Court Order, Wire Says No Notice Yet" *Newslaundry* (24 February 2022) <https://www.newslaundry.com/2022/02/24/bharat-biotech-defamation-case-a-day-after-court-order-wire-says-no-notice-yet> accessed 24 May 2022.
65. *The Functioning of The Central Drugs Standard Control Organisation* (n 29).

Epilogue

Minutes before the formal launch event of the first edition of this book on 15 October 2022, both authors of this book received a menacing legal notice via email from the CDSCO threatening us over an interview we gave to the press, where we raised legitimate questions regarding the role played by the CDSCO in regulating a pharmaceutical company whose cough syrups had been identified by The Gambia and the WHO as the cause of deaths of approximately 70 children.

The timing of the legal notice, which was sent to us via email at 6:00 PM on a Saturday, an hour and a few minutes prior to a launch of our book, a public event, was an attempt to intimidate us against speaking about the cough syrup controversy. There was no merit to the arguments in the CDSCO's legal notice and we never withdrew our comments. Ultimately, the CDSCO never sued us.

In the weeks that followed, the "spin-masters" within government spread elaborate canards claiming that the deaths in The Gambia were caused by E-coli and not the cough syrup exported from India. This despite laboratory tests commissioned by the WHO revealing alarming levels of poisonous DEG in the cough syrups. Further, the children who died showed signs that were entirely consistent with DEG poisoning. Our research also revealed that the pharmaceutical company accused of manufacturing the adulterated cough syrup had a terrible track record and was blacklisted by many government procurement agencies in India because its products, including syrups, had failed quality testing.

None of these facts appeared to make any difference to the Indian government, which appeared to be more worried about the reputation of the Indian pharmaceutical industry than the public health implications of adulterated cough syrup being sold here and exported to other countries. With no remedial action being taken by the government, it was no surprise when two months later, in December 2022, Indian cough syrups manufactured by a different company were accused by Uzbekistan of causing the deaths of 20 children.

One would have expected that after two major international incidents, the Government of India would tighten the drug regulatory framework. Instead, quite incredibly, in the last week of December 2022, the Ministry of Commerce announced that as part of a new initiative, it was introducing a legislation in Parliament named the Jan Vishwas Bill, 2022 to decriminalize minor offences across 42 laws. One of the offences being decriminalized was a provision in the Drugs & Cosmetics Act, which prescribed mandatory imprisonment for the manufacture of substandard drugs. The Government was proposing through this bill that pharmaceutical companies could now escape a criminal prosecution and imprisonment for the offence of manufacturing substandard drugs by paying a fine of ₹20,000. This was a shocking move on part of the government given the mounting complaints against the pharmaceutical companies and the fact that the existing law was barely enforced. The pharmaceutical industry had been lobbying for such an exemption for a very long time. Parliament voted in favour of passing the Jan Vishwas Act in August 2023 without the opposition raising any objections since it had already staged a walkout from Parliament. The Bill passed via a voice vote.

The ease with which this law sailed through the parliamentary process without any real scrutiny serves as a stark reminder of the lobbying power of the pharmaceutical industry in India. In no other democracy would the legislature reduce punishments for an industry at the time when it was in the dock for causing the deaths of more than a hundred children across the world.

In the same month that the Jan Vishwas Act was passed by the Parliament, the pharmaceutical industry received a stinging rebuke from the medical community in the form of a revolt against a new rule imposed on them by the National Medical Commission (NMC) requiring all doctors to prescribe drugs only by their generic names, instead of their brand names. Doctors protested loudly against this rule primarily on the grounds that they had no faith in the quality of all drugs sold in India and that they preferred to prescribe certain brands which had demonstrated consistent results in their clinical practice. The NMC had to ultimately withdraw the rule. That the doctors in the supposed "pharmacy of the world" had no faith in the quality of all generic medicine should have been a wake-up call for the government.

Towards the end of 2023, we were pleasantly surprised when we received invitations from the Prime Minister's Economic Advisory Council, as well as the National Human Rights Commission for consultations on how the drug regulatory system could be reformed. In both meetings, we received a patient and receptive hearing as we advocated for specific reforms. Just as we thought that we were making some progress, a malicious disinformation campaign painting Dinesh as an "anti-national" was launched in January 2024 by an anonymous website with a track record of spewing clownish conspiracy theories against persons critical of the Government of India or the ruling political party. A senior advisor to the Ministry of Information & Broadcasting, as well as the ruling party's troll army amplified the disinformation campaign on social media.

The attempt of these conspiracy theories is to delegitimize and intimidate critics of the regulator and the Indian pharmaceutical industry. While we continue to advocate for reform in the national press and social media, the campaign to intimidate has been successful in chilling speech by others. For example, we were once contacted by a team of documentary film makers who were interested in making a docuseries based on the first edition of this book, except they were worried that if the focus was on criticizing the government, none of the major online platforms would agree to screen the series for fear of a backlash from the government.

Despite these and many other setbacks and threats over the last two years, the silver lining in our opinion is the support that we have received from many doctors and citizens who have been convinced by our arguments in this book about the myth that is drug regulation in India. The battle for reform will ultimately have to be fought and won in the court of public opinion.

Acknowledgements

Books like this one are typically difficult to write in a country like India, given the opacity with which much of the drug regulatory structure carries out its duties. The main instrument of our research was therefore the RTI Act, 2005. We have filed more than 400 applications under the RTI Act with drug controllers and other government departments across the country to elicit information tucked away in the dark corners of government offices. While we are aware that the RTI Act has been the subject of many an obituary in the recent years, it does deliver results, often after a mind-numbing and frustrating process. It takes patience, some good luck, and the occasional public spirited "Public Information Officer" to ensure a meaningful reply but we have been able to collect hundreds of pages of useful information that form the basis of this book. This book would not have been possible without the RTI Act and for that we are grateful to the many ordinary and extraordinary people who made the RTI Act possible. We are also very grateful to those Public Information Officers who provided us with honest, helpful information in a timely manner, complying with both the letter and spirit of the RTI Act. Many of their colleagues were less than helpful and we continue our endeavour to hold them accountable.

The second set of people we would like to thank are the many law students who worked with us as research assistants on this project. Top of the list is Balaji Subramanian, who is now a lawyer in London. While a student at NALSAR University of Law, he helped strategize and execute a pivotal round of RTI applications. It is thanks to Bala that we were able to corner the Ministry of Health and CDSCO on the missing Mohapatra Committee report. Both of us authors had missed key clues on the existence of the report until Bala's eagle eyes spotted a document that opened the can of worms for the government. The second research assistant to whom we are especially grateful is Harsh Tripathi, a student at NALSAR University of Law, who was our main pillar of support during the course of writing this book. Apart from being able to dig up obscure documents for us, including dated notifications published in the *Gazette of India*, Harsh also helped extensively with the referencing for every chapter of this book. We are also very grateful to Gayatri Gupta and Vishal Rakhecha, who while students at NALSAR University of Law, painstakingly read through a few hundred judgments of trial courts that we had collected from the e-courts website, to plot trends in prosecutions under the Drugs and Cosmetics Act 1940 and the Drugs and Magic Remedies (Objectionable Advertisements) Act 1954. It was a tough assignment and they executed it flawlessly. Vishal also helped with strategizing and filing RTI applications. We are also thankful to Khushi Mittal, a law student at NALSAR University of Law, for her research assistance on the tricky question of the rights of practitioners of traditional medicine and also for her assistance in digging out data on pharmaceutical trademarks in India. Lastly, we would like to thank law students Nipun Kalra, a student of NLU Delhi for his research on similar pharmaceutical tradenames and Revathi Thushara, a student of NLU-Orissa for her research on the rights of traditional medicine practitioners when it came to prescribing modern medicine.

We also thank Bhavesh Kaachhadiya for helping us scrape judgments related to the Drugs and Cosmetics Act 1940 off the e-courts website. We were able to read judgments from across a number of states thanks to his efforts. Studying these judgments gave us excellent insights into how the law is actually implemented in India.

A special thanks to our lawyer, Harsh Parashar, who apart from providing us with legal counsel and representation before the Delhi High Court also sportingly agreed to let us use his office address as the destination for replies to our many RTI applications. We owe an enormous debt of gratitude to his law clerk, Dharmendra Mishra, who diligently scanned and emailed us each RTI reply received from government offices across the country. We are also grateful to our lawyer Sai Vinod Nayani, who has helped us with pursuing many appeals under the RTI Act before the

Central Information Commission and some lawsuits against the drug regulator.

Conversations, on different occasions, with Prof. Ajay Shah, Harleen Kaur, Priyanka Pulla, K.L. Sharma, Dhvani Mehta, and Shreya Shrivastava helped shape some of our thoughts and arguments in this book. We are very grateful to them.

We are also most grateful to Professor Lionel Bently at Cambridge University, a world-renowned academic in the field of intellectual property law, for providing us a copy of an old British law—the UK Food and Drugs Act, 1938—which we were unable to procure from any online sources. An email out of the blue asking Prof. Bently for advice on how we could access this old law resulted in his offer to personally look for it in the libraries at Cambridge and send us a copy. We are thankful for his generosity with his time.

We would also like to thank Gavin Morris for the wonderful cover that he has designed for this book. It was one of many fantastic covers that he sent us. Last but not the least, we would like to thank our editors at Simon and Schuster—Himanjali Sankar, Megha Mukherjee, and Sayantan Ghosh—for tolerating many busted deadlines, hand-holding us through the process of publication, and bringing out the book to the market in record time.

- From the authors

~

This book wouldn't have been possible but for my co-author, Prashant. As an Overseas Citizen of India, I am not allowed to file RTI requests in India (I have challenged this restriction before the Delhi High Court). Much of the data we collected and analyzed in this book was led by him. The analysis we present to bolster our views and the conclusions we draw are largely his work product. On many a occasion, his counsel and advice to temper my expectations given how bad the situation is with our drug supply was instrumental in the recommendations we make.

The credit for genesis of this book has to go to the Supreme Court of India and its former Chief Justice, T.S. Thakur. He dismissed two PILs that I had filed, after a year of painstaking research, on the grounds that it dealt with "academic issues"; this was the prime motive to prove to the citizens of India that this issue is anything but academic. Credit also should go to Dr Harsh Vardhan, the former Minister of Health, Union of India who agreed to meet with me, made me wait for hours outside his office and was distracted watching television for the brief time he gave me. Both these incidents informed me that the only way to affect change in the country was to educate its people, especially doctors, who prescribe medicine, not repose my faith in either the administration or the judiciary. I haven't been proven wrong during the last two years while authoring this book.

Lastly, this is an attempt to address the law-making process in the country. Much of the process of framing laws has become pedantic and ideological of late. We do not invest in empirical research, we don't frame regulations based on facts from the ground. Not only has the drafting process become perfunctory, much of the regulation is driven by lobbying from vested interests. No wonder we end up with laws that undermine each other and create loopholes for exploitation. This is an effort to educate the law makers, doctors and other stakeholders; an attempt to show why understanding how we got here is important in charting out the path for where we need to go as a country.

– *Dinesh S. Thakur*

~

My initial interest in drug regulation began in the context of pharmaceutical patent litigation since in India much of it gets embroiled in regulatory issues. The gamechanger in 2012 was a defamation lawsuit against my friend and mentor Prof. Shamnad Basheer, by a leading Indian pharmaceutical company in India for some of his comments about a patent infringement lawsuit involving the company that were published on SpicyIP, a leading blog on intellectual property law founded by him. As a fellow contributor to the blog, I believed that no "good deed" should go "unpunished", least of all a defamation lawsuit. Knowing that the pharmaceutical company in question had some skeletons in its "regulatory closet" I convinced Shamnad to extract the relevant information from the Ministry of Health using the RTI Act 2005. While the process took time, once we received the information from the government, we realized to our horror the absolute chaos of drug regulation in India. Based on this information, Shamnad, Sai Vinod Nayani, and I published a report, on SpicyIP on this issue. That report led to a long conversation on drug regulation in India with Prof. Amir Attaran at the University of Ottawa, who was then working on drug quality issues. Subsequently, Amir introduced me to Dinesh who was looking for a lawyer to help him dig into the chaos of Indian drug regulation. I ended up quitting my position at a law firm to work full time with Dinesh to unearth the dark secrets of India's drug regulatory system. If it was not for that pharmaceutical company suing Shamnad, it is unlikely that I would have paid much attention to drug regulatory law in India!

The main inspiration, though, for my decision to try and write more, including this book, has always been Shamnad. Several years my senior from law school, I had the privilege of writing with Shamnad on a number of issues pertaining to intellectual property law and I got a front-row seat to his style of thinking and writing. While Indian law schools can be exceptionally cynical places, too often seeding students with unhealthy cynicism, Shamnad was that rare Indian legal academic who, through his scholarship and advocacy, could inspire law students and lawyers alike into believing that the law, even in India, can be used for the greater good. I think working with Shamnad made me less cynical. It was shortly after we lost him in 2019 that I quit my job at a think tank and joined forces with Dinesh to work full-time on this book, fuelled by the memory of many conversations with Shamnad on drug regulation and the Indian pharmaceutical industry. I suspect he would have enjoyed reading this book.

A second academic figure I would like to thank is Professor Hank Greely at Stanford Law School. During the course of my LLM at Stanford, I got to take his courses on drug regulation and the intersection of law and the biosciences. As a student fellow at the Centre for Law and the Biosciences, headed by Prof. Greely, I also got exposure to a number of brilliant scholars who used to lecture at the university. This was the first and only formal education that I received on issues pertaining to drug regulation and it proved to be very useful while thinking through many of the issues in this book with Dinesh.

I am very grateful to my family and friends. Writing a book outside an academic institution during the worst pandemic in a century can be an isolating and uphill venture, even if it is with a co-author as wonderful as Dinesh. My deep gratitude to Laasya and Suhas, who were my flatmates at different times in Bangalore during the first phase of the pandemic when we had just begun writing this book. They provided the company, food, and liquids to keep my spirits high. Also, thanks to my wonderful friends from law school: Harsh, Mukul, Subramanian, and Apurva for keeping me entertained on calls and messages, especially during the forced isolation of the pandemic. A special thanks to my school friends in Hyderabad—Aman, Kailash, Shashank, Kashyap, Keerti, and Abhishek who provided a much-needed respite from the book-writing process, after I shifted back to the city.

Amongst family, I am very grateful to my wonderful parents, Satya and Sudhakar, for ensuring I got all the opportunities in life that were not available to them. Mostly though I am just relieved that they have been surprisingly tolerant of my "trajectory-less" career spanning three universities, two law firms, one think tank, one whistle-blower, one philanthropic foundation, two books, and one masters program over a period of 14 years. I am also grateful to my brother Vikas and his wife Mrudulata. I have spent many comfortable, lazy Sunday family lunches with them, arguing over politics even when we agree with each other. Also, my gratitude to my lawyer niece, Shanu, who has done wonders in building my reputation amongst my extended family and hopefully she convinces all of them to read this book. A professional PR expert could not have done a better job.

Last but not the least, I am grateful to my co-author Dinesh Thakur. Co-authoring a book is never easy, especially with me, and especially on a topic as frustratingly complex as the working of India's opaque drug regulatory machinery. It takes a good deal of patience, coordination, optimism and a whole lot of trust. His bravery and integrity in blowing the whistle at Ranbaxy inspired me enough to give up a career in a law firm. It was a decision that I never regretted. While progress in effecting change to India's drug regulatory system has been slow, there has nevertheless been progress.

– Prashant Reddy T.

About the Authors

Dinesh Singh Thakur is a trained chemical engineer. He turned whistleblower against Ranbaxy after witnessing large-scale data fraud at the company. His efforts led to Ranbaxy pleading guilty to violating American law before an American court in 2013. The company agreed to pay a penalty of $500 million dollars as a part of its guilty plea. For his actions, he received the Joe A. Callaway Award for Civic Courage and the ACFE Cliff Robertson Sentinel Award. Since 2014, he has advocated for reform of India's colonial-era Drugs & Cosmetics Act, 1940 and has founded an advocacy group called the Citizens for Affordable, Safe & Effective Medicine (CASEM). He is also the founder and President of the Thakur Family Foundation, a philanthropic organization that provides grants for research on public health and health journalism in India.

Prashant Reddy Thikkavarapu studied law at the National Law School of India University, Bangalore and Stanford Law School, California, as a J.N. Tata Scholar. After a stint in the litigation teams at two Delhi-based law firms specializing in intellectual property law, he worked in academia and think tanks in New Delhi, Hyderabad and Singapore. Over the last few years, he has been advising Dinesh Thakur in his advocacy campaign for the reform of drug regulatory law in India. Prashant is also the co-author of *Create, Copy, Disrupt: India's Intellectual Property Dilemmas* (OUP 2017).